Seeking the Best

Psychological Service to Veterans

By

A. Jack Jernigan

1663 Liberty Drive, Suite 200
Bloomington, Indiana 47403
(800) 839-8640
www.AuthorHouse.com

AuthorHouse™
1663 Liberty Drive, Suite 200
Bloomington, IN 47403
www.authorhouse.com
Phone: 1-800-839-8640

AuthorHouse™ UK Ltd.
500 Avebury Boulevard
Central Milton Keynes, MK9 2BE
www.authorhouse.co.uk
Phone: 08001974150

First published by AuthorHouse 2/23/2006

ISBN: 1-4208-6450-5 (sc)

Printed in the United States of America
Bloomington, Indiana

This book is printed on acid-free paper.

Table of Contents

Acknowledgements

I am grateful for a Nation that provides benefits to those who have served during times of war. As a World War II veteran I became a recipient of the GI Bill of Rights, and was trained by the Veteran Administration as a Clinical Psychologist to assist in the treatment and rehabilitation of veterans.

Psychological and medical mentors patiently taught me in graduate school and in the classrooms of the Veterans Administration. Given the opportunity to train graduate students, I continued to learn from them. Hopefully they profited from the experience. I did.

My thanks go to the hundreds of veterans who shared their innermost thoughts and feelings in the hope of achieving a more wholesome adjustment. In an effort to serve them, the veterans helped me become a more sensitive clinician.

I thank my family for encouraging and sharing the assembly of this book: Daughter, Beth and wife, Jean for suggesting the autobiography (see Chapter 21); son, Austin for his technical assistance; and son, Richard for the creative book cover. I am especially grateful to Jean for her suggestions and careful editing, and her summation: "This is 'our' story." The errors are mine.

Most of all, I thank a loving God who makes all things possible.

Preface

A World War II assignment with Aviation Psychology's Aircrew Selection Program introduced me to the field of psychology. After the war the Veterans Administration offered employment as a payroll clerk and it was at the Veterans Administration I met my wife, Jean. A few months later the Veterans Administration presented an opportunity through the GI Bill of Rights to become a Clinical Psychologist.

This story is a journal of thirty-three years of Psychological Service for Veterans of four wars, an adventure with a loving wife, and the birth, growth and development of our three beautiful children. It is a personal, professional, and spiritual blend.

An act of Congress established the Veterans Administration in 1930 to care for the needs of those who offered their lives to serve our nation. Sixteen years later, WWII Ashburn General Hospital became the McKinney Veterans Administration Hospital, McKinney, Texas. Ashburn General was one of many WWII Service Hospitals designated as a Veterans Hospital at the end of the "big" war.

The book gives a glimpse of duties at four Veterans Hospitals: McKinney, Texas; Lexington, Kentucky; Waco, Texas and Dallas, Texas. I began as a Payroll Clerk at McKinney VA in 1946, later served as an Educational Therapist and Assistant Vocational Advisor before resigning to enter graduate school under the GI Bill of Rights in 1947.

The enticing announcement stated: "A Training Program for Clinical Psychologists Associated with Part Time Work in V. A. Stations where Neuropsychiatric Patients are Treated." It caught the eyes of an engaged couple in McKinney, Texas. This is the story of how they followed their bliss and became a part of the nationwide Psychological Service for Veterans.

Chapter 1 - 1946 - 1947

Elizabeth Jean Gibson and I began to explore graduate school possibilities before our marriage in Melissa, Texas on July 5, 1947. We resigned our positions at the Veterans Administration Hospital, McKinney, Texas, packed the 1940 Plymouth with all worldly possessions, and departed for Kentucky September 17, 1947. We spent the night in Little Rock and the next morning dropped a card to Austin and Blanche Jernigan. 1

"Wed. Morn.
Dear folks,

Left McKinney at 1:30 Tuesday arrived in Little Rock at 9:30 last night. We got everything cleared up at McKinney and can't think of a thing undone. We are looking forward to the trip to-day for it will be new scenery entirely. Just finished breakfast and are on our way. Next card will be from Kentucky.

Love,
Jack and Jean"

The racing season was in full swing at Keeneland when we arrived in Lexington, Kentucky September 18, 1947. The motel offered only one night's lodging. All Lexington motels were booked for the rest of the week. The next day the University of Kentucky Housing Office directed us to 343 Oldham, home of Charles H. Shepherd, a WW I veteran. He and his young wife offered for rent a front bedroom with shared bath and some kitchen privileges for $50 a month. Jean and I immediately moved in and found the Shepherds to be a generous, giving couple.

But I am getting ahead of the story. How did Jean and I meet? What decisions led to graduate school in Kentucky?

Post War Adjustment

I lived with my parents during the February-March 1946 interim after discharge from WW II, and joined the "52-20 Club." The "Club" was a 52 week provision in the GI Bill of Rights that gave returning Veterans a stipend of $20 a week until employment was found. The veteran was required to report job search efforts to the Texas Employment Commission.

Employment came in five weeks when the word went out that veterans received employment preference at the new Veterans Administration Hospital in McKinney. During the war the facility was known as Ashburn Army Hospital. I qualified for the position of Payroll Clerk, and received the following announcement:

"Confirming verbal order given March 30, 1946, covering training period April 1, 1946 through April 6, 1946, you are hereby authorized and directed to proceed by the most direct practical route as a passenger accompanying Mr. Davis W. Taylor, from your residence in Van Alstyne, Texas to the Veterans Administration Branch Office No. 10, Mercantile National Bank Building, Dallas, Texas, daily and return, for the purpose of training in finance activities. No per diem authorized.

E. H. H. FOSTER, M. D.,
Acting Manager"

Davis W. (Windy) Taylor, Chester Howell of Anna and I were the selected payroll clerk trainees and among the first employees of McKinney Veterans Administration Hospital (VAH). Windy was married and lived in McKinney. Ches Howell and I stayed in the Bachelor Officers Quarters (BOQ) on the VAH grounds. We were soon joined at the BOQ by Recreational Therapist Jouette Hunter. We three single World War II Veterans ate at the Nurses' Dining Room, became close friends, and also friends of some cute nurses. We played the Hospital's nine-hole golf course and occasionally dated one of the nurses. As none of us had an automobile, we walked from the VAH along Church Street to downtown McKinney for a movie or malt at one of the drug stores. I attended worship services at the VA Chapel where Chaplain Harris, a pipe smoking Presbyterian, presented thoughtful spiritual messages. He told of his interest in the writings of Psychologist Gordon Allport who later inspired my interest in personal documents.

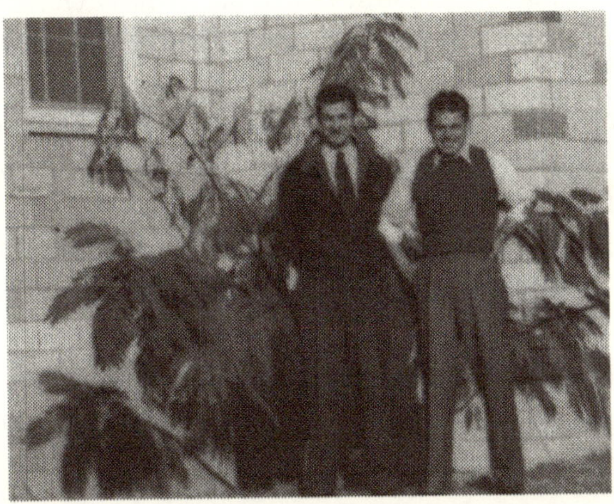

Bachelors Jack Jernigan and Jouette Hunter stand at side of one of the wards of the McKinney VA Hospital, fall 1946.

The finance office expanded and another veteran, Johnny Whisenant, joined the Fiscal Office, but soon left to enter the field of banking, subsequently becoming President, Collin County National Bank. Johnny and all the men mentioned became life long friends.

The rapidly expanding Veterans Administration system offered a variety of opportunities for advancement and in August, I applied for and was accepted for a "position in field for which trained" as an Instructor, Education Retraining with the department of Physical Medicine and Rehabilitation Services (PMRS). This opened up a host of new experiences, new friends and the meeting of someone special.

A "Divine" New Beginning

Elizabeth Jean Gibson graduated with honors in June 1946 from North Texas State College, Denton, completing her B.S. degree in three years while financing her education as student assistant to the Dean of the College, twenty two hours of work each week. After graduation, Jean accepted a Social Services position at the State Hospital in Austin, Texas, but in early October 1946 became dissatisfied with the work environment and returned home.

Jean's father, William Marvin (Jake) Gibson and mother, Mary Chambers Gibson lived in Melissa on old Highway 75 as the road turned west going out of town. Civil War Veteran Capt. John Fitzhugh Gibson, Marvin Gibson's father, moved from Missouri to that site in 1880, and accumulated 280 acres of land. Jean's parent's first home was destroyed by Melissa's 1921 tornado, five years before Jean's birth. The Gibson's "new" home had a wrap around front porch on the north and east with banisters wide enough to sit on.

The Gibson's seven children were John, Frances, Marian, Doris, Billy, Margaret, and Jean. All were married by 1946 but Doris and Jean. Jean's brother, John Gibson had a daughter, Iva Gene who was almost the age of Jean.

Church at Melissa First Baptist on Sunday was followed with Mrs. Gibson's great fried chicken and delicious lemon pie. The family gathered after lunch on the front porch and continued their fellowship of visiting. Any wayfaring relative or stranger was always welcome to this house-by-the side of the road.

During my early childhood, our family drove by the Gibson's house most every Sunday after church at Westminster on the way to McKinney to have lunch with my maternal grandparents, Perry and Sally Coffey. It is possible that we saw a precious little girl on the Gibson front porch during the period, 1926-1932 (Jean's birth and Mammy Coffey's move from McKinney).

Two of Jean's brothers-in-law were also VAH McKinney employees. Fred Waller, World War I Veteran, husband of Frances was a Refrigerator Mechanic. Clyde Tilton, World War II Veteran, husband of Margaret was a Manual Arts Therapist in PMRS. These men encouraged Jean to apply for the vacant position of secretary to C. D. Taylor, Chief PMRS. Clyde told me about this cute sister-in-law who might be coming to work at the VA Hospital.

However, I was in the hospital as a patient on the Orthopedic Ward that October day Jean reported for duty. A group of us were playing volley ball after work, and on spiking a ball I made a twisting motion that produced back pains more severe than those felt at Randolph Field in 1945. I became immobile and was admitted to the hospital.

After discharge from the hospital, I rested at my parent's Sedalia home a few days, returned to work where I met the beautiful girl who was to become my wife. I became painfully aware of the need for an automobile. The only way to get to Melissa was to ride the interurban or walk the six miles or borrow my parent's 1940 Ford. Desperate, I found a used automobile on sale for $275 at Melvin Close's Gulf Service Station, a "late model" 1931 Chevrolet two-door, black with yellow wheels. Jean was to report years later she almost didn't marry me because of the automobile that Clyde and the other VA men described as "smooth-mouthed," e.g. worn out - like an old horse. It was better than that.
2

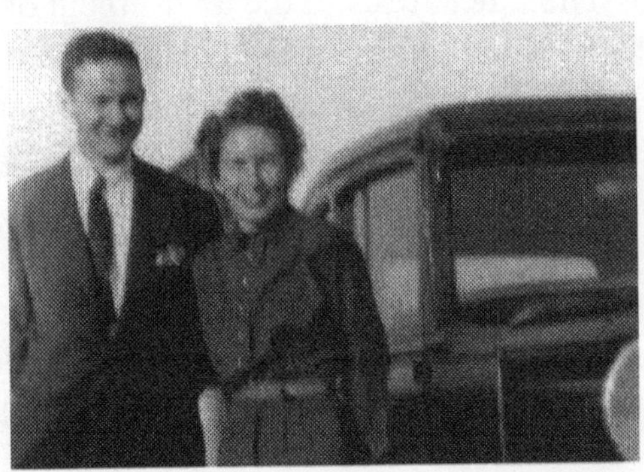

Jack & Jean beside '31 Chevrolet

At last I had "wheels." Jean never complained. One of our first dates was an unscheduled visit one night to her Aunt Pearl Strother's home in McKinney. The '31's gas gauge was broken and we ran out of gas a block from Aunt Pearl's home so Jean suggested we go there to call for gas. This delightful old aunt asked what kind of car I drove. Jean quickly ended the inquiry with, "It's a Chevrolet." Sweet Aunt Pearl responded, "Oh, that's nice."

The twenty mile drive to Sedalia to visit my folks was the longest trip we ever made in the 1931 Chevrolet. There were few entertainment possibilities in post war McKinney. Church on Sundays at Melissa or Westminster or a movie in McKinney could certainly be handled by the '31. We both enjoyed Chaplain Harris' sermons at the VA Hospital Chapel. Jean had a wealth of Collin County relatives to visit and I remember one night we baby sat young Bobby Tilton.

Much of our courting was in the Gibson's living room and it was just a skip and a jump from the BOQ to Melissa in the '31. For me the 1931 Chevrolet was a godsend for it made possible the courtship of one truly sent by God.

In December I accepted a new VA position, Vocational Advisor (Psychometrist), basing my qualifications on WW II Aviation Psychology experiences. The Personnel Officer accused me of being an opportunist. (And I was.) The Psychometrist administered psychological tests in the advisement of veteran patients whose rehabilitation required new vocational choices. William D. Pollan, Chief, Vocational Rehabilitation and Education, somewhat older, divorced was also a resident at the BOQ. He and I were the only staff of the section.

Jean and I drove to Sedalia one night during the Christmas season, and Jean was introduced to my brother Jamie and his wife, Frances. Jean graduated from McKinney High School in 1943 and knew oldest brother, Stewart who in 1943 was McKinney High School Band Director.

Jamie interviewed Jean in great detail about family, education, goals, etc., and this bright, clever young lady gave the future inquisitive brother-in-law "tit for tat." My family fell in love with Jean as I already had, but not yet expressed to them. And I don't remember when I told Jean but she and I soon knew we were meant for each other.

We borrowed the 1940 Ford and took in the Cotton Bowl Game on New Years Day, 1947. It was a miserable, misty-rainy, at the freezing mark day, but we thought we had a good time. The mist froze on the windshield when we drove back toward McKinney as the '40 Ford, like the '31 Chevrolet, had no heater. During the winter I always carried a blanket, and too, we sat close together.

Spring came and so did an engagement ring along with permission from her father to marry his youngest daughter. We found so many common interests, even down to the burial site of ancestors. We volunteered to clean the graves at Highland Cemetery in preparation for Spring Decoration Day, and discovered the Coffey and Gibson gravesites were adjacent, as if our joining together was established many years before. While cleaning the graves a large snake slithered out of the grass, I ran, Jean took her hoe and chopped off its head. My bravery was established.

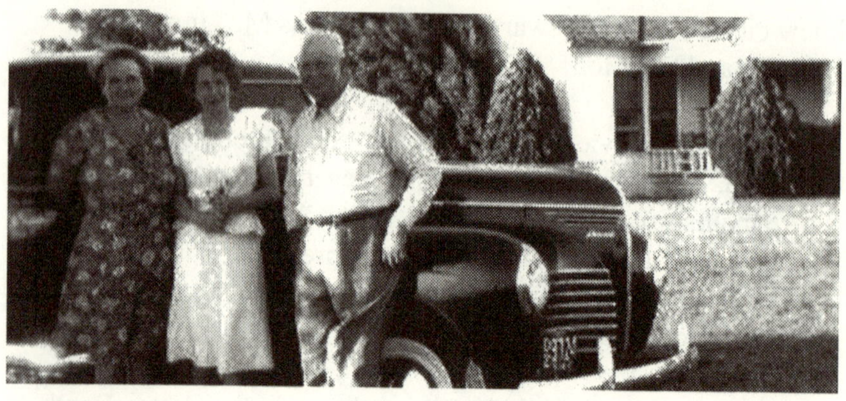

Mother and Daddy Jernigan with Jean, and 1940 Plymouth at Sedalia, Texas summer 1947

The time came to upgrade the 1931 Chevrolet. I contacted an employee with Davis Motor Co. in Denison, World War II Veteran, S. H. (Dick) Montgomery with whom I entered the Air Force at Perrin Field in 1942. Dick had a low mileage, 1940 two-door, black Plymouth with heater for sale. We traded automobiles plus $950 to boot. Jean was delighted, and I was pleased to be driving an acceptable automobile.

We began to make wedding plans, and rented a garage apartment on Hunt Street June 9, 1947 for $46.83 a month. As housing was scarce, we loaned the apartment to Mr. Wallace, a V A Hospital Rehabilitation Instructor for a few weeks so he could invite his wife to McKinney for a visit. Check stubs indicate we paid rent to Mr. H. D. Gamble through September 12, 1947.

As invitations went out to relatives and friends there was a drama playing on another stage of our future life. But first, let's go to the wedding.

Mr. and Mrs. W. M. Gibson
request the honor of your presence at
the marriage of their daughter
Elizabeth Jean

to

Mr. Austin Jackson Jernigan
on Saturday evening July the fifth
Nineteen hundred and forty-seven
at eight o'clock
Melissa Baptist Church

I asked Floyd Everheart to be best man, but at the last moment he had to cancel and Windy Taylor became an excellent replacement. Jean's bridesmaid was Diane Schrader, a close North Texas State College friend, Ches Howell and Jouette Hunter were ushers.

Those were not the days of video or complex cameras. No one in the two families owned a camera with flash so only a few daylight-hour black and white photos documented our marriage. But the scene is etched in memory: My beautiful bride, dressed in white coming down the isle of Melissa Baptist Church. Jamie sang "Because" and Frances accompanied at the piano, Chaplain Charles D. Harris led us in the wedding vows. Five year old David said, "She looks just like Jesus."

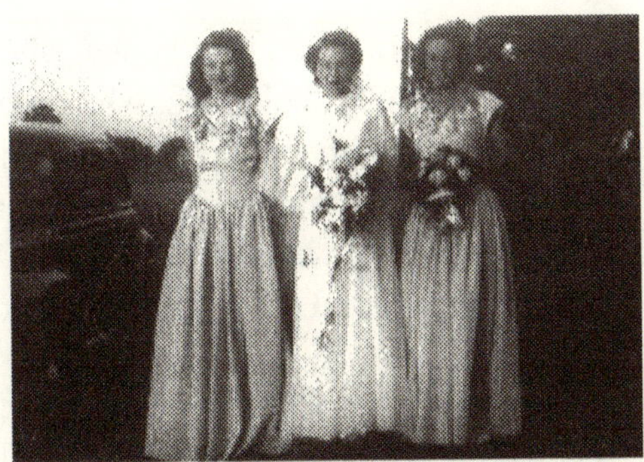

Elizabeth Jean Gibson Jernigan

Nineteen hundred and forty-seven, following wedding with attendant Iva Gene Gibson and bridesmaid Diane Schrader.

There was a reception afterwards at the Gibsons.

We honeymooned at Hot Springs Arkansas, spending our first night at the Grayson Hotel in Sherman and driving from there the next morning to Paris, Texas where we attended worship services at a convenient Presbyterian Church before proceeding to Hot Springs.

We returned to our small apartment on Hunt Street in McKinney and to our positions at McKinney VAH, as we waited the possible development of other vocational plans.

Graduate School Opportunity

In April 1947 my attention was drawn to VA Circular #105 posted on the Personnel Bulletin Board. The Circular announced a most interesting opportunity, a "Training Program for Clinical Psychologists Associated with Part Time Work in VA Stations where Neuropsychiatric Patients are Treated." I contacted Dr. J. J. Blasko, Acting Chief, Neuropsychiatry, VA Branch #10, Dallas, who when told of my Air Force experience, replied he was acquainted with Col. Arthur Melton.

Veteran applicants were given preference. The goal of the program was to train Clinical Psychologists, who on completion of the doctorate could remain with the Veterans Administration and serve in the treatment and rehabilitation of veterans. Students selected for the training program were hired by the VA and detailed to VA Hospitals near an approved University. The student was to work 1056 hours a year (22 hours a week for 48 weeks). First year Interns received 22/40 of the full time salary of $2644.80, plus a married veteran received a $90 a month subsistence allowance, tuition, and books and supplies up to $500 a year. As the student progressed through the four years the annual salary rate increased to $4490.60. The starting salary plus monthly GI Bill assistance was almost equal to my current VAH salary of $3390.

Although the program was designed for men with a bachelor's degree in psychology, there were some possible options. I believed minimum academic requirements were met in that my bachelors included 18 hours of Education, 6 of which were in Educational Psychology.

This sounded like a great opportunity for the engaged couple, and Jean began to help prepare correspondence to learn more about the program. Thirty-three Psychology Departments were listed as approved for VA – University joint training. The Lexington VA Hospital affiliated with the University of Kentucky was the nearest to Texas.

Air Force buddy, Jack (Jockey) Baker of Lexington, Kentucky, and Dr. Arthur Melton at the University of Missouri were contacted. The letter to Dr. Melton was forwarded to Ohio State University where he was then Professor of Psychology. Dr. Melton wrote that Ohio State was affiliated with the program but all the "training slots" for 1947 were filled. He sent an impressive letter of recommendation, as did Dr. Glenn Finch, my superior officer, when I was Chief, Psychomotor Testing, Medical and Psychological Examining Unit 5, Miami Beach, Florida, 1943-1944. 3

Jack Baker was most encouraging about the University of Kentucky, as he was an assistant to then Chairman, Department of Psychology, Dr. W. W. White soon to be designated Dean of the University. Jack Baker sent application details, necessary forms, and reported that Ed Harris one of our former SAACC enlisted psychologists was already in the VA program at Lexington as fourth year graduate.

I forwarded to Dr. W. W. White, Department of Psychology, University of Kentucky all necessary forms and papers as applicant for the position of First Year Psychological Intern. We wrote the Dean of Men on June 16, 1947 and requested application forms for married couple quarters at "Cooperstown or Shawneetown." Jack Baker paved the pathways for becoming established students.

Notification of acceptance for graduate training came from the University of Kentucky Graduate School June 25, 1947. The next step: Be approved by the Veterans Administration. Nine days before our marriage, Dr. Frank A. Pattie, recently appointed Chairman Department of Psychology from the same position at Rice University, wrote that the application was forwarded to Washington, D. C., ". . . . first on the list."

There is an interesting anecdote associated with being "first on the list" of ten approved candidates. Some years later, Jamie as Dean, Texas A&I visited with Dean White, University of Kentucky, at a national meeting of University Deans. Jamie remarked he had a brother in Graduate School at U.K. Dean White commented, "Oh yes, your brother was ranked first in the class of 1947." He went ahead to explain that my application arrived after the completion of the 1947 rankings. At the last moment, the applicant ranked #1 informed Kentucky of his decision to attend another university. My name was conveniently substituted in the # 1 slot. Jack Baker's endorsement was another gift in the Jack-Jean saga of 1947.

There were some other cliff hangers. While on our Arkansas honeymoon, Dr. E. Lowell Kelly, Project Director for the Research Project on the Selection of Clinical Psychologists, University of Michigan wrote I was scheduled to attend an assessment class in Michigan commencing July 22, 1947. I asked to be rescheduled for the August 9 class. Dr. Frank A. Pattie, Chairman of the Psychology Department, University of Kentucky wrote that attendance was not required.

James G. Miller, M.D., Chief, Clinical Psychology Section, Neuropsychiatry Division, VA Central Office wrote July 29, 1947 that attendance would be inappropriate, and indicated notification would arrive within the next two or three weeks. Dr. Pattie wrote

August 27 I was accepted ". . . for internship in the program in clinical psychology sponsored by the Veterans Administration. Registration begins here on September 25, classes on the 29. The housing situation is bad, especially for married couples. We will be glad to see you here in September."

A September 9, 1947 TWX from VA Branch Office, Columbus, Ohio gave official notification of my appointment as a First Year Level Clinical Psychology Intern.

And that is why Jean and I were in Lexington, Kentucky September 18, 1947 searching for a place to live at the start of the racing season. The mystery of tomorrow follows.

Chapter 2 - 1947 - 1951

We contacted Air Force friend, Jack Baker after getting settled in our room at the Shepherd's September 19, 1947. Jack was most helpful in orienting us to the campus. I met Dr. Frank Pattie, Chairman of the Psychology Department, and visited Dean White's University Office.

We drove to the VA Hospital on Leestown Road, and met the Chief of Psychology Service, Dr. A. Dudley Roberts. Jean interviewed for a position with the VAH Personnel Office, and was given a temporary position. She later became the Secretary to Personnel Officer Duggan.

Jack Baker told staff at the Dean's Office of my psychological testing experience with Air Force Aviation Psychology, and I was asked to group administer the admission tests to incoming 1947 UK Freshmen. It was a nice experience with a small stipend to boot.

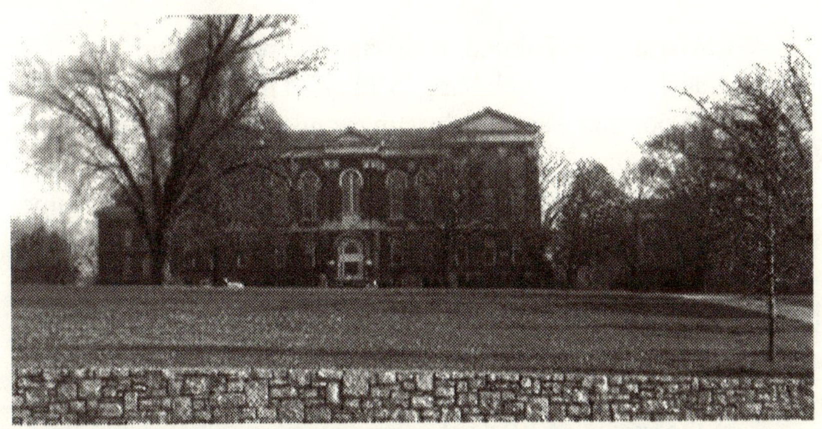

Administration Building, University of Kentucky, Lexington, Kentucky, 1947.

The 1947 class became a close knit group: Cecil and Joan Peck, Dick and Hatter Thomas, Bob and Evelyn Ferguson, and single men Ed Baggs, Elmer Wingrove, Harry Feamster, and Ray Durham. The Elgie Smiths had a child, and Charlie and Jane

Leiman became parents before graduation. Ours was the second class of the nation-wide, joint Veterans Administration-University training program for clinical psychologists.

Others within the VA program during the four graduate years were the Dick Griffiths, Arnold Krugmans, and Lou Feigenbaums. We became close friends with Mac, Judy, and little Mike Sterling from Dallas. Mac was in graduate school at Kentucky when we arrived in 1947 and a year or so later Mac received a VA psychology trainee appointment.

University courses and part time assignment at the VA Hospital were quite challenging. Jean worked 40 hours a week in the VAH Personnel Office, but we found opportunities for rest and relaxation. We enjoyed the ambience of Lexington and the Kentucky horse country. On a visit to Calumet Farm and Man of War's grave we wished for a paneled room as nice as the stalls of the race horses. We attended the Trots (our preference) and the races at Keeneland, making a bet on one occasion. We had picnics with the psychology families at Moore's Mill.

Christmas 1947 found us driving the reliable and comfortable 1940 Plymouth back to Texas. Thus began a pattern of returning to our homes each Christmas and a visit in the summer. Stewart, Mary, David and Susan were able to make only one return visit to Texas while in graduate school in California, and at a time we were unable to coordinate visits. We met Jamie and Frances on several occasions at Sedalia, and visited with them once at the University of Chicago. They in turn came to Lexington from Chicago.

In the spring of 1948 we moved from our one room - share bath - kitchen with the Shepherds to an upstairs apartment with bedroom, living room, and private bath at 161 Chenault in the lovely home of Mrs. Greenwood "Cokie" Cocanougher. Mrs. Cocanougher, a Powder Puff Derby Pilot, a UK college student, and the mother of a married son in Oklahoma, adapted an upstairs alcove sewing-room into a semi- kitchen with a Magic Chef apartment-size stove and a small Servel gas refrigerator, but no kitchen sink. Our dishes were washed in a pan on a small table and waste water carried across lovely pegged oak floors to deposit in the commode. The rent was $90 a month.

We made inquiry of the Office of Price Administration, a carry over agency from WWII, with authority to regulate rent. Five months later the OPA established the rent at $65 a month and we received a refund of $175. "Cokie" was very unhappy - we denied we "turned her in" - she didn't ask if we had made an OPA inquiry. We felt a little guilty, but happy the rent was reduced.

I used John Knight Motors, Chrysler-Plymouth outlet for maintenance of the 1940 Plymouth. By September 1948, new post-war automobiles became plentiful, and my eye was attracted to the showroom's four-door Deluxe, black 1948 Plymouth. Jean and I decided we could afford to trade as we had the necessary funds in Postal Savings at McKinney.

John Knight offered $567 for the '40 Plymouth toward the $1867.70 cost of the new 1948. As it would take several days to get the balance from our McKinney savings account and fearing the loss of this "great" trade, we made the following sales agreement on September 7, 1948: "$300, cash plus $567 for '40 Plymouth trade-in, plus unpaid balance of $1,000, plus 167.12 insurance, finance charges, etc. payable in 12 monthly installments of $97.26." Over anxious to buy - we agreed to borrow the money from Commodity Credit Corporation (whom the dealer recommended) until WWII savings from McKinney came. When the Postal Savings money arrived a week later, discovered we had to repay a "finder's fee" of $50 plus interest, a total of $97 to clear the use of funds for one week.

It was a good lesson. That was the last time we borrowed money from anyone but ourselves to purchase an automobile. However, later Jean would feel she worked only to pay for a new car as we began our family pattern of monthly payments to replenish funds borrowed from the savings account.

A Calling

There was strong motivation to succeed in graduate school and become a professional psychologist. The void in basic background courses in psychology was bridged within a year, possibly accelerated by subliminal learning from the associations with WW II psychologists. The immediate practical application of University academic training to assignments with psychotic veteran patients was an excellent learning experience. I enjoyed the detailed diagnostic evaluations, graduate courses, case conferences, supervised training, and the opportunity to be of possible help to a disturbed individual. I had found my calling.

The Kentucky program followed the pattern of a thorough grounding in the assessment of intelligence and development of the clinical skill of evaluation of a patient's intellectual and emotional functioning. One of the first clinical assessment instruments mastered was the Wechsler-Bellevue Intelligence Test consisting of six Verbal sub-tests and five non-verbal Performance sub-tests. I always thought of Jean when administering question 16 of the Information Test sub-test: "When is Washington's birthday?"

In our early 1946 courtship-getting-acquainted days I asked Jean for her date of birth. She responded that it was the same as George Washington's birthday, and I failed the Wechsler-Bellevue question.

I was able to keep pace with the four year training program as outlined in VA Circular #105. When our class entered the more advanced stages of clinical assessment, e. g., the Rorschach, Thematic Apperception, etc. we began to better understand some of the complexities of mental illness. Dr. Graham B. Dimmick, our key Clinical instructor, seminar leader, and mentor spent one afternoon each week at the hospital leading a teaching seminar where each student rotated in the presentation of case material. He was a master of the Rorschach and identified by Samuel J. Beck, Ph.D. as his best student.

Dr. Dimmick announced he was attending a Samuel J. Beck seminar on "Affective Reaction Patterns in the Rorschach Test" to be held at Michael Reese Hospital, Chicago June 6 -10, 1949, and stated the seminar was open to graduate students. Four of us, Cecil Peck, Charlie Leiman, Dick Thomas, and I, prepaid the $40 tuition fee and attended. Fifty-five people registered for the opportunity to listen to Dr. Beck's detailed analyses of Rorschach protocols. A former Air Force psychologist associate, Harrison G. Gough was also in attendance. At that time Dr. Gough was a member of the faculty of the University of Nebraska.

There were fifteen to twenty University-VA trainee students each year at Lexington VAH during the four years of graduate study. Advanced VA students were given supervisory responsibility for first and second year graduate students. Graduate student role models were men like Ed Harris (also a 1942 Veteran of Psychological Research Unit #2), and Dick Griffith.

Relaxation came with such activities as keeping the yard at Cocanougher's and tending a small vegetable plot behind the garage with Jean. Large shade trees limited vegetable growth, but we had some excellent bib lettuce.

We transferred our church letters from Westminster-Melissa Baptist Churches respectively to Immanuel Baptist Church. The church was only a couple of blocks from our Shepherd "apartment" and we walked to services except in bad weather. Later we occasionally visited the First Presbyterian to hear their scholarly Ph.D. minister. We and the Sterlings were the only Baptists in our group. The Leimans were Methodists from Maryland and the Pecks were Lutherans from Minnesota. Jack Baker was a devout Catholic.

Family Correspondence

Communication with our extended families was limited to correspondence through the U. S. Postal Service. My parents did not have telephone service at Sedalia, and recall only one telephone call to Jean's parents in Melissa: When Marian's husband, David Wallace died in 1950.

To conserve our time for academic studies, yet maintain communication within the Jernigan family, a "Round Robin" (RR) letter was initiated that followed the pattern: From the AJJs to Chicago - JCJs to Oakland - JSJs to Sedalia - AWJs to Lexington - AJJs. Each family received a packet of four letters to be kept no more than a week before forwarding to the next family, first removing their previous letter and adding an updated letter to the RR packet. In addition, Mother usually wrote each family separately once a week. An August 1949 RR letter told of Jean's plan to enter graduate school at the University of Kentucky.

The extant Kentucky letter preserved by Mother was undated, but the content suggests it may have been mailed in early spring of 1949. Excerpts from this and subsequent letters give examples about our every day life in Lexington.

"Today has really gotten away from me. I cooked dinner and washed the dishes while Jean typed my experiment and by the time we were finished it was four o'clock.

"Jean took off one day last week and went shopping with her income tax money. She bought some beautiful material (silk) for a new dress. She got it cut out, but nothing else. Jean's boss' wife had a birthday Friday and the girls in the office gave her a surprise birthday supper at the Duggan's (boss) home. Mr. Duggan bought the ham and Jean baked it. She also baked a cake, it was the prettiest cake I ever saw, and tasted good too. We all had a big time.

"... We washed yesterday morning and Jean ironed yesterday afternoon and last night. I sat up last night to listen to the basketball game. Kentucky played Oklahoma A&M at Seattle, Washington for the National Championship. The game started there at 9:30 P.M., 11:30 P.M. here. Kentucky won which made it worth while to sit up until 1:30.

"... We haven't decided yet whether we will go up and see Jamie and Frances at Easter. It is a long trip, but we hate not to go for they won't be there much longer.

"... I have to get in some more studying this weekend. Have test this week."

A week later I wrote that Jean finished her "lovely" dress. The University dismissed classes for the return of the National Basketball Champions, the "fabulous" Kentucky Wildcats from Seattle. Jean and I saw most of the home games that basketball season in the UK coliseum "that Coach Adolph Rupp built."

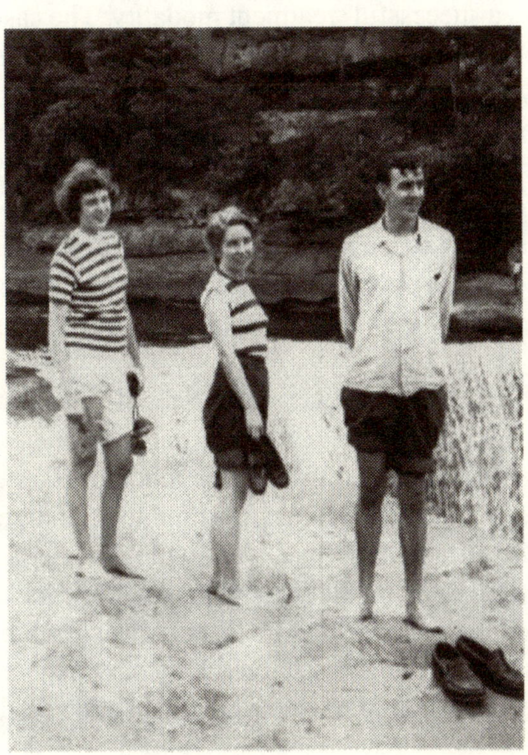

Dick and Hatter Thomas went with us to Cumberland Falls State Park in the southwest corner of Kentucky for a July 4, 1949 weekend. It was a relaxing mini-vacation for all four of us. Years later we took our three children there for another weekend visit as part of our Tennessee-Kentucky vacation tour.

Surgery Seminar

One of my assignments the summer of 1949 was research clerk to the distinguished philosopher-psychiatrist, Dr. Irwin Strauss, a WW II-era, German Jew immigrant from the University of Berlin. Dr. Strauss coordinated a lobotomy study and my task was to collect data regarding progress made by the patients since their surgery. VAH Lexington was host to a regional conference on the subject and we attempted to locate case-subjects to present to the conference

The seminar presenters made an effort to demonstrate that lobotomy was a successful treatment modality. The case-history of each patient, pre and post surgery was presented at the seminar. A guitar playing Kentucky World War II Veteran made gentle by the operation was selected as a star patient example of a successful lobotomy. The psychiatrist introduced the former patient as a positive example, and at the conclusion of the interview invited the young man to play the guitar for the doctors. The lobotomized veteran sang (off key) as he strummed a ballad with the single preservative theme, "Oh Look What You Have Done To Me."

Jean to Graduate School

It was during preparation for the lobotomy conference that Jean resigned her VA Hospital position to attend graduate school, and the girls in her office, wanting to give her a surprise party, called and asked me to bring Jean to a home located in the country. I used the pretense that Dr. Strauss was unable to receive a response from one of the discharged lobotomy patients, and I was to go the next night to interview the man and asked Jean to go with me. The office girl giving the party lived in the boondocks. After driving around the Kentucky countryside one night for two hours, I finally located the "patient's house," and persuaded Jean to accompany me to the interview. The door to the "patient's home" opened with the shout, Surprise, Surprise!" We had a good time.

After returning from the August vacation in Texas, both of us entered graduate school the fall of 1949. Jean registered as a two-year Kentucky resident, and was challenged by the registrar that she was an out-of-state graduate student. The fee was several hundred dollars more than we had expected to pay. She explained she had been working at the VA Hospital for two years and paying Kentucky taxes. But the registrar's office replied that Jean was married to an out of state graduate student under the GI Bill.

That did it! She forcefully argued that her husband's graduate school status had nothing to do with her enrollment at Kentucky. She won her case. We failed to recognize her graduate degree plan should have been changed to law school instead of business education with a minor in sociology.

Jean registered on the occasion of Kentucky's first admittance of African-American students to graduate study at UK. The University limited the number of African-American who could enroll for graduate study, and the individuals were asked to sit in back of the room. An African-American graduate student registered for Jean's Education class, taught by Dr. Frank Dickie (later President of UK), and complied with the regulation to sit in the back of the room. Dr. Dickie's first response was to ask the student to come and take the front seat, "that such back room seating would not be allowed in his class."

Jean was eternally grateful for having classes under this distinguished educator. Many years later upon reading of an award given Dr. Dickie, Jean wrote him a congratulatory note and thankfully reminded him of that first day in class. She received a gracious reply from Dr. Dickie that he too remembered the historic day. Dr. Dickie enclosed a sample of his art work as an example of his retirement activities.

We drove to Texas our third Kentucky Christmas. When we left Texas to return to school, Mr. Gibson asked if there was room in the trunk for a sugar cured ham. Did we?! Back in Kentucky, the ham was swung on a rafter in the attic store-room just off our bedroom. The unheated attic became a cool "smoke house" storage space. A January 1950 letter told of a ham and eggs breakfast.

"We cut our ham last week and are really enjoying it. This morning we had ham, eggs, biscuit and ham gravy for breakfast. We ate just before we went to church and consequently weren't hungry when we came home, so decided to go for a ride. We drove over to Frankfort and went through the Capitol building. It is a very beautiful and impressive building and we enjoyed it a lot. Jean pointed out a number of historical facts she had learned in her history course."

In that same letter, I thanked my parents for the gifts bought at the first of year sales with their money gift to Jack and Jean: Side-view mirrors for 1948 Plymouth for $1.98, Arrow shirt, marked down from $3.60 to $2.00 and a pair of gloves for $1.95, originally $3.95. Jean was making molasses cookies from molasses received or purchased from Weldon Lane. Grades had arrived for the previous semester - - 2 A's and a B+.

Jean received her grades the next day: All A's! And that pattern continued throughout her graduate school days at UK - a "straight A" student.

For the next semester, Jean took courses in Education Psychology, Health Education, Curriculum Development and Teaching General Business. Her graduate advisor was also instructor in two of her courses and a co-author with one of Jean's former North Texas State College professors of the text book used in one course. It was anticipated she would do well that semester, and did.

I enrolled in three courses: Theories of Learning, Psychology of Language, and Practicum, a course taken each semester as a part of VA training. Between semesters the University professors and VA Chief of Psychology, A. Dudley Roberts reviewed each VA graduate student. In a personal interview, the Chairman of the Department, Dr. James Calvin, an Experimental Psychologist, said my work at the hospital was reported outstanding and that every professor reported I was doing very good work. It confirmed my belief (and hope).

Later one of the graduate students stated that Dr. Roberts explained the scale he was required to use in rating each student. One scale item listed characteristics of emotional adjustment and professional ethics. Dr. Roberts told them, "Now there aren't many men I can rate high on those qualities, but someone like Jack Jernigan I could and would feel justified in doing so." My perception of Dr. Roberts' psychological stature increased significantly. Actually, was surprised and humbled by the evaluation.

Uncle Jim Hoyle

There were two family deaths during our four years in Kentucky. As previously mentioned, Jean's brother-in-law, David Wallace died in November 1950, and my Dad's brother-in-law, James Felix Hoyle, husband of Claudya Jernigan Hoyle died in February 1950. Aunt Claudya preserved the letter I wrote March 1, 1950. A paragraph is quoted in part:

". . . .I wish I could have been with you and Alton and Anita today. Not only to offer what little comfort I might give but to pay homage to a person whom I loved so much. . . . his friendly, jovial and kind and loving association will live on in our hearts forever and ever. He was such a fine person and I have always been so proud of my Uncle Jim."

University Guest

Hodding Carter spoke at the University on the subject, "Is the South Really that Bad?" This newspaper man-author from Greenville, Mississippi used his home town as a typical Southern town, and told of all of the good things people had done for one another and for the nation. During the question period a member of the audience asked Mr. Carter if he thought Greenville, Miss. was really a typical town, and did people react that way. I wanted to tell them that such cooperative community spirit was not uncommon in Sedalia and Melissa.

One Friday night we rewarded ourselves with a movie and saw Lionel Barrymore in "Down to the Sea in Ships." A preview of a coming attraction was a movie adaptation of the radio program, "The Life of Riley."

Doctoral candidates were required to have a reading knowledge of two foreign languages and the exams were reported to be superficially administered to "comply with tradition and an outmoded requirement." But it was a worrisome hurdle and I began to prepare by studying a book written by a Dr. Pollard of the University of Texas on how to read German. Pollard established 12 basic rules and claimed anyone could learn to read German in no time by following his advice. I was told of another route many students used to pass the German exam.

The candidate selected psychological books in French and German for the examination that had English translations. The language examiner randomly selected a passage from the foreign language book selected by the student and the student completed a written translation of the passage. The graduate school grapevine reported German exams could be passed by memorizing an English translation of the first page of several chapters of a candidate's choice of a German text. The student hoped (prayed) the examiner would select a memorized chapter. I selected a translation of Freud's writings on dreams, and remember my great joy when I saw the selected chapter, recalling to this day Freud's opening sentence: "A dream then is a psychoses."

The language department was most cooperative in that they did not want a doctoral candidate to fail graduate school because of a language deficiency, and invited students to bring dictionaries and other resources to the exam. Though not consciously planned, I discovered that the English translation of my French text was one of the resources I took to the exam. And I looked - and have forever felt guilty for cheating. God has forgiven me, but the scar remains - as is true for most all sins. Hopefully we learn from such experiences, and I did.

While Mac Sterling was at the VA Hospital, Louisville collecting data for his dissertation (as I would a year later), Jean invited Judy and little Mike for lunch and I took a break from studies to join them. It was a fun experience to play with the three year old instead of studying at the library, and later wrote home that I wondered how Stewart could study with two children to occupy his time.

During one of our rest breaks we drove to Berea, Kentucky to visit Berea College where students from Kentucky hills worked their way through college on farms and industries run by the college. Berea students were/are encouraged to return to his/her home community upon graduation to teach others. One of Berea's many industries is broom making. We sent gift brooms to our mothers from Berea for Mothers Day. Jean continues to order brooms and other products from the College.

Qualifying Examinations

My oral examination for admittance to doctoral candidacy was successfully completed on May 17, 1950. The previous week all candidates were given written examinations over seven fields in Psychology: Clinical, Experimental, Comparative, Statistics, Industrial, Child, and Systems. There was a two hour exam over each field except the major field, Clinical which was an eight hour, all day examination. A "B" average was required to pass the written comprehensives. I made an "A" in the major field, Clinical, and an "A" in Industrial, thus offsetting "C's" in Experimental and Statistics, and a "B" in the other three fields. I recall being so keyed up by Friday night that I did not sleep and, read TIME magazines missed during the weeks of preparation.

The orals were considered a mere formality as a rule, but Chairman Dr. Frank Pattie warned that some of the experimental professors weren't pleased I passed with such low grades in their fields and might try to flunk me on the orals. But they were gentle with their questions.

I hoped for a "halo effect" in Statistics. The Statistics professor was an Air Force buddy whose course I had taken the previous semester, and made the highest grade in the class. However, papers were coded and the names weren't revealed until the day the staff met to decide our fate. He might have stretched the grade to a "B" had he known. Ten graduate students took the exam, three passed. I felt happy and sad at the same time because fellow students who failed had to wait until January 1951 to take the next scheduled written exam.

Respites

Jean learned that a Summer Stock Company was to present "Claudia" at a former WW II army hospital theater in Danville, Kentucky. We attended with Cecil and Joan Peck.

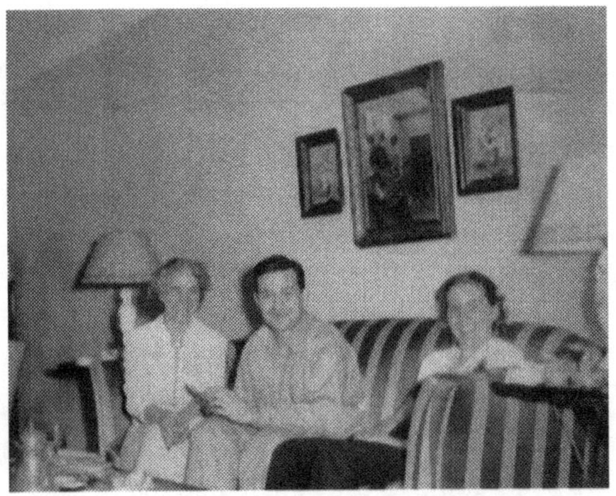

"Cokie" and her renters

We took a break from studies one Saturday to attend a Kentucky auction of the household effects of a local funeral home. We bought a table lamp for $1.50 and a silver coated serving dish for $1.00, and having found the auction so enjoyable returned in the afternoon where I became reckless, bidding on several items.

An antique marble top table with Mahogany base, twenty by thirty inches, and about thirty inches tall came up for auction. Estimating it would go for $20, I bid $12, got into a 50 cent bidding war with a lady - I bid $15.50, and the auctioneer said <u>Sold</u>. He added, "I can tell how happy you have made your wife, look how she is smiling." Actually, she was laughing that I had overplayed my hand.

Another lady offered us $20, and we later shared the story with Mrs. Cocanougher who estimated the table to be worth $75. It was the first piece of furniture bought in our three years of marriage, and it graces our home today.

Dissertation

It was possible to graduate by June 1951. August 1951 seemed a more attainable goal. But the final hurdle of selecting a unique dissertation subject seemed overwhelming. I noted that psychiatric patients were required to submit their written letters to the Nursing Station for staff review before being posted. My research idea was to study psychiatric patient's letters, and measure treatment progress through changes in a patient's intellectual and emotional functioning as reflected in letters. I read Gordon Allport's 1942 publication on "The Use of Personal Documents in Psychological Science" in preparation for a pilot study.

VA staff supervisor, Dr. Morris Roseman became intrigued with the personal document research idea, encouraged me, and was disappointed when I came to the conclusion the research would be a risky venture. We had begun to think of starting a family, and wanted to complete graduate school in 1951. Interest in personal documents remained dormant for a few years. 1

58th American Psychological Association Annual Meeting

In an effort to change direction in the search for a dissertation subject, we decided to attend the American Psychological Association (APA) annual meeting at State College, Pennsylvania. Fellow graduate student Bob Ferguson and wife, Evelyn rode with us to Pennsylvania in the fall of 1950. The trip was documented in an eight page letter to my parents. 2

It was the last year an APA meeting was held on a University campus. We were housed in a Penn State dormitory and up early each day to attend seminars and paper sessions. Throughout the first day I met former Air Force friends, many of them established in post-war psychological positions. Two friends offered an immediate position, and believe others would have done so had I been in the market for a job. I hoped opportunities would be as prevalent the following year.

We four attended several meetings together. Jean and Evelyn went to some meetings on their own while Bob and I selected presentations thought helpful to the completion of graduate studies. We discovered that an APA convention covered almost every conceivable subject a student might wish to attend. Two presentations were of special interest: That of Carl Rogers of U. of Chicago on Monday night and the Presidential address by Dr. J. P. Guilford on Tuesday night. Jamie took a course from Dr. Rogers at the University of Chicago and the convention offered an opportunity to hear Dr. Rogers discuss his client-centered psychotherapy.

During the seven day, 1600 mile drive to Penn State and return we experienced the Pennsylvania Turnpike, visited Gettysburg, Washington, D. C, the Lincoln and Jefferson Memorials, Washington Monument, Arlington Cemetery, Mt. Vernon, the Capitol Building, visited Sam Rayburn's office (he was in Bonham, Texas), Bureau of Printing, Smithsonian, Shenandoah National Park, Lexington, Virginia, and White Sulphur Springs, West Virginia.

Fourth Year

In October 1950 we moved into a duplex at 309 Transylvania Park in a redesigned house owned by Mr. Lyle Phelps. For the first time in three years we had an apartment with a complete private kitchen.

On October 12, 1950 the Board of Directors of the American Psychological Association announced my acceptance as an Associate of the APA effective January 1, 1951. The certificate was signed by Fillmore H. Sanford, Executive Secretary. Fillmore Sanford was an interesting psychologist. 3

An anxious search for a dissertation problem continued. Dr. Dimmick dropped a hint in a lecture about a Rorschach experiment he thought would be of research interest. He gave me permission to explore the idea. Jean told of this and her excellent graduate school progress in an October 14, 1950 letter to the AWJ's.

"I meant especially to write you last week on your anniversary, because I have more reason to be glad you decided to marry and produce such a fine husband for me. Although I don't say so, I am grateful for the fine upbringing you gave him and I will try not to spoil your results too much!

"This has been a busy week. Jack has been working awfully hard and consistently on his problem. I think he has found something that he can turn into a dissertation, and I surely hope so. I think this part of trying to get started is the hardest part of all. Once he knows where he is working toward, it shouldn't be so worrisome, although it will be lots of work.

"I completed the driver-training part of my course yesterday -- fortunately I didn't run into any ditches or anything, so I passed. It has been hard to put in the time it has required, but I have learned so much I think it is worthwhile.

"Today I took the National Teachers' Exam. It is a test that has been developed for teachers all over the country. It lasted from 8:30 until 12:15, then Jack met me for lunch, and then I went back for the last part from 1:15 until 3:00 this afternoon.

"The test this morning covered the general field of education and English expression. The latter included spelling, vocabulary, grammar, and then gave paragraphs to read and answer questions about. We also had what they call "non-verbal reasoning" - a series of figures which have a pattern and we were to supply the missing parts. This afternoon the test covered "General Culture" - general information, world affairs, arithmetic, literature, art and music. I surely did wish that Jack could have taken that part - he keeps up with current events so much better than I, and his math is good where mine is very poor. I don't expect to make a good score, but I think I passed.

"I am enjoying my student teaching. I haven't done much actual teaching - just helping individual students who are having trouble, grading papers, and helping out generally. I have taught bookkeeping two days - I'm afraid the class didn't learn much, but I surely did. Both my supervising teachers are very nice, and they seem to be interested in seeing that we get the most from student teaching. I like the pupils, too. We haven't had much trouble with discipline - of course, in short-hand and typing their hands are so busy they haven't time to get into mischief. We have a "homeroom" of sophomores. They meet every day for the rest of the time they are in school with the same teacher, and Mr. Sims is supposed to give them help any way they need it. He has different students assigned to read from the Bible every day, and then they repeat the Lord's Prayer, or call on someone to pray. I thought of you, Mother J., the first day they started it, because I knew that was one thing you always did at school.

"We had a letter from Mac Sterling, the boy who finished here in August and went to Dallas. He says it is wonderful to be out of school and back in Texas. He is working at the Lisbon VA Hospital in Dallas, and was to go to McKinney one day a week to give some tests. Made us realize that it will be possible for us to get back to Texas, too, before long.

"Take care of yourselves. So you gathered corn again on your [44th] anniversary. Is that your annual celebration? We're glad you are able to do so, but glad that it is all in and you won't be doing any more.

"Love to you both, Jean."

In a few days Jean received the results from the National Teachers' Exam. The University's policy was that scores falling within the upper fourth of the national norms excused the degree candidate from final orals. Jean was shooting for that score but she over shot her mark with a score at the 98th percentile on the national norms, the highest ever made by a student at the University of Kentucky. We went out to dinner that evening to celebrate!

Jean's sister Marian called on Thanksgiving Day 1950 that her husband, David Wallace died. David was a rural mail carrier in Rockwall and Marian had taught at Rockwall High School. David had been ill for sometime but we really didn't expect his death. He had some 16 operations over the years for a lung condition. David was a very fine person and we were saddened by his death.

The University brought to campus a number of excellent numbers for the concert series that fall, James Melton, Charles Laughton, and the Royal Philharmonic Orchestra of London, Sir Thomas Beecham conducting. The latter especially was quite a treat. However, my favorite was Charles Laughton's reading and acting out the "fiery furnace" and "lions den" scenes from the Book of Daniel.

The chairman of my dissertation committee, Dr. H. H. Humphreys withdrew from the University the first of December 1950. The Dean of Graduate School, Dr. Herman E. Spivey wrote Dr. Frank A. Pattie and asked him to accept appointment as the "chairman for special committee." Dr. Pattie was an excellent choice.

We returned to Texas for Christmas, 1950. Mother invited the Mac Sterlings for supper one night. Both sets of parents filled our car with preserved foods including another ham and sack of sausage from the Gibson smoke-house. Jean wrote a thank you letter January 2, 1951 to the AWJ's.

"We have surely been enjoying the sausage, pickles, eggs, cake, candy, lard - and I'm sure that isn't all the things that kept falling out of sacks when we got home. I can't fuss at you, Mother J., for giving them to us, for we surely do enjoy your good cooking. (Thanks too, for the preserves and ham - I'll probably keep thinking of things as this letter progresses.). . . Thank you too, for the beautiful quilt. It would certainly be nice if the two of you were near enough to come for a visit - at least I'd have cover for you.

". . . Last night we had the Leimans (with whom we had Thanksgiving dinner) and the Thomases (who lived at Mrs. Cocanoughers [in the basement]) over for scrambled eggs and sausage. We used one jar that you gave us and a part of the roll Daddy gave us. I just wish that you could have been here to see them eat. We had the "party "pickles and some of the plum preserves (or is it jam), too. They surely did enjoy it all. They said for us to be sure to thank you for them, too! We'll save the rest for ourselves - actually we hated to give away even that part of it, it is all so good."

Four couples of our Clinical Psychology trainee group gathered at the Pecks for a New Year's Eve watch. Elmer Wingrove dropped out of the program and began selling hearing aids, married a Southern Belle, Mary Ann from Russellville, Kentucky and rented the duplex next door. Mary Ann and Elmer returned from their Christmas at Russellville with pounds of fresh ribs and invited us over one night for barbecued ribs. The Wingroves were a delight. One time on their return from Russellville, Mary Ann brought along a live baby goat.

Kentucky won its first major bowl, the 1951 Sugar Bowl. Lexington turned out en masse for a big celebration at the new coliseum. The governor was there and designated each member of the squad a Kentucky Colonel. Former governor Happy Chandler was present along with other Kentucky big-wigs to acclaim and honor Coach Bear Bryant and the team. School was out for the day.

That January I concentrated on preparing for the presentation of the dissertation subject at the graduate seminar. Doctoral candidates assisted each other along the way and John Love, an older Texan from Corsicana asked me to serve as a rater of some of his data. John came one January night bearing two cans of Wolf Brand Chili along with a group of tests to be judged. He brought back a case of Wolf Brand when he returned from Corsicana at Christmas. It had "been too long - podner" since we ate Wolf Brand Chili, so we consumed a can that night and John explained to Jean how to make a Frito-pie with the other.

John Love returned on Sunday with another rating request that took all afternoon. I began to regret the offer to help as it was taking time from research, but felt rewarded when John took us to dinner one night at Richmond.

The research seminar presentation on the last Friday in January was favorably received by faculty and students. Several stopped by to compliment the presentation. 4

Jean completed student teaching and pupils brought gifts: The typing class a compact and the shorthand class a set of ear rings. The teacher, whose place Jean took temporarily because of the teacher's illness, gave Jean a sterling nut spoon. Jean was more thrilled by their responses than her excellent straight-A record. We attended Rubenstein's wonderful piano concert at the University that evening.

Family

We decided toward the end of 1950 to begin our family, and each consulted physicians. Jean's physician said she was in perfect physical health prescribed thyroid and she soon became pregnant. By January we were certain, but waited a month to announce. A "Special Addition" letter to all family members:

"On or about September 20, 1951 some of you will become cousins, some of you will become Uncles, some of you will become Aunts, and some of you will become Grandparents (again). No doubt you will be pleased, but you won't be as enthusiastic as we are."

I was inexperienced in observing expectant mothers but noticed that Jean was a little woozy once or twice. But an example of her good health was demonstrated by our walking in the snow in

15 degree weather to attend the Kentucky-Georgia Tech basketball game. Our duplex was near the campus.

It was about this time that we had the "really big snow." The deep cold made

to start the 1948 Plymouth, but fortunately it was parked along the side of the house near the bathroom window. John Knight Motors explained the starter "solenoid" was frozen and to apply heat. We turned up the bathroom heater to full heat - placed our new Electrolux cleaner near the gas heater - reversed the cleaner hose to the blower end of the Electrolux - extended the hose through the window and directed hot air onto the frozen starter. In no time, the starter thawed and transportation was available for the drive to the Lexington VA Hospital.

Jean began to make baby and maternity clothes. We visited another expecting couple and saw all of their baby clothes. There were five VA trainees whose wives were on the expectant list. Ex-GI's were eager to begin families.

Incentive increased a hundred fold for completing graduate school. With the research proposal approved, the focus turned to data collection. The "normal" veteran population came from Louisville's General Medical VAH and Dick Thomas and I made the trip together to Louisville. Hatter Thomas stayed with Jean while we were away from home testing patients. Collecting data from Lexington VAH population was a slower process. I was in a hurry to get to the analyses and write.

Job Search Begun

I wrote the Executive Secretary, Committee of Expert Examiners, Veterans Administration, Washington, D. C. on March 24, 1951, enclosed an application for preliminary processing for a Clinical Psychologist Position, and stated, "With the exception of my doctoral dissertation, I have fulfilled all requirements for the Ph.D. degree. I hope to have met all requirements by August,

1951." A courtesy copy of the letter went to Area Chief, Clinical Psychology, Dr. N. Norton Springer of the Columbus, Ohio Area to inform him of an interest in appointments to VA Hospitals in Temple, Marlin, Houston, or McKinney, Texas.

In turn, Dr. Springer referred me to Dr. W. S. Phillips, Area Chief Clinical Psychologist for the Southwest at St. Louis, Missouri. A letter to Dr. Phillips was the first of many communications with that helpful psychologist.

A letter to Dr. Harold M. Hildreth, Chief, Clinical Psychology Section, Veterans Administration Central Office, Washington 25, D. C. on April 2, 1951 informed him I was in ". . . the final stages of collecting data for my dissertation problem," and expressed an interest in Texas for first VA assignment.

We attended the University's fine arts number to hear the Russian-born American, Jascha Heifetz and "his famous violin." The last performance of that great fine arts season came from the Dallas Symphony Orchestra. 5

Mothers Day found us at a roadside park eight miles outside Kentucky. It was a warm day in May, so while I studied Jean prepared a picnic lunch. "Jean wanted to get out of the house." Wrote our Mothers as we basked in the sun after the picnic lunch.

All data for the doctoral dissertation were collected and statistical analyses begun by June. Jean completed her studies for the Masters and attended Sunday afternoon Baccalaureate Services, but because of pregnancy did not walk across the stage for the diploma at June 1, 1951 graduation exercises.

The Electrolux Vacuum Cleaner purchased in January 1951 was designated by Jean as her graduation gift. I learned the hard way in 1948 not to take such a statement at face value. She bought two pair of shoes at the January clearance sale and said that would be her 22nd birthday gift February 22, 1948. The day arrived and I reminded her she received her gift in January. That was a mistake!

Smarter, I encouraged Jean to buy a new dress for graduation and she said we couldn't afford it. Library research was interrupted on graduation day to order a corsage of two gardenias to be delivered while I studied at the library. She was quite pleased and decided the new dress was necessary to go with the corsage. So we drove down town about 10 minutes before the stores closed and purchased a lovely dress. She never looked prettier than she did that Friday night at graduation. Everyone complimented her.

By June 3, 1951 the struggle began to find words for the opening paragraph of the dissertation. The gas heaters were stored, the window fan installed, and furniture rearranged so there was plenty of space to write. Yet, the search for words continued, and finally, an opening statement.

Clyde, Margaret, their two children, Bobby and Kathy, and Marian came for a two day visit in mid-June. Manual Arts Therapist Clyde came to Lexington to represent the McKinney VAH at a regional Physical Medicine conference.

It was a good time for Jean to have a visit from relatives. She prepared lobster for one of the meals. A number of photographs documented the mini-vacation. We toured Calumet Farm, visited Man of War's statue, picnicked at Moore's Mill, and made a trip to Richmond. Jean and I were pleased to have relatives visit from Texas, and receive a break from writing.

Jean typed a letter June 27, 1951 to Dr. Ruth Hubbard, Chief, Clinical Psychology Section, Waco V.A. Hospital, enclosed a Standard Form 57 (application), and inquired about possible future openings. Dr. Mac Sterling, a recent staff member of the Waco VA Hospital, was given as reference. A copy of the letter was sent to Dr. Phillips.

A Marchant Calculator and Royal Typewriter were sophisticated equipment in 1951. The graduate school required an original and three carbon copies of a letter-perfect, typed dissertation. My beautiful pregnant wife, with excellent typing skill waited patiently as each page slowly evolved. Consultation began with dissertation Chairman, Dr. Frank Pattie with completion of the first draft in July.

We took time off one evening to hear an interesting talk by Senator Paul Douglas of Illinois who spoke on the Korean problem. He was being "talked" as a possible presidential candidate.

Dr. Ruth Hubbard wrote July 9, 1951 of her interest in the application and invited me to visit Waco. Dr. Phillips wrote the same day saying the application was ". . . receiving favorable consideration," and suggested Dr. Will Rogers of San Antonio might have a possible opening at the Mental Hygiene Clinic. Dr. Rogers was contacted July 30, 1951, and responded August 8, 1951 requesting a Standard Form 57, mailed August 18, 1951. These details are presented to document some of the job hunting activities as the dissertation writing continued.

All those professional letters were typed by Jean as she waited to type the slowly evolving dissertation chapters. The GI Bill paid $75 for the typing of a dissertation. Jean bought an antique walnut desk with her $75 at Bernice's in Waco.

A Bound Dissertation

The dissertation was submitted August 9, 1951 with these acknowledgements:

"The writer wishes to express his appreciation to the members of his committee: Dr. Frank A. Pattie, Dr. Graham B. Dimmick, Dr. James S. Calvin, Dr. Morris Roseman, and Dr. Irwin T. Sanders. Without their interest, advice, and generous help, this study could never have been carried through. Dr. A. Dudley

Roberts, Chief Clinical Psychologist, Veterans Administration Hospital, Lexington, Kentucky, Dr. Joe L. Lawson, Clinical Psychologist, Nichols Veterans Administration Hospital, Louisville, Kentucky, and the personnel of these two hospitals contributed in many ways to this research, especially in screening the patients used as subjects in this study. The author is deeply grateful to Dr. Graham B. Dimmick for the idea of the Rorschach test-retest technique employed in this experiment. Above all, he desires to express his obligation to Dr. Frank A. Pattie, under whose direction this study has been made, for his continued interest and criticism during the course of the work. To my wife, Jean Gibson Jernigan, who participated in all stages of the development of this study, goes my immeasurable gratitude for the countless ways in which she provided inspiration and encouragement." 6

I don't recall the Dissertation Committee's oral examination or the defense. I wrote my parents an undated letter on or about August 20, 1951 that it was a two hour defense, but . . ."I out talked them, Daddy. My phenomenal luck is still holding up." During World War II my Dad often made the comment, "Jack is the luckiest fellow I ever saw" referring to my premium duty assignments, promotions, leave privileges, etc. I have come to the conclusion it was "Divine luck."

Seventy-five dollars was deposited August 21, 1951 with the University of Kentucky Office of the Comptroller for "Dr's Degree & Deposit." That same day we wrote the Executive Secretary, Committee of Expert Examiners, Washington, D. C., "I have now completed all requirements for the degree of Doctor of Philosophy at the University of Kentucky, with a major in Clinical Psychology. A statement to this effect from the Graduate Office is enclosed . . . To date I have worked approximately 4,296 hours as a Clinical Psychologist Trainee at the VA Hospital, Lexington, Kentucky. . . .Please address any correspondence to me in care of W. M. Gibson, Melissa, Texas."

Dr. Phillips made a special detour through Lexington on a return trip to St. Louis especially for an interview. He recommend a temporary transfer to McKinney VAH. The Columbus Area Chief, Dr. Springer, approved Phillips' plan to transfer me as a fourth year trainee to the McKinney VA Hospital, until a position could be established at Waco.

We immediately began to plan the move, Jean by plane, as recommended by her obstetrician, and I to follow later by car pulling the trailer we bought especially for the trip. Our 1947 Kentucky landlord, Mr. Charles Shepherd, wired the trailer for lights and their connection to the 1948 Plymouth. One of the first items loaded in the trailer were the shelves Mr. Shepherd helped build for storing books, canned goods, etc. in our one room with kitchen privileges. The shelves were our first piece of furniture, and continue to give good service.

I drove Jean to Louisville on Wednesday of our last week in Lexington for her 10:45 A.M. American Airline flight to Dallas by way of St. Louis. Clyde met her plane at Love Field. I returned to Lexington to pack and load the car and trailer. We had completed a fruitful four years. I am eternally grateful for the gift God gave us.

Chapter 3 - 1951 - 1956

Jean flew to Texas carrying a Master's Degree – pregnant with our soon to be delivered baby. I followed in the '48 Plymouth leading a 4 x 4, two wheel trailer, and carried a letter from the Dean of the University of Kentucky Graduate School stating that all requirements had been fulfilled for a Ph.D. in Clinical Psychology. There was a promised Psychology position waiting at the Veterans Administration Hospital, Waco, Texas

A few hours of sleep in a Memphis motel and I was on the road again driving toward Texas. The car rolled to a stop the afternoon of the second day at the Gibson's home in Melissa, Texas. The floating, tattered tarp slowly settled over the trailer's contents. Jean said she was never so happy to see anyone.

A brief visit with Jean and all the relatives, and on the road again to Waco for an interview with Dr. Ruth Hubbard who confirmed a position as soon as the Committee of Expert Examiners verified the GS 11 rating. I accepted a temporary appointment as a Fourth Year Level Trainee at Waco VAH that insured income during the interim. Mac and Judy Sterling offered a cot for the night. The next day I opened a bank account with $500 borrowed from Daddy, as our funds were still in a Kentucky bank, and rented a two bed-room house at 3641 North 25th Street for $75 a month. I returned to Melissa August 29, 1951 for a rapid move to Waco.

The four wooden boxes of wedding gifts stored in the Sedalia attic since 1947 were loaded on the trailer. Jean had periodically checked the boxes and their contents during our 1947-1950 visits to Sedalia. One Christmas night she asked that the box containing crystal be brought down to the living room for examination. The box was packed in straw-like material. Later that night Jean discovered her engagement ring was missing. So-o-o, the box was brought back from the cold attic to the fireside of the living room and Austin, Blanche, Jamie, Frances, Jean and Jack carefully searched the straw-packing. The ring was found.

We purchased a sofa and chair from Marian and borrowed a half-bed from Grandma Gibson to add to our marble top table and a bookshelf. Jean and I moved to Waco August 30, 1951, assisted by Grandpa (Jake) Gibson and Clyde Tilton. The furniture was placed on Grandpa's 1948 Ford Pickup, and the repacked trailer attached. Clyde drove Grandpa's pickup pulling the loaded two-wheel trailer covered with its tattered tarp. Jean and I followed the caravan in the Plymouth filled with the balance of our personal possessions.

When the convoy reached Waco at noon, Grandpa directed Clyde to pull into Youngblood's Fried Chicken parking lot. We bought chicken, found a beer for Grandpa, and all four of us sat in our loaded vehicles eating lunch. Jean, in her final month of pregnancy was most eager to move into the new home and rest.

We bought an apartment size Magic Chief stove from R. T. Dennis for $159.50 the next day, a duplicate of the stove Jean admired at 161 Chenault, Lexington. We also purchased a refrigerator from Sears for $289.95 with the stipulation that it be delivered before the Labor Day weekend. After four years of marriage we "set up housekeeping." I took a mini-vacation. We selected an obstetrician, and continued the search for furniture, old and new.

A letter to the Secretary, Committee of Expert Examiners in Washington on September 3, 1951, asked for ". . . expeditious processing of my Standard Form 57." A letter that same day to Dr. Phillips, Area Chief Clinical Psychologist informed him of the decision to continue as a trainee effective September 10, 1951 at Waco VAH.

Jean's letter on September 13, 1951 to Austin and Blanche Jernigan summarized those first few days in Waco.

"Dear Mother and Daddy J.,

"We've enjoyed *your daily postals*, and hope that you're enjoying the cool weather.

"We have had two good rains this week and are hoping that it will make the bermuda grass grow. Jack got the yard all hoed [of tall Johnson grass] (but not raked), and it is nice to be able to see out!

"Jack seems to be very well pleased with his work so far. He has been busy every day, and that certainly does make a job more pleasant. He eats at the Mess Hall, like he did in McKinney [VAH 1946-1947], at noon each day, and he says he's going to get fat, the food is so good. I guess I'll have to start skipping supper since the doctor has told me not to gain any more. I went to him the Tues. after we got here and again last Saturday. He said everything was fine, except I've gained a little too much, and he seems to be very conscientious and thorough. I will go again Saturday, and I'm hoping that will be the last time. I feel fine - just clumsy. 1

"We still haven't found any living room furniture, although we've been running down the second-hand ads in the paper. I guess we may have to wait until we can go to Dallas later on, since there just isn't much selection here.

"We got a rocker from one of the ads. It's a small antique-ish affair with arms and a sort of cane seat (round). We thought it was very pretty even if it does squeak with hard rocking. Some people were moving to Colorado and it was the man's Mother's chair.

"Jack has been waxing the floors and washing woodwork at night. I hate for him to have to do it after working all day, but he insists.

"We have some very nice neighbors. The girl across the street is a nurse - her husband is an officer in the Air Force Headquarters here. She gave me the names of some women who take baby cases, and I've gotten in touch with one. She seems very nice, but isn't sure she will be available, since she is keeping her daughter's baby while she is sick. She said she thought she could tell me this week-end whether she could help or not. She is a practical nurse, and has taken care of a lot of her own grandchildren, as well as other cases.

"Oh, about the pillows: We will surely appreciate them. We have two Mother fixed 4 years ago, so haven't bought any more. We can certainly use another pair, and appreciate your making them up. We like rather small ones. I'd rather have pillows I think than a bolster. Hope you are both well. Don't work too hard.

Love, Jean"

We purchased a maple bedroom suite from R. T. Dennis and Company Furniture for $278.40. We paid "a Mrs. Tucker" $18.50 for the Mahogany "Grandma" rocker and "a Mr. Quinn" $45 for a walnut dining room suite. 2

Birth of a Baby

Beth Ann Jernigan was born September 26, 1951. Beth's safe arrival concluded her exciting development in her mother's womb while the parents raced to complete graduate school. It was a gloriously happy ending!

I wrote at 7:15 AM, September 26, 1951:

"Dear folks,

"Mr. Terry should have the news to you by now. Your grand daughter is beautiful, cold black curly hair about 1/2 inches long. Perfect features, not a mark on her, and has a good set of lungs. She certainly does favor her paternal grandmother. Name, undecided. 7 lb -12 oz.

"Jean felt some pain yesterday morning. Since we had a phone, I went on to work and called back every couple of hours. Last night her pains were coming every 30 minutes. At 10: PM they got down to 5 minutes and we went to the hospital [Hillcrest]. They prepared her and around 1:30 gave her sedatives; at around 4 AM she went to the delivery room and sometime between 4:30 and 4:45 the baby was born. The nurses told me, 'She is a wonderful patient - never a peep out of her - she's the sweetest thing, etc.'

"The doctor [Dr. Traylor] came out after it was over and said it was remarkable how easy it was for her since this was the first one. I waited until she got to her room and then saw her only a minute. Came home, called the Gibsons, Jamie, wired Stewart, and then called Sedalia [Mr. Terry's grocery store] at 7. I'm still all keyed up, but thank God everything turned out so well.

"I'm going back over at 8:30 to see how Jean feels. Also want to try to get her in a more private room. Ours was the 6th baby last night at the hospital, the maternity ward is full and Jean is in another ward. There were 3 more to come when I left.

"Jamie called last night. He had received my card in which I told Frances that we might take her up on her offer to help. At that time we didn't have anyone to stay with Jean when she returns. (We do now - a motherly woman, widow, seems nice.) I really believe Frances wants to come and we still may decide we need her. Maybe the second week, just to keep Jean company. I thought it was sweet of her to offer.

"Now, when are you coming? I called the M-K-T. Only one train out of W.W [Whitewright] each day. Leaves W.W. 8:22 PM -- Waco 1:30 AM. Round trip $9.66. That means overnight, but we have a new bed for you to sleep on. Now, if you can't do that - let me know - I'll drive to Sedalia either early Sat. or Sun. morn.

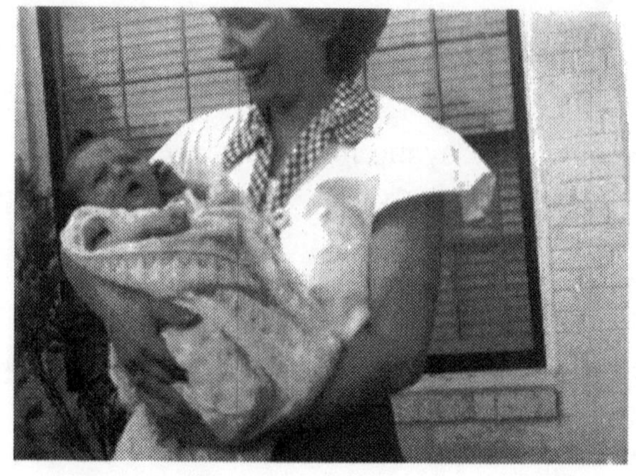

- bring you down, take you back same day.

"Jamie said this morning that they will probably come up this weekend. I'm sure some of the Gibsons will come too. If you could come sometime while Jean is in the hospital (prob. 7 days) it would probably be easier on you.

"Got a number of things to do.

Love, Jack"

Later, Jean mailed Hallmark announcements to relatives and friends.

"Announcing A New Edition - Title - Beth Ann Jernigan - Co-Editors - Jack and Jean Jernigan - Published At - Waco, Texas - Date Sept. 26, 1951 - Weight 7 lb., 12 oz.

An unabridged description would fill a great big book. But if you want complete details just come and take a look!"

Many in the Gibson family came to Waco to see their new granddaughter and niece that weekend. Frances Jernigan stayed with us for a week after Jean and Beth came home.

Among Beth Ann's visitors was Mr. and Mrs. Biggs, our next door neighbors. Large "Mr. Biggs," a retired telephone employee looked at Beth, peacefully asleep in her crib and remarked, "Oh, what I would give if I could sleep like that."

Uncle George and Aunt Bernice brought my parents to Waco October 7, 1951, date of their 45th wedding anniversary.

Most VA employee couples had only one automobile, and car-pooling was a necessity. Such was not easily arranged those first few months in Waco, and Judy Sterling, along with little Mike and new sister Sandy, drove Beth and Jean for Beth's "four week's check-up" with Dr. Flowers.

That October 24 Jean wheeled Beth in her baby carriage across the vacant lot to a small grocery store, bought ingredients, came home and cooked a chocolate cake for my 31st birthday. What a family!

Church

Check stubs outlined our search for a church home in Waco. We consistently gave a $10 offering to the churches visited: September 17 - Calvary Baptist; September 24 - First Baptist; October 21 - Highland Baptist; November 5 - Columbus Avenue Baptist; November 12 - Westminster Baptist; November 25 - Columbus Avenue Baptist. The pastor of Columbus Avenue Baptist was the gifted Dr. W. W. Melton. It was there Beth Ann received her first introduction to church, and was our church home the five years we lived in Waco. Jean joined a Sunday School class. I identified with a Bible class led by prominent Waco lawyer, Frank Wilson. Two other VA Psychologists, Mac Sterling, and Don Gorham, also attended Frank's class.

Work

I felt warmly welcomed to Waco VA Hospital by Manager, Dr. George T. McMahan (native of Van Alstyne), Personnel Officer, H. L. Beckam, and especially the Psychology Staff led by its Chief, Dr. Ruth Hubbard, and staff, Drs. Verner Baugh, Don Gorham and Mac Sterling. I entered duty as if a staff member, but was technically a 4th year trainee (and so paid) until September 28, 1951. Again, in looking back, there was a miraculous blending of events not only in the development of our family, but in the post-doctoral work assignment.

The Waco Veterans Hospital of the 1950's had a capacity of 2,000 + beds. It was larger than the Lexington VAH, but the two hospitals were similar in their approach to treatment. Psychology Service had its offices in the basement of Building 11. Patients were brought to a large office-reception area managed by Secretary to the Service, Mrs. Doris Newman. A group therapy room with one-way mirror and observation room wired for sound joined the reception area. Staff Psychologists and trainees' offices were to right and left along a hallway that ended with Dr. Hubbard's office and conference room at the end of the hall.

The Hospital had a large Psychiatric Staff some of whom were Drs. Goode, Segal, Ross, John R. Shawver, Mitchell, McElroy, Tom Frank, and Director of Professional Services, Walter L. Ford. The psychologists perceived most all the psychiatrists to be "organically oriented." That is, patients' illnesses were primarily medical in origin, treatable by electric shock therapy, water-soak treatments, some medications, and in extreme cases, lobotomy. Psychopharmacology was in its formative stage. With the advent of Insulin Coma Therapy, Dr. Don Gorham introduced Group Psychotherapy as a necessary component, and I assisted as a group therapy leader.

Weekly Psychiatric teaching-staff conferences led by a staff psychiatrist always included a Social History reviewed by a social worker and a comprehensive psychological study by a staff psychologist. The psychiatrist usually interviewed the patient and presented the concluding diagnoses.

One of the psychiatrists gave an orientation tour of the hospital wards and I had the good fortune of correctly identifying a Huntington Chorea patient when the psychiatrist asked for a diagnostic opinion. The opinion was based on academic studies for I had never observed a person with this dread diagnosis. It was a good start for the "new psychologist on the block," and was respectfully received when soon afterwards my turn came to present at the Psychiatric Staff meeting.

Dr. Ruth Hubbard was a child psychologist prior to her appointment as one of the first female Chief of Psychology Service with the Veterans Administration. She came to the VA with a strong academic background. Her father had been President of Oberlin College - her sister was a Psychiatric Social Worker, and her brother a Psychiatrist, a "family" Mental Health team. Ruth was a good psychological role model for a post-doctoral psychologist and I profited much under her supervision.

Though never married nor a mother, Ruth Hubbard was very interested in our new daughter, Beth Ann, and I was always pleased to tell about Beth's growth and development. Ruth's Child Psychology explanations of Beth's behavior were helpful, but not always practical.

Family and Work

Beth was a delightful baby and Jean was a wonderful mother. Those were the days when mothers were encouraged to place babies on formulas instead of nursing the infant. I was quickly taught to prepare the formula, sterilize bottles, and all the other details of caring for an infant. Dr. Spock was the popular authority. We worked a feeding arrangement that Jean usually gave Beth the bottle in the wee small hours of the night and my time came on weekends. I can recall how thankful we were when Beth began to sleep all night.

Precocious Beth Ann sent her paternal grandmother a birthday card December 6, 1951, "For You, GRANDMA DEAR, on Your BIRTHDAY." Jean added that I was in Austin attending (my first) annual meeting of the Texas Psychological Association. Beth Ann and mother "were batching."

Soon after becoming comfortable with the professional role as a Staff Psychologist at the Waco VA Hospital, Area Chief Psychologist Phillips began exploring my interest to help establish a psychology position at McKinney VAH. I wasn't, and diplomatically attempted to so respond in a November 25, 1951 letter to Dr. Phillips suggesting a transfer would be more appropriate when McKinney VAH decided to open a Psychiatric Service. Nevertheless, the McKinney VAH Manager and Dr. Phillips asked me to visit the hospital for an interview.

The visit took place December 14, 1951 and a lifelong friendship began with VA Manager, Dr. W. H. Buckholts. It would be five years before a transfer occurred, and that to Dallas VAH Hospital after Dr. Buckholts was appointed joint manager for McKinney and Dallas VA Hospitals.

Christmas 1951

On return to Waco after the McKinney VAH visit, I stopped at the new A. Harris Store in Oak Cliff and purchased a Philco radio-record player, a Christmas gift from my parents. Plans were outlined for Beth Ann's first Christmas with her four grandparents.

Blanche's January diary entry summarized the 1951 Christmas season. Stewart was still in California working toward completion of his doctoral studies.

"Diary - January 1, 1952

We had a very happy Christmas. Jamie and Frances, Brother and Bernice, Jack, Jean and Beth Ann were with us on Sunday aft. Dec. 23. . . . The children stayed with us until Tues. Morn. We had our Christmas Dinner Dec. 24."

Our First Home Purchase

We made a $550 down payment February 20, 1952 for a new house with two bedrooms, central heat, single bath, one-car attached garage in Belmont Gardens at 3913 Colcord. The $9,000 house was purchased from Corwin-Brazelton Co. through their agent Sig Dickson, a North Texas State friend. The GI Bill of Rights secured the 4 ½% Prudential Insurance loan of $8,450 with monthly payments of $56.21.

Soon after moving to Colcord we paid $5.00 to a man with a team and turning plow to break up our back yard so we could begin a garden and sod the lawn. We had begun a vegetable garden at North 25th Street and returned to dig up the onion plants. Mr. Biggs observed that never before in his lifetime had he seen a family take a garden when they moved.

Mr. Biggs offered to locate excess telephone poles, cross beams, and wire for clothes lines for our new home on Colcord. He instructed that a four foot hole for each pole be dug, and "rack them slightly off center" so that when he came to string the wire the lines would remain taut. He laughed when he saw the exaggerated "rack" of 15 degree off center. He said tilt them and I tilted. But the clothes line wires always remained tight.

Dr. Verner Baugh and family lived on a farm and Verner plowed Bermuda grass sprigs from his pasture to sod our barren yard. Jean and I planted the sod and soon had sufficient lawn to require purchase of an "Eclipse" push-lawnmower from Cogdill's Hardware.

Stewart to Texas A&M

Stewart and family returned to Texas in August 1952 to accept a faculty position with the English Department of Texas A&M. Stewart experienced the dread of all doctoral candidates, a disruption in the dissertation committee. His committee chairman took a year's sabbatical in Europe.

Stewart left the student ranks with an additional Masters Degree in English and resumed his teaching career. They came through Waco to meet the new niece and cousin before driving on to Bryan. David and Susan stayed with us for a day or so while Stewart and Mary drove on to Bryan to locate a house. What a delight it was to be with these two beautiful children again.

Beth's first birthday was celebrated at Sedalia September 26, 1952 with Uncle George and Aunt Bernice also in attendance. A week later Jamie and Frances adopted an infant son, James William Jernigan. The family of three visited with the Sedalia grandparents, and the proud parents came through Waco on their return to Kingsville. We were so happy for them.

Grandfather Austin was not feeling well the day little Jim visited, and a few days later Blanche wrote in her diary that "Austin had a spasm." He was hospitalized on October 14 at McKinney Hospital, and a downward health trend began. Being the son living nearest to Sedalia-McKinney, it was necessary to make many trips north during the following forty months.

Professional Opportunities

Opportunities for professional growth were enhanced by Waco VAH Psychology's close tie with the APA approved Clinical Psychology Training Program at University of Texas, Austin. A variety of UT-VA Clinical Psychology Trainees were assigned to our training program and a host of faculty consultants visited Waco, among them being Drs. Wayne Holtzman, Phil Worschel, Austin Griggs, and Ira Iscoe. There are only a few extant documents, but some of the trainees were: Tom Ray, Philip Roos, Earl Wilkinson, Carl Young, Buzz O'Connor, and Ed Kuekes, all of whom went on to become leaders in the field of psychology.

Dr. Phillips made annual visits to the Waco VAH and Jean and I usually volunteered to assist in his off-duty hours entertainment. Jean invited Sharm for dinner during one of his "official hospital visits", and to his delight she served a "country supper" that included blackeyed peas. He asked for more cornbread to "sop-up the blackeyed pea pot-liquor", said it was the best part of the dish. Jean was a charming hostess, loved, and respected by all professional friends. On another "Sharm-visit" a group of us gathered at Ruth Hubbard's one night for coffee after attending a Baylor lecture.

We also entertained the psychology trainees, and sometimes made and served home-made ice cream. One Christmas, Beth was old enough to go caroling with the group. She called Phil Roos, "Pill Roos", a brilliant trainee, but not so gifted, musically. When he chimed in as the group sang "Silent Night" the dogs of the neighborhood began to bay and howl. Phil responded in his deep Belgian accent at the end of each verse of the Holy song, "Dammed dogs!"

Waco Summary - Form 57

An extant Form 57 submitted in 1957 as an application for promotion to a higher grade summarized the Waco VAH years, September 30, 1951 - October 7, 1956 as a "Supervisory Clinical Psychologist." It must be remembered that all Form 57's are written to enhance one's qualifications.

"Descriptions of Work: From September 1951 to March 1953 I served as staff psychologist with service equally divided between psycho-diagnostic testing and individual and group psychotherapy. Most of this assignment was with the Admission Service for acute intensive treatment. In addition, I helped inaugurate a group psychotherapy program for the Insulin Coma Service. A doctoral dissertation for one of the Clinical Psychology Trainees [Phil Roos] developed out of this work.

"In March 1953 I was promoted to the position of supervisory psychologist in charge of training. In this capacity, I was responsible for formulating policy relating to the training in clinical psychology.

"I also was responsible for evaluating the competence and training progress of trainees. I was responsible for the clinical supervision of from one to four trainees assigned to the station at any given period of time. Trainees were usually assigned for periods of six months or a year. It was my responsibility to outline a program for each trainee that would foster the trainee's growth in the areas of diagnosis, psychotherapy, and research. The program was individually outlined so that each trainee received an opportunity to work with members of all disciplines. I supervised the trainees in psychological testing, individual and group psychotherapy, and research; and followed closely the supervision of the trainees in these areas by other members of the staff.

"In addition to the specific training responsibilities, I assisted in the group psychological testing program for all newly admitted patients, did individual diagnostic studies, interviewed all patients referred for psychotherapy by the psychiatric staff of the Admission Service to evaluate a patient's appropriateness for psychotherapy, and in consultation with the psychiatric staff, conducted both group and individual psychotherapy. I assisted in the psychological research of the hospital. The hospital research program was primarily a coordinated program involving several disciplines. I served as Acting Chief of the Clinical Psychology Service in the absence of the Chief."

Group Psychotherapy

Don Gorham introduced group psychotherapy to the hospital and I became one of his first associates. Patients were brought to the Clinical Psychology Office for the group therapy hour, and met in the room designed for teaching and supervision of trainees with an adjacent observation room, a one-way mirror and wired for sound. Waco VAH was a Veterans Administration pioneer in group psychotherapy, and the hospital management occasionally requested permission to bring visiting Washington dignitaries to sit in the observation room.

We carefully explained and demonstrated to each incoming patient the purpose of the one-way mirror. One day a patient waiting for group therapy slipped into the observation room and left this note on the one-way mirror: "Mirror - mirror on the wall who is the most psycho of us all? The Mirror answers back, 'There are no psychos in that class - the psychos are all behind the glass.'" We left the note to remind visitors of the sensitive nature of our work.

I was invited to University of Texas one spring to describe our group psychotherapy program to the Psychology Department. One bright person assumed to be a student asked a number of stimulating questions. The person was not a student, but young faculty member, Dr. Ira Iscoe who became an outstanding leader in Texas Psychology, and a very good friend.

Baylor University

Dr. Verner Baugh developed an affiliation with the Psychology Department of Baylor University and in 1951 told of a possible teaching assignment the next semester with the Department. Verner, Don Gorham, Mac Sterling, and I taught in the night school, but Dr. Hubbard did not elect to teach.

Baylor University's graduate psychology program was in its infancy and I taught only one graduate night course. Beginning in 1952 I taught one or more semesters each year at the undergraduate level in the area of psychology and mental health. Full time Baylor students could take night courses, but most of the students were from the daytime employment ranks.

I enjoyed the Baylor affiliation, but never felt called to full time teaching as did Mac Sterling. He resigned from his VA Psychology Staff position while we were in Waco to accept a professorship at Baylor and was subsequently Chairman of the Department of Psychology for many years.

Jack and Jean cooperated in a letter, Easter Sunday 1953, quoted in part.

"Dearest Mother and Daddy,

"Jean is typing; Jack is telling her what to type; Beth Ann is sitting on Jack's lap helping both!

". . . Daddy, the other night Jean was reading Beth a story, and when she turned to one page, Beth started saying, "Paw, Paw." It was Santa Claus! . . . When Jack came home [from Baylor] that night she had called Santa Papaw, Jack asked her to bring him the book about Papaw, and she did bring the one about Santa. I guess she knows who Santa Claus really is.

". . . Jack went to Austin Friday to a meeting of psychologists and philosophers. They were dedicating some new buildings. Dr. Phillips, from St. Louis, came and will be in Waco all this next week. Don't guess we will have him out since we did last time, but there probably will be a picnic or something for him.

"Our garden is doing very well. Beans are up now and the second row of lettuce, radishes and spinach. Planted some squash and okra yesterday and set out some more tomato plants, and we both cleaned up the yard. Wish you could see it, since it looks very pretty. Uh, Beth is distracting me. (Quote)"

Counseling Psychology Enters Training Program

Dr. Phillips wrote following his annual visit in April 1953 urging me, "to submit a Form 57 to Board of Examiners for rating as a GS-12 on the Counseling Psychologist (Vocational) register." His reason was that I could be temporarily detailed to "cover that brother program at Waco should the incumbent (Mr. Evans) take another non-VA job." He added, "Thank your wife again for me for the after-Warren coffee - but not for her highly literate charade titles. It was a lot of fun and I now occasionally look at Pogo. Incidentally things look so good at your station I'm afraid I'll never have the nerve to ask you to move. It's a top notch program."

The VA staff entertained Sharm by inviting him to a lecture at Baylor by Earl Warren. Afterwards all came by our house for coffee and then charades. Pogo was a popular cartoon figure of the day.

Waco Tornado

The Waco Tornado of May 11, 1953 killed 114, and injured 597 people. It was Don Gorham's car-pool day. Hospital personnel were authorized to leave work early because of possible turbulent weather. As Don drove toward home our eyes focused to the southwest as tornadoes traditionally came from that direction. Had we looked to the right the tornado might have been seen as it entered downtown Waco.

It was a Baylor teaching night, and Jean had an early supper. I first heard the news of the tornado and its destruction on the car radio. One could view downtown Waco from the top of the hill after turning right on to Fifth Street. The city lay flattened. It reminded me of Manila, 1945.

The R. T. Dennis Building where we purchased most of our household items was completely destroyed. Many of the Dennis employees were friends through our church. Coffins were lined up in the Chapel of Columbus Avenue Baptist Church where Dr. Melton gave one memorial service after another. It was a sad, sad time, and Waco opened hearts and pockets to the hurting.

1954

My Dad was hospitalized for a week in January at McKinney Memorial Hospital. We made two trips, as Mother wrote in her Diary, "Jack, Jean and Beth have been home twice since Christmas. Beth gets cuter and sweeter all the time."

In due time a pregnancy occurred that brought a new burst of joy into the lives of Jack, Jean and Beth. Whereas there are a number of extant pre and post documents, surrounding Beth Ann's birth, the extant pre-birth document was a Diary entry by Mother: "August 20. We've been hoping to hear we had a new grand baby at Waco for several days."

Jean began to experience labor pains Friday night, August 20. She asked for something to help distract. The psychologist in me suggested she take the Rorschach and concentrate on what she saw in the inkblots. Somewhere there is an incomplete, invalid Rorschach protocol given by a mother in the early stages of labor. As prearranged, Beth Ann was taken next door to spend that night with Ben and Lulu Torrence.

The Hillcrest Memorial Hospital, Waco, Texas birth certificate states:

"Austin Jackson Jernigan, Jr. was born to Dr. & Mrs. Austin J. Jernigan in this Hospital at 3:10 A. M. Saturday the Twenty-first day of August A. D. 1954."

After visiting with Jean and Jackie in the early morning hours of August 21, I returned home and began making telephone calls. Later, Beth and I went to a restaurant for breakfast, and she listened to the latest news about her brother. Beth was excited about the new sibling, and had many questions.

The Blue Cross Hospital Service statement indicated Jean was admitted at 12:25 A. M., 8/21/54 and discharged 8/25/54 at

11:00 A. M. The total hospital service cost was $126.80 ($14 rate per day), $69.05 paid by Blue Cross, balance by patient. Oh, for the good 'ole days!

Jean recalls I took a weeks leave of absence from the VAH to care for her and the two children, and that neighbors and friends brought much food to help in the responsibility. August was hot, we had no air conditioning, and only a hassock fan for cooling Jackie's room. He broke out with a heat rash.

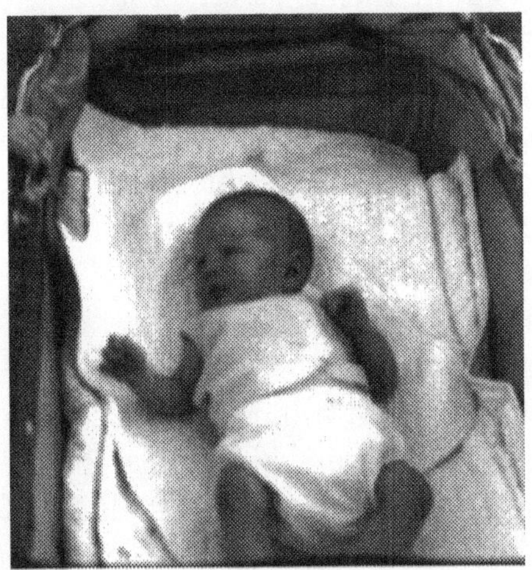

Announcement

"Announcing
A New Arrival
Hillcrest Memorial Hospital Waco, Texas

To Announce
Austin Jack, Jr.
weighing 6 lbs. 7 ozs.
arrived 8-21-54
to The Jack Jernigans"

Mother wrote in her Diary that Jim, Jamie, and Frances, "Made a flying trip more to see Jackie than anything else. . . Spent the night . . . September 2."

1955

We needed a larger house so Beth and Jackie could have separate bedrooms and began to search for a new home. Sharm Phillips' antenna picked up the signal and sent a written note to "Ruth & Jack" February 1.

". . . Tell Jack hold housing open a bit. I have understanding from C. O. (Hildreth, etc.) on his use as a Texas Chief and something may develop soon. It would be an attractive billet. I can not make any commitments as yet on such. The future of the hospitals, indeed are of interest to as important a person as Sam Rayburn and matters are simply not decided yet. I would recommend Jack as Chief of a new hospital (new bldg. of 500, plus old) in Texas and such may be possible soon. I can only say any discussion of such by either of you may well get out and again work adversely to carrying this out."

The next day he added a second note that ". . . word has come through Dr. Buckholts will be Manager of Dallas." Sharm again emphasized, "You are of Chief caliber that C. O. and I would concur on." He also mentioned Temple VA if Dallas didn't materialize, and encouraged us not to buy a new house.

Later that month I attended the "Seventh Annual Institute in Psychiatry and Neurology" held at the Veterans Administration Hospital North Little Rock, Arkansas, February 24-25, 1955. Dr. Hubbard took three of us to the meeting in her 1954 Pontiac.

Sample topics for discussion at the Institute: "Some Relations of Psychiatry and the Law; Sciatica; Some Aspects of Cerebral Vascular Disease; Evolutionary Basis of Sexual Behavior; Recent Advances of Psychoanalytic Therapy; Current Trends in the Study of Personality; Forms of the Family Romance, etc."

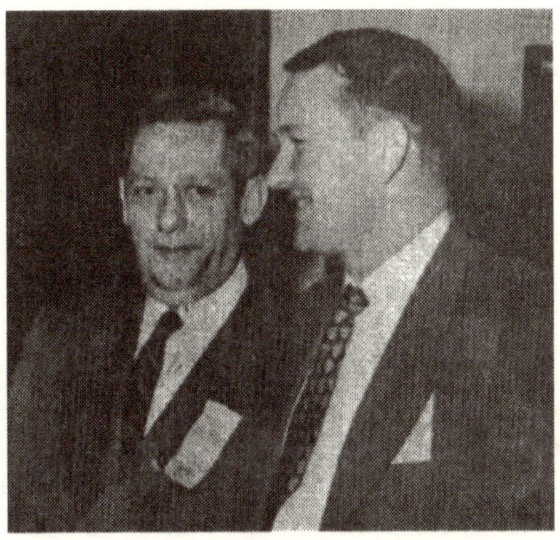

Dr. W. S. (Sharm) Phillips and Jack Jernigan

These and many other topics were summarized in a thirty-six page publication, HILL ECHOES. Sharm and I had a long discussion about the Dallas VA Hospital.

Dr. W. H. Buckholts wrote in March 1955, and offered the psychologist position at the Dallas VAH ". . . when the Psychiatric Service opened." An exchange of letters between the two of us began, interspersed with frequent letters to and from Sharm Phillips. This correspondence covered an eighteen month period. In addition letters and verbal inquiries were received from psychologists about a possible staff position in Dallas.

I wrote Dr. Phillips August 9, 1955 about a four hour personal tour given by Dr. Buckholts in Dallas' new hospital building where the Manager outlined his vision and dreams for Dallas VAH. The hospital opened shortly thereafter. Dr. Buckholts also introduced me to the designated Counseling Psychologist (Vocational), John Geers and his wife Bea. Dr. Buckholts apologized for filling the position before bringing me on board, but was fearful some one would recruit Dr. Geers, a former trainee at McKinney with a recent Ph.D. from University of Missouri. I wrote Dr. Phillips, "John seems to be getting in the harness and strikes me as a person who will be pleasant to work with. I gather that Clinical and Counseling will be independent services in the organizational framework."

In August 1955 Dr. Buckholts said January 1956 was the "upper limit date for opening the N.P. Service." He counseled, ". . . that our house not be put on the market until September 1955."

Family

Jean wrote the AWJ's on Jackie's first birthday. The "McKelvains" were nearby neighbors on Colcord. John was a VAH Social Worker. His wife, Jean, and my Jean were both pregnant at the same time, and their premature baby demanded much extra attention. We became close friends.

"Sunday, August 21, 1955

Dearest Mother and Daddy Jernigan,

"Jackie has had quite a nice birthday. Your check came Thursday. I got him some really cute house shoes at Sears . . . We surely do thank you. Mother and Aunt Ella sent money and we'll get him a peg board or something else with it. Several of the neighbor children came by with gifts - a pull toy cricket, a wooden train, and some blocks. The McKelvains gave him a Davy Crockett t-shirt; Jamie and family sent a darling ferris wheel made of blocks, Beth gave him one of those push sticks with blocks in it, and we all gave him a rocking horse. Beth has enjoyed his toys as much (maybe more) as he has. She said it was just like Christmas. We went to SS this morning and the McKelvains are coming by later to eat cake.

". . . We are going to start advertising our house next week. Jack talked with the real estate man who sold us our house and he advised that we try to sell it ourselves and that he would get a loan set up for us. Then if we left town, he would sell it. I am dreading trying to keep it straight enough to show!

". . . Jack is Acting Chief at the hospital while Dr. Hubbard is gone for six weeks. It is extra work, but I do believe he enjoys it. He has been thinking about buying a power mower, but can't quite make up his mind to do it now or wait until next year. They aren't putting them on sale the way he hoped."

A letter to Dr. Phillips October 19, 1955 informed him we had sold the house and final papers would be signed about the first of December. The sale failed to develop. However, Dr. Buckholts was unable to locate a suitable Chief Psychiatrist for Dallas' Psychiatric Service, and the "imminent" transfer was again extended.

In looking back this was one of those times the hand of God was present in the incomplete house sale. It allowed us to be stable when sadness came to our family in January 1956.

1956

The four of us visited the Gibsons and the Jernigans Christmas 1955. I recall a Christmas time, living room night scene of Daddy holding Jackie's hand doing an Irish jig.

Mother wrote that our dear black friends, Sedalia's respected citizens, Jim and Emma Jones lost their house by fire on January 5, 1956. There was an outpouring of helpful responses from people from miles around. Jean referred to the incident in a January 1956 letter, and also told of purchasing curtain material for the AWJ living room.

"We surely do enjoy your letters, although I so rarely say so.

"We had a real nice note from Jim Jones. It was unexpected and gave us such a good lift.

". . . . We had the trainee [Pat Kuekes from U. T.] Jack supervises and his family to dinner last night. They have children 10 months and 2 1/2, so we had a crowd. The children did very well, we thought. Beth kept things organized!

"Jackie and Beth had their second polio shots Friday. They are fine and had no reactions. The norther just blew in. Jack and Beth are playing paper dolls. She tells him what to say. He just repeats and changes clothes.

"I believe this is all. Love, Jean"

"The Life Went Out"

Mother wrote, after the fact, all the details she could remember about her day, January 30, 1956. The final paragraph of that Diary entry stated:

"I had fish, hot corn bread, coffee, canned peaches and cake for lunch. Austin tried to get Weldon [Lane] to stay for lunch with us but he said Grace was waiting but he said he'd be back to take us to the clinic Tues. morning. After he left Austin decided to take a dose of Sal Hepatica. Then we sat down, he returned thanks as always. He enjoyed his lunch, said the fish tasted good. We talked about going to the clinic - he did not want to go to the hospital as he said he wanted to be at home at night. I asked him if there was any one in the list of obituaries that we knew - he said there weren't but were several listed. I asked him about our bank statement. He asked me if I wanted to know how we stood. I told him I was afraid to ask. He laughed and said it wasn't so bad but that we'd spent a lot as we always did. I do not remember what he said as he left the table but am pretty sure he told me he enjoyed his meal as he always said something of the kind. I told him I'd put the fish in the refrigerator as he'd enjoy it for supper. I followed him immediately but he had sat down on the couch and was gone when I got to him. Then the life went out of our happy home."

The word of my Dad's death came to us later that day through a telephone call from the Sedalia store. We drove to Sedalia late that afternoon, and I recall crying for the first time when I sat on his bed.

Many cards and letters were received by the A. W. Jernigan family. The first letter received following Daddy's death was from Jim and Emma Jones.

Jamie initiated, and the three of us contributed to a tribute published in the Van Alstyne Leader, February 17, 1956.

TRIBUTE TO A FATHER

Austin Wallace Jernigan was born January 12, 1882 at Sedalia, Texas, the son of Mr. and Mrs. A. J. Jernigan, pioneer citizens of North Texas. He married Miss Blanche Coffey of Westminster on October 7, 1906. To this home were born three sons, J. Stewart Jernigan, now professor of English at Texas A. & M. College, James C. Jernigan, dean of Texas College of Arts and Industries at Kingsville and A. Jack Jernigan, psychologist at the Veteran's Hospital at Waco.

He leaves his wife, his sons and their wives, whom he loved like his own daughters, six grandchildren, David, Susan, Beth Ann, Jim, Jackie, and Laura; and three sisters, Mrs. L. E. Rosser, Mrs. J. F. Hoyle, and Mrs. Pansy McDougal of Dallas.

He joined the Westminster Baptist Church in 1907, and had been a deacon of that church for nearly fifty years.

This man was a Christian gentleman in the fullest sense of the word. He demonstrated the fact that a man can be a leader without obviously leading; that a man can preach without ever standing in the pulpit; that a man can leave a rich endowment without vast holdings of material goods. His life was a life of service, first to his God, second to his family, third to his fellowman.

He left to his sons a name unblemished. His word was recognized as his bond. He left to his wife a love that is undying. He left to his friends an example of Christian humility.

On Monday, January 30, 1956, after lunch with his beloved wife, he walked into the living room, sat down, and quietly left to join his Maker. He died as he lived -- quietly and with no bother to anyone.

By His Sons

All three families stayed until Friday of that week. Stewart and family returned to Bryan. It began to snow. Jamie and I found boxes to make "sleds" so the four little children could slide down the snow covered "storm cellar." Later they would remark, "Didn't we have fun when Grandpa died."

Frequent trips were made from Waco to Sedalia during the next nine months, usually alone, but often the four of us would visit. Mother took driving lessons in her '40 Ford during these visits. She subsequently learned "to herd" the Ford toward Sedalia store and Westminster church. Through the months I participated in the probation of the will, purchase of a monument, suggested business responsibilities not previously assumed, took her to Van to buy groceries, etc. She was determined to live alone and succeeded along with the help of a community of neighbors, especially Weldon and Grace Lane.

A New Life

Clyde and Margaret visited one weekend in May 1956 and he and I built a redwood picnic table that is still in use by our lakeside. That summer, back pains began to radiate to one leg, I sought review of symptoms at VA Regional Office, and was told that it was not believed to be a disc problem. I recall sleeping on the floor many nights that summer.

We announced a pregnancy. The wheels began to turn again on the transfer to Dallas VAH. Jean added a P.S. to a letter to Mother:

"We all are feeling much better. Beth is anticipating having a sister to 'dress alike.' Her comment - we have enough boys! We are glad it will be a Dallas-ite so you will be close enough to help us out. At the rate you're going you'll have to put us on your calendar - you have so much going to do.

"Don't worry about us, we are making it fine."

Dr. Buckholts wrote in July and asked me to make a "protocol" visit to Dr. McCranie, acting Chairman, Department of Psychiatry at Southwestern Medical School, and Drs. Carmen Michael and Harold Crasilneck of the Psychology Division. Dallas VA was a "Deans Committee Hospital", and Chiefs of Service participated in education of medical students assigned to the VA Hospital. Dallas VAH Personnel requested personal references, one of whom was Dr. Ruth Hubbard who shared a copy of her letter to Dr. Buckholts. 3

I wrote Mother in August, ". . . the back and leg are much, much better. I still have some pain but I can tell that the symptoms are moving away. For instance this morning I put on my pants without having to hold on to something.

". . . Jean is feeling fine. She said the other day she didn't ask you if you would like to help when she goes to the hospital - she just assumed you would. I know when she learned she was pregnant we were talking about plans. One of the first things she said was how good she would feel if you could be with Beth and

Jackie while she is in the hospital. The baby will come on the anniversary of a sad memory and I think that will be good for all of us. We got the appraisal back on the house Friday, $8900. That is an increase of $150 over last time but $100 less than what we paid. We were quite pleased. Also we had another bit of good luck: Prudential Insurance will finance the loan and charge us 2%. Most of the sellers pay 5% or more. We are running an ad right now. If we have no luck within a week we are going to turn the house over to an agent. He plans to have the house open for inspection this next weekend." 4

We signed a contract August 21, 1956 with Pelt and Foley Builders of Dallas to build a three bedroom, living room, den-kitchen, one and one-half bath, two-car attached garage house on a tree lined lot at 1808 Swansee, Dallas. 5

Beth Ann and Jean wrote Grandma and Grandpa Gibson September 29, 1956.

"Dearest Grandma, Grandpa, & Doris,

"Thank you for the money. I haven't spent it yet, but I am going to.

"Daddy has gone to Dallas to rent us an apt. We will move the last of next week. Is it all right if we bring Frisky up there until we move in our new home?

"I had a wonderful party at Jack and Jill School. Wish you could have come. I have a new bride Ginger doll and telephone switchboard.

"Love, Beth"

Jean was pregnant when we moved to Waco in 1951 and pregnant when we left Waco for Dallas in 1956. However, it was a much different scene: We were parents of two children, I had a position, our household goods were moved by the Federal Government, and a home under construction

Chapter 4 - 1956 - 1959

Dr. Buckholts decided a Clinical Psychology Service was needed at Dallas' General Medical and Surgical (GM&S) Services Hospital with or without a psychiatrist. The transfer as Chief, Clinical Psychology Service (179), Dallas VA Hospital became effective October 7, 1956. 1

We rented a Southern Oaks Apartment accessible to the VA Hospital for $47.75 a month. Although somewhat cramped for space there were playground swings for the children. Lovable black Cocker Spaniel, Frisky was invited to stay temporarily with Grandpa and Grandma Gibson.

Jean's Waco obstetrician, Dr. Clayton J. Traylor referred Jean to Dr. W. K. Strother, Jr., whom she saw October 31, 1956.

The move, documented by Mother in a diary note, came at a significant time for her.

"On Oct. 5, 1956 Jean and Jack moved to Dallas. They came on and spent the night with me. The next day I went home with them. On Oct.7, our 50th wedding anniversary, Jack and Beth Ann brought me home. We'd stopped at Coffman's [Florist] on the way down and ordered flowers, picked them up the next morning and brought them to the cemetery and Jack cleaned his Daddy's grave, would not let any rocks or gravel show covered it with black dirt. It looked so peaceful and sweet when he'd finished and placed the lovely spray on it. He and Beth stayed until about 3 o'clock."

Getting Started at VAH

Dr. John Geers, the same age as my brother Jamie had been on duty at Dallas VAH for more than a year as Chief, Counseling Psychology Service (175). John was educated at SMU and University of Missouri with a Ph.D. in Counseling Psychology. His primary psychological focus was the Vocational Rehabilitation of

Veterans. John was well acquainted with the professional staff as he had worked with them as a trainee at McKinney VAH, enjoyed his role as the only Psychologist for Dallas VAH. John and his wife Bea interacted socially with the Manager and most all the former VAH McKinney professional staff.

Much need for patient care was discovered awaiting the opening of a Clinical Psychology Service (179). Dr. Geers graciously welcomed me. His good rapport with the hospital staff was helpful, but at the same time somewhat competitive. The Manager always referred to me privately as his Chief of Psychology, correctly identified John as responsible for Vocational Rehabilitation, yet, Dr. Buckholts' strong personal relationship with the Geers may have influenced his continuation of two independent Psychology Services. Consolidation of the two services into one Psychology Service (183) came approximately five years later after much encouragement by Central Office.

Clinical Psychology was assigned two offices with secretarial assistance through Social Service's Secretary. The offices were on the first floor in the new nine-story hospital building, identified as Building 2. Adjacent Building 1 was constructed in late 1930's in the Lisbon suburb of Dallas, and the hospital was called the "Lisbon VA Hospital" for many years thereafter. 2

Social Service had two staff members, Chief of Service, Louis DuMall and Social Worker, Dorothy Warwick. Jean met Ms. Warwick in 1946 when they both worked at Austin State Hospital. Mr. DuMall soon resigned to join the Hogg Foundation in Austin, and was replaced by Douglas Torrie.

Louis DuMall, (later Doug Torrie), John Geers, and I developed a wholesome professional working relationship as we each wished to serve the hospitalized veteran to the best of our abilities. I found Chiefs of Medicine (Friedman) and Surgery (North) and their staff eager to make referrals. Nursing Service quickly sought psychological assistance for those emotionally disturbed patients "mistakenly" admitted to Dallas VA. The hospital staff welcomed my years of training and staff duty with psychiatric patients.

It was 1956 hospital policy to confine psychiatric patients to the locked security room on the unopened Ward 7A of the projected Psychiatric Service. The isolated patient communicated via an intercom with the Nurses' Station on Ward 6A, one floor below. The patient was frequently the only patient on the 7th floor wing of the building.

Referrals from Medicine and Surgery for psychiatric consultation came directly to Clinical Psychology. I modified the group assessment battery developed by Waco VAH, and followed with an individual interview. A more comprehensive psychological assessment was conducted where indicated. The approach made it possible to assess many patients and give rapid consultation turn-around. All patients confined to Ward 7A were referred for evaluation and follow-up.

Medical and surgical residents responded positively to the clinical services. Psychological assessment information was also shared with John Geers and the Social Workers. I initiated a psychotherapy group and also offered individual psychotherapy to selected patients.

Dr. Grady Niblo, a Dallas Psychiatric in Private Practice was the hospital's only Psychiatric Consultant. I screened most all psychiatric consultations and verbally summarized findings with Dr. Niblo before he interviewed a patient. Grady Niblo gave strong support to Clinical Psychology and helped pave the way for the establishment of a sound Psychological Service.

One morning Dr. Niblo complimented my communication with a schizophrenic patient we jointly interviewed on 7A. Grady observed, "You have learned to speak the schizophrenic language." The pharmacological era of psychiatric drugs had its beginning in the mid-1950s and to be theraputically supportive required development of a special type of verbal rapport with psychiatric patients. Nine years of training at NP hospitals were helpful.

Family – Church

Before we left Waco, I borrowed John McElvains's movie camera and took a three and half minute film of Beth's fifth birthday party. We were hooked, and purchased a spring-wound Kodak 8mm Movie Camera with lights. One of the earliest Dallas movie scenes was the children dressed in Halloween costumes preparing to make the rounds at our apartment.

We attended Grace Temple Baptist Church October 22 according to a 1957 check-book entry. Cousin Rena and Jethro Banks were members of Grace Temple. We attended Cedar Crest Baptist Church November 26 where Cousin Alton Hoyle was a devoutly active Cedar Creek member and deacon.

The first "Cliff Temple Baptist Church" check book entry was December 9, 1957, and weekly thereafter. The morning we transferred church membership to Cliff Temple Baptist Church, Dallas, Education Director Dr. Earl Mead invited me to teach in Sunday School.

I became acquainted with Cliff Temple as a young lad in the 1930s while visiting Dallas relatives. All my Aunts: Ella Johnsey, Belle Matthews, Claudia Hoyle, Pansy McDougal, Lizzy Rosser, their spouses and children were members of Cliff Temple Baptist Church. Aunt Lizzy Rosser organized Cliff Temple's first church orchestra, taught piano to many members including Pastor Wallace Bassett's children. The church had a membership in excess of 3,000. We became members of a church that also had family heritage for Jean as some of her cousins were members. In addition, most Westminster Baptist families who migrated to Oak Cliff in the early 20th Century joined Cliff Temple Baptist, and some were still there in 1956.

Although the time probably passed slowly for Jean and the two children, we moved from the apartment into our new home at 1808 Swansee the first week of December. A letter of appreciation mailed December 4 to Texas Fireproof Storage thanked them for the storage and safe delivery of "4,440 pounds of household effects." That same day one of the children visited Dr. Tobolowsky who became the family's Pediatrician.

Christmas 1956 was the first Christmas after Daddy's death. Mother wrote in her Diary December 26, "Stewart's family came the 23rd and left Christmas Day. Jack's family came last night and spent the night." Our first Christmas at 1808 Swansee was documented with many pictures around the tree. Then we drove north for the Gibson tree, and later in the afternoon, to Sedalia. No photographs were taken at Sedalia that year.

One of the first purchases for our new home was a Sears' clothes line. We did not own an electric dryer. We contracted with Atlas Fence Co. to build a combination redwood and chain link fence in early January 1957. The fence divided our lot from our neighbors, the Gaddos on the east, and the Terrells on the west, two very nice and congenial families. The two Gaddos children were much older than ours, but the four Terrells were same age or younger.

Family Complete

Jean patiently waited for our third child. She prearranged with Mother to come and stay when time came to deliver. Clyde and Margaret Tilton lived in Melissa and volunteered to bring Mother to Dallas when Jean's "time came."

Jean woke early on March 3, 1957 with labor pains, called Dr. Strother, but he did not recommended immediate hospitalization. We telephoned Clyde. Clyde was at home with Bobbie, Kathy, and Jim as Margaret had nursing duty that day. Clyde and the three children left for Sedalia and brought Mother to

Dallas. In the meantime, Jean cooked a roast so that when the five arrived there would be good food available. Later, Jean and I drove to Baylor Hospital where the thirty-one year old mother gave birth to Richard Gibson Jernigan.

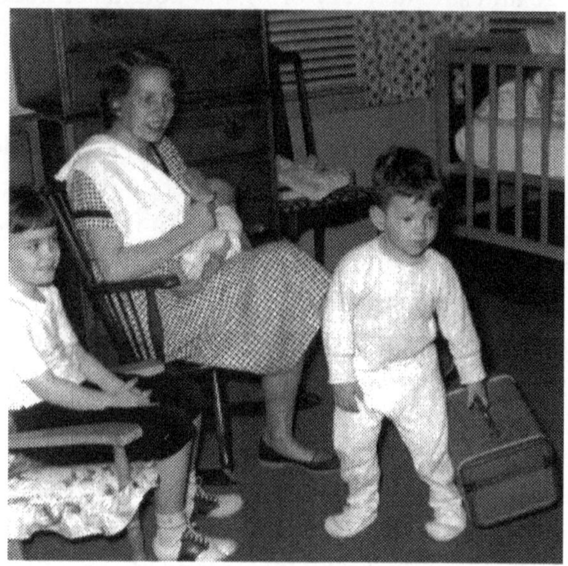

Beth – Jean – Richard – Jackie

Mother stayed two weeks. Excerpts from a letter mailed in March 1957:

"Dear Mother,

"We made the weekend fine but we certainly do recognize what all you have been doing. Jean really was bragging on you yesterday morning at breakfast. She said she didn't believe you could have come in and did what you did and she felt so free and relaxed. She was also talking about how much effort you put out to insure everything ran smoothly. Also, she was wondering how you kept your humor under all conditions.

"Richard is sleeping most all of the night. Jean got up at 3 last night and he was still asleep when I left. He sure is a fine baby. If he keeps this up of not keeping us up at night it will be remarkable.

"... The children and I went to SS yesterday morning. . . We do appreciate every thing you did so very much.

Love, Jack"

Organizing a Psychology Service at Dallas VAH

Psychology and Social Work Services were relocated to the ninth floor. John Geers was assigned the Chief of Psychiatry office suite. Chief of Clinical Psychology office suite had an adjacent office for a secretary, and to the left, an office with one-way observation mirror for supervision of trainees.

Professional Staff Dallas Veterans Hospital 1957

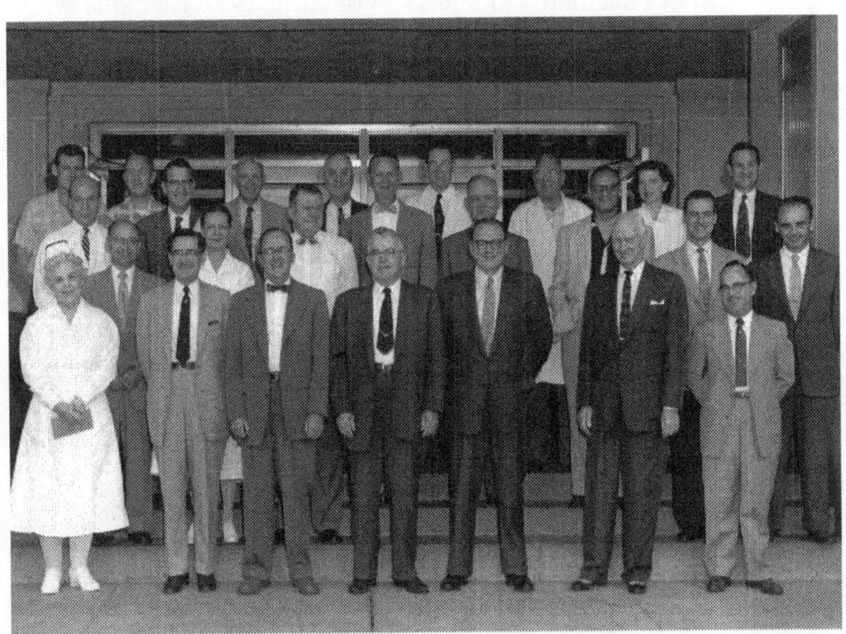

Front row: (Ch. Nurse), Ross, Gaubert, Buckholts, Moran, Wade, Modisett; Second row: Walker, (Dietician), Williams, Nelson, King, Torrie; Third row: Eisenberg, McCullough, Geers, Cohen; Fourth row: Sullivan, (?), (?), (?), Hayes, (Laboratory), (Dietician), Jernigan

When the Veterans Administration accepted Counseling Psychology at the doctoral level for staff positions in the early 1950s it also opened up the VA Psychology Training Program for Counseling Psychology trainees. As reported in Chapter 3, Sharm Phillips urged me to apply for the Counseling Psychology Register in 1953 to serve, supervise and train others.

John and I jointly selected Mrs. Helen Dennis as secretary for the two services. Mrs. Dennis assisted in scheduling and recording the work of psychiatrists for the Psychiatric Consultation Service, coordinated by Clinical Psychology. Consultants came first to our office to review new consultation requests before interviewing a patient.

Southwestern Medical School (SWMS) recruited Dr. Robert Stubblefield from Colorado's Medical School as Chairman, Department of Psychiatry in late 1956 or early 1957. He came with a vital interest that Dallas VAH become a teaching facility for his Psychiatric Residents. Dr. Stubblefield made weekly consultant visits to the VAH and became acquainted with the needs of the Medical and Surgical Services. He and I met frequently to discuss psychiatric consultations as well as to inform him of the hospital's readiness and\or reluctance to accept psychiatry as a part of the medical team.

Soon after Richard's birth, Bob Stubblefield expressed interest in meeting Jean and our new son, Richard. He and I drove to our home, seven miles west of the Hospital one afternoon, to visit Jean and the baby briefly. He wished to become better acquainted, and perhaps evaluate.

A letter to Dr. Phillips on August 19, 1957 summarized developing plans.

"Dr. Stubblefield and I have devoted considerable time in the last month thinking through some of the future plans for the hospital. Our working relationship is good and apparently he is quite accepting of my present role. He wants me to continue to coordinate the psychiatric consultant activities. We now have three psychiatric consultants: Dr. Niblo, Dr. Fred Hinman and Dr. Stubblefield. . . Dr. Hinman is an attending, and follows Dr. Stubblefield from Colorado. . . Dr. Stubblefield will make three visits each month (one per month to McKinney). He is placing himself in the role of teacher and through discussions with Drs. Friedman and North has set up two staff meetings each month. . .The first meeting using Social Work, Psychologist, Psychiatrist and medical resident was held this week for the medical staff and went quite well.

". . . . I continue service to the nurses and nursing assistants. They are quite emphatic in saying these group discussions are bringing about changes in attitudes and leading to better patient care. The fact that the 4-room closed section has been opened for only a one week period within the last seven months lends some validity to their evaluation."

Dr. Stubblefield recruited a personable and gifted Psychiatrist, Dr. Dave Fuller, for the Medical School Faculty. Dr. Fuller was assigned responsibility for teaching psychiatric residents as they rotated through the VA Psychiatric Consultation Program. Administrative coordination of the program continued to be delegated to Psychology Service.

Dave Fuller, Jean and I became good friends. Dave's sister, Aletha Fuller was a Baptist Missionary to Nigeria. Once when Aletha was home on furlough, Dave invited us to his apartment for dinner, and included a mutual friend of his sister and Jean, a Baptist Student Union acquaintance. We exchange Christmas greetings with Dave each year.

First-cousin A. J. Hoyle, a Club Director of the South Oak Cliff Lions Club invited me to address the Lions Club members April 4, 1957 at Arthur's Drive-In Restaurant, 3103 S. Lancaster

Road. A Dallas newspaper covered the event with the headline, "VA Methods Described - Emotionally Disturbed Given New Treatment." The article focused on my discussion of group psychotherapy as a new treatment modality. The talk also included a brief overview of Clinical Psychology's role as a member of a Mental Health Team, and the public's need to be aware and accepting of mental illness.

Family Matters

In the summer of 1957 Beth began what would become an annual event for one or more of the children: A few days with Grandma Blanche on the farm. Beth dictated a thank you letter to her grandmother on July 29, 1957.

"Dearest Grandma Blanche,

"I had fun at your house. Grandma [Gibson] and Aunt Doris came back with us, and Daddy bought a new barbecue at Melissa. We cooked wieners one night. Judy had a birthday today and we all went to the zoo - not Jackie, just the 5 and 6 year olds.

"Jackie and I have just been swimming at Patty's. She has a pool. I shared the cookies and everyone liked them. We enjoyed the cake, too.

Love, Beth"

We were desperately in need of another automobile to supplement the 1954 Plymouth and in September 1957 purchased a two-door, gray 1950 Plymouth from Mr. J. E. Morgan, an elderly Cliff Temple Baptist Church deacon who dabbled in car sales. The 1950 Plymouth brought cheap transportation for a bit over $100 plus insurance and gas, and Jean had the 1954 at her disposal.

Family Life and the VA

In Waco we lived across the street from Price Perrill, an industrious insurance salesman from whom we bought three term insurance policies to insure my life, Jean's, and the family. The rationale was the need for coverage during the family's formative years. Price encouraged an education policy for Beth, but calculation indicated a systematic monthly savings of $5.00 to a savings account in her name paid better returns.

A like fund was initiated for (Austin) Jackie in 1954, and for Richard in 1957. A $5.00 deposit in Richard's name was made at Oak Cliff Savings and Loan on April 8, 1957. All three accounts remained at Oak Cliff Savings until Clyde Tilton and I were selected by the VA employees to help organize the VA Hospital Federal Credit Union.

VA Hospital Dallas Federal Credit Union

In late 1957 or January 1958 the hospital employees nominated a group to organize a Credit Union. Clyde and I were among the employees nominated to form the first Board of Directors, who in turn selected Clyde as Treasurer and me as President. The earliest extant document is a Memo to the Board of Directors, written March 24, 1958 following a weekend study of the Federal Credit Union Bylaws and the Handbook. Excerpts:

"Our first two months have been successful ones. Each of us is learning something new every week. We are all making errors, but these are honest errors. Our Credit Union will grow through being aware of our mistakes and making intelligent corrections of these. Each of us has been honored by being selected by our fellow employees to direct the affairs of the Credit Union. The membership's trust requires considerable study and thought from each of us to live up to the trust.

". . . First, read the Bylaws and the Handbook in their entirety. . . I am amazed how neatly all phases of the organization blend together. . . Every person's position is of equal importance. . . Learn what the by-laws say about your position."

The first year Financial and Statistical Report, dated December 31, 1958 for Charter No. 12038, VAH Dallas Federal Credit Union, 4500 South Lancaster Rd., Dallas 16, Texas gave a Total Assets balance of $7,591.50. There were 152 accounts [$5 deposit to open an account] - 83 loans made during the year for total amount of $10,124.00. At end of year there were 50 current loans in amount of $5,281.07; 2 of the 50 were delinquent. The report was signed by Clyde Tilton, Treasurer.

I served only one year as President, but continued to have a vital interest in the Credit Union as indicated by my membership on the Nominating Committee to recommend candidates for the Board of Directors and Credit Committee for 1969. Mine was a great opportunity to serve fellow employees with their financial needs.

Family Happenings – 1956-1958

Each Thanksgiving we ate dinner at both "grandparents house" and were always well-stuffed by the end of the day. Christmas morning opening of presents was celebrated at our home. Later in the morning, after the children completed their initial interests in Santa Claus' gifts we traveled north to share Christmas with the Gibson Family and Grandma Blanche.

The Gibson family "drew names" at Thanksgiving, so that each person had a Christmas present under the tree. In addition, dear Mrs. Gibson had a talent for coming up with inexpensive, but practical-precious gifts for each member of the family.

It was a tradition that when all the Gibson-tree gifts were distributed, Mr. Gibson would slowly reach for his weathered billfold stuffed with papers and dollar bills. As he sat in his chair, Mr. Gibson called each grandchild to his side and handed him/her a dollar bill. The little girls hugged him, avoiding the pipe that swung from his lip, but only the smallest of the boys hugged. The older boys, Bobby Tilton, Freddie Waller and Billy Waller give him a sly grin and a "thanks."

Richard received a Grandpa Gibson dollar in 1957.
The previous Christmas, Grandpa gave silver dollars to each grandchild, and at the end of the ceremony called for his youngest daughter, Jean full of child. He gave her a 50 cent piece for yet the unborn Richard Gibson.

Grandma Blanche usually sent Christmas checks to her three sons and their families, but always had gifts for each child and grandchild under her Christmas tree. The Sears Catalogue was Blanche's primary shopping resource.

Mother became self-sufficient as documented in her voluminous correspondence. But we frequently made the sixty mile trip north to "do things" for her, being the nearest relatives, geographically. The trips took me away from family when the other members were unable to go along. Mother always sent food and special items to the children. Jean wrote after a visit in March 1958.

"Dearest Mother J.,

". . . Beth and Jackie are just about over their "spots." They feel fine, but are getting restless. . . .Jack enjoyed his visit with you. The children enjoyed the cookies and money. They all 3 have started eating eggs for breakfast now, and they always make sure they're Grandma's eggs.

"Richard has shown no signs of measles. He is walking across the room now, and seems so proud of himself.

Love, Jean

"P.S. We are enjoying the delicious jelly."

Current Events - 1958

Larry Powell, Dallas Morning News feature writer, summarized highlights of News articles for May 21, 1958.

"President Dwight Eisenhower urged Americans to pull together in lifting the economy to higher and higher levels . . . New York held a ticker-tape parade for Fort Worth's Van Cliburn, the first American to win Moscow's Tchaikovsky International Piano Competition . . . Chrysler Corp. . .lost more than $15 million in its first quarter and asked 'executives earning from $10,000 to $15,000 to sacrifice one week's pay' . . . at the Southwestern men's apparel market in Dallas, a 'radical innovation' - Velcro closures for men's and boy's jackets . . . Madame Alexander dolls cost $8.95 . . . 1958 Ford Edsel $1,988 . . .'South Pacific's' Southwestern premiere was at the Wynnewood in Oak Cliff (tickets were $1.75 to $3.95) . . . on TV: Captain Kangaroo, American Bandstand, The Mickey Mouse Club, I Love Lucy . . . regular gasoline sold for 19.9."

Excerpts from an August letter to Grandma Blanche:

Dear Mother:

". . . Richard's Sunday School teacher had to come get Jean this morning. He just wouldn't quit crying. I'm in hope his moving to a new class this next month will help him get readjusted.

"We certainly did enjoy the day with you Saturday . . . thank you for each item you gave us.

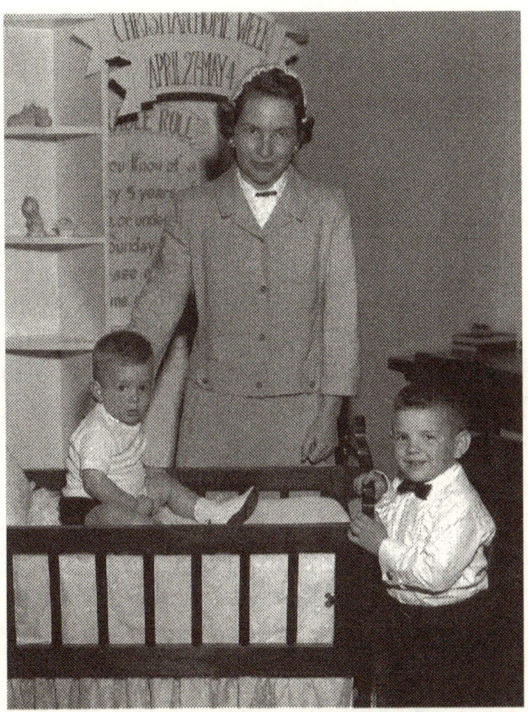

Richard, Jean, Jackie at Cliff Temple Nursery

"The okra was still frozen hard when I put it in the refrigerator last night. We had your good jelly for breakfast. We appreciate the fresh food but especially all of the work and planning that goes into it. And it helps out on our grocery bills too.

"When Richard got in last night he wanted his 'Grandma Blanche gum' and has referred to it today also. Jackie's Sears package had come during the day. He was thrilled with the Tinker-Toys. You know one gift was aplenty. If I recall, back in the summer you said you were going to limit birthdays to $2. What ever happened to those plans?

". . . I think it is remarkable the way you keep everything looking so pretty and nice. I know you put out hours of work to do it. I hope your hip continues to improve.

Love, Jack"

We hired a contractor to pour a shuffle board court adjacent to the west redwood fence. We had many happy games with hospital staff, Sunday School classes, and our family. Dr. Buckholts required close monitoring that he not "step over the line" to improve his scoring position.

Psychology Training Program 1957 -1958

As a beneficiary of the nationwide Veterans Administration Psychology Training Program, I was eager to add Dallas VAH to the list of participants in the University of Texas-VA internship program. Six Veterans Administration training sites shared the pool of VA Psychology Trainees: Waco, Houston, Temple, Dallas VA Hospitals and the VA Mental Hygiene Clinics in San Antonio and Austin. Representatives from each of these VA installations made up the Regional Psychology Training Committee for placement of Psychology Trainees recommended by University of Texas Departments of Clinical and Counseling Psychology. The American Psychological Association later added University of Houston and Texas Tech University to the approved list.

The Regional Psychology Training Committee evaluated trainees' progress, scheduled their assignment to hospitals, and helped to maintain training standards. The Committee attempted to schedule their review during the annual meeting of the Texas Psychological Association in December, or the Southwestern Psychological Association in March or April. Occasionally, the Committee met at one of the VA stations. Joe Rickard, Chief, Psychology Service at Temple VAH was Secretary of the Regional Training Committee for many years.

The Veterans Administration adjusted its training program to include individuals with an Ed. D or Ph. D. degree in psychology but had not completed an internship. The post-doctoral candidate followed the training schedule of a fourth year level trainee: To be sponsored by an APA approved university and accepted by a Veterans Administration facility.

The first Dallas VA Psychology Trainee was a post-doctoral Counseling Psychologist sponsored by the Educational Psychology Department, University of Texas. Dr. Byron W. Johnson, a former Junior College Dean of Students was accepted for a year of training September 1957. Dr. Gordon Anderson was University consultant and Dr. John Geers the trainee's supervisor.

Our second trainee, Donald W. Giller of the University of Texas Clinical program, began training three months later as a Third Year Level Trainee. Don promoted to Fourth Year Level in 1958, and began a study on stress collecting doctoral research data using surgical patients as subjects. Dr. Ira Iscoe, chairman of Don's doctoral committee, made frequent consultant visits from Austin to Dallas. Ira was always a stimulating visitor, full of psychological information. Don required only minimal supervision in his final year, and assumed the responsibility of a staff psychologist. He completed the training program in January 1960, and later became Chief Psychologist at Terrell State Hospital.

Staffing Changes 1957

The first opportunity to recruit staff came in the fall of 1957. Projected plans called for the transfer of the downtown Dallas Regional Medical Office to the VA Hospital. Before the move took effect, the Mental Hygiene Clinic Psychologist position became vacant and I was asked to recommend replacement.

The first recruitment letter went to former Waco trainee, Phil Roos, then a member of the faculty at T.C.U. I met Phil's private plane at Red Bird Airport and from there by auto six miles to the hospital and a review of the vacant position. It was one of the many unsuccessful recruitments of Phil.

Former trainee, Earl Wilkinson, a member of the Waco VAH staff was also contacted. Psychologists at Austin MHC, Sherman Whaley and Reese Kinser of San Antonio MHC became interested in the Dallas vacancy. Sharm Phillips encouraged the selection of Reese Kinser. However, the Regional Office Director's choice was Earl Wilkinson. It was my first recruitment experience.

The news that Dallas VAH was an attractive teaching hospital brought many letters of inquiry. Some were generated by Sharm Phillips in his effort to give hope to graduating psychologists. Dr. Ralph Robinowitz, a member of the U. S. Army Hospital's Mental Hygiene Consultation Service, Fort Gordon, Georgia wrote in February 1958 stating he would be leaving service in the fall of 1958 and would like to move to Dallas. It was the first introduction to someone who would become a trusted, life long friend, and associate.

Letters inquiring about possible psychology positions at Dallas VA were always answered even when we were not actively recruiting. The Hospital Manager's office was informed about attractive prospects to remind the front office of our need, and the availability of a candidate.

The Medical School appointed Irwin J. Knopf, Ph.D. as Chairman, Division of Psychology in 1958. He brought Maurice Korman, Ph.D. with him from the University of Iowa. Jay resigned in 1964 and Maurice replaced Jay as Chairman. Both men consulted at the VAH, but it was Maurice through whom we developed stronger ties with the Medical School psychology program.

A Letter from the Manager

Documentation is no longer extant as to why a personal letter was sent to the Hospital Manager, Dr. W. H. Buckholts, but the tone of his response on February 16, 1959 suggested he was encouraged by the communication.

"Dear Jack:

"I shall always remember and appreciate your thoughts and letter of Feb. 11.

"In my humble and inadequate way I strive to conduct my personal and official life in such a manner so as to be a Christian witness at all time. I am the first to admit my failure far too often.

"You have no idea how much I value your letter.

Most Sincerely,
W.H Buckholts, M.D."

Psychiatrist Candidate Interviewed

The recruitment for a Chief Psychiatrist seemed to be a never ending challenge for the Medical School and hospital management. Dr. Stubblefield invited a former resident of the Denver Medical School, Dr. Ben Goodwin to visit the hospital in March 1959. I was requested to escort Dr. Goodwin during his three day visit. At the conclusion of the visit, Dr. Goodwin asked to be sent names of people contacted. I responded March 23, 1959.

"Dear Dr. Goodwin:

"You requested a list of the people you talked with during your visit to our hospital on March 16, 17, and 18. I will attempt to give them to you in the order in which you saw them. On Tuesday morning you met with Dr. Earl B. Ross, Director of Professional Services. You also met with the Chief Nurse, Miss Jeanne E. Riddle, Assistant Chief Nurse, Miss Florence S. Schroeder, Assistant Chief Nursing Education, Miss Helen M. Murphy, and Mrs. Agnes Elmore, Supervisory Nurse. The latter, Mrs. Elmore, is the nurse earmarked for the Psychiatric Service. You met with Mr. Rufus Dupree, Chief of Pharmacy, and we had lunch with the Manager, W. H. Buckholts, M.D., and the Assistant Manager, Mr. A. L. Gaubert.

"Tuesday afternoon you met Dr. A. Earl Wilkinson, the Clinical Psychologist assigned to the Mental Hygiene Clinic. You met the following people as we returned from the Mental Hygiene Clinic: Mr. Robert E. Williams, Chief of Special Services, and Dr. Charles Pearce, Chief of Outpatient Service (you may recall he was in the process of introducing to the hospital the physician who is to be responsible for the Outpatient Tuberculosis Clinic at that time). You met a number of physicians in the admission office, but the two names you will probably want to remember at this time are Dr. A. S. Brussels, Assistant Chief, Outpatient Service, and Dr. Kenneth G. Moore, one of the two examining psychiatrists in the Outpatient Service.

"On Wednesday afternoon you met with Douglas E. Torrie, Chief of Social Service. You also talked with Dr. John B. Geers, Chief of Vocational Counseling Service. You visited briefly with Robert W. Darnall, Registrar, in his office on the first floor. I believe you also met sometime during your visit Dr. Ben Cohen, Chief Neurology Service. You were unable to meet with either Dr. Ben Friedman, Chief of Medical Service, or Dr. John P. North, Chief, Surgical Service. Nor did you meet Chaplain George A. Nelson, and Dr. T. W. Wade, Chief of Physical Medicine and Rehabilitation.

"This was your itinerary as I recall it. I might add the response has been most favorable and I have had a number of people stop in the hall inquiring of your decision. I appreciate the opportunity of getting to know you and go with you on your tour of the hospital. I am looking forward to working with you. Please feel free to call on me if there is any way in which I can be of assistance to you in the coming months.

"Sincerely yours,

A. J. Jerngian, Ph.D., Chief, Clinical Psychology Service"

There were a number of letter exchanges with Dr. Goodwin during the spring and summer. Ben Goodwin also sent copies of his correspondence with other hospital staff, and made a sincere effort to communicate his thinking.

During the time of the Ben Goodwin correspondence, Joe Rickard and I also conferred on the possibility of his transfer from Temple to Dallas to assist in psychiatry and develop a Research Psychology position. There was a nation-wide effort to develop VA Psychology as a service independent of Psychiatry. I quietly struggled to bring about psychology's independence from psychiatry. Dr. Stubblefield wanted psychiatric supremacy - Dr. Niblo had psychiatric loyalty, but agreed to support psychology. Fortunately, we received management's support that Clinical Psychology should be under the direct supervision of the Chief of Professional Services.

A quote from a letter to Joe Rickard May 4, 1959:

". . . Psychology at Dallas is strongly supported by Management. The possibilities are unlimited in one sense, and yet there are real limitations, many of which are comparable to those at your station. We fight an uphill battle on budget and the immediate possibility for funds for a research psychology position is remote. I believe we will be able in time to sell the Powers on a research program. We certainly will get support from Southwestern Medical School on this."

I attended the American Association for Rehabilitation Therapy for Physical and Mental Rehabilitation at the Statler-Hilton Hotel in Dallas April 17, 18, 1959, and served as a workshop group leader on the subject, "Fundamental Areas for Research Development."

Caduceus Investment Club,

Fifteen members of the hospital staff met May 1, 1959 to form the Caduceus Investment Club, each person contributing $50 to be invested in the stock market. The Club met monthly with each member investing $10. The group discussed the stock market, and voted to purchase a stock through Merrill Lynch, Pierce, Fenner and Smith. 3

The Club was educational, social, and financially helpful. Jean and I used the accumulated funds in the purchase of a new home seven years later.

Psychiatric Service to Open

An August 14, 1959 Hospital Bulletin reported that Ben Goodwin, M.D., Chief, Psychiatry Service was assigned office space in the Mental Hygiene Clinic in "Room 31, Ground Floor, Building No. 1." The Bulletin also stated: "Requests for psychiatric consultations will continue to be routed as at present, i.e., to Chief, Psychology Service." (This Bulletin was issued two years before the title "Chief Psychologist" became official.)

A 20-bed Psychiatric Service opened October 8, 1959, with Ben Goodwin as Chief of the Service. Former Waco VAH Nurse, Agnes Elmore was designated Chief of Nursing for the Psychiatric Service. Psychology was authorized to recruit a psychologist for the service.

Family-Professional Decision

There is no recollection of when or why Central Office invited me to be their candidate for Area Chief Psychologist, Columbus, Ohio. Excerpts from two personal letters to H. Max Houtchens, Ph.D., Chief Clinical Psychologist, VACO:

July 13, 1959: "After carefully weighing all factors, I do not wish to be considered for the Area Chief Psychologist position of the Columbus Area. There are two reasons. . . The Dallas VA Hospital is approaching closure on many of the areas of projected expansion . . . have a strong identification with the objectives . . .

would prefer to remain . . . see through to completion. Secondly, my family is quite young and an Area Psychologist assignment would necessitate frequent absences. . . would require me to redirect a part of my primary family responsibilities. . . express my deep appreciation for being given the opportunity to consider such an excellent assignment."

The letter brought calls from two other members of Central Office, Bob Waldrop, M.D. and classmate, Cecil Peck, Ph.D. They thought they ". . . read between the lines that I really wished to accept such a challenging and attractive offer." They argued against two objections: responsibility and family (travel). They believed the Dallas obligations had been fulfilled - C.O. interested in moving me along as fast as possible - time to take on more rewarding challenge. "And regarding travel through the five states of Ohio, Michigan, Indiana Illinois, and Kentucky, the incumbent Chief, Earl Brown was able to cover by being away from home only one or two nights at a time, only a third of time on the road, unlike the St. Paul or St. Louis Areas in that respect. Columbus offered many wonderful opportunities for professional growth."

Following are excerpts from my second letter, July 17, 1959:

"Since talking with Cecil and Bob on Tuesday, I have gone over and over my reasons . . . the trauma of relocating family . . . current responsibilities in the present job."

". . . As you know, I have had something of a unique role at this hospital, attempting to give leadership in the general area of psychological factors in illnesses. An important facet of this has been assisting the hospital to move toward the establishment of a psychiatric service. A Chief of Psychiatry has been selected and is to come on duty in August. . . I am not an indispensable person, but feel that we psychologists have been delegated certain responsibilities and it would be unsound professionally to not follow through on our obligations. . . this obligation I speak of will be markedly reduced a few months hence. . . I have given my word to Management that I would assume certain responsibilities, and feel leaving right at this moment would be a breach of contract.

". . . I dislike very much saying no to such good friends . . . thank you for giving additional time to review your proposal."

Some 1959 Family Happenings

In the spring we bought a large upright piano for seven and half year-old Beth. She began piano lessons with a lady living in our neighborhood.

Jackie Jernigan, age 4 years, 9 months, spent a few days with Grandma Blanche in June. She wrote his parents after the first night.

"I asked Jackie what he wanted me to tell you and he said to tell you he went to sleep real fine and that he was <u>real</u> fine up here. He did go to sleep early . . . never woke up until nearly 5 o'clock. . .Then we talked a little but he didn't go back to sleep.

"We had our breakfast. He fixed his toast on the Scotch oven - ate it and a piece of bacon - pear preserves and drank his milk - takes care of himself - <u>is no trouble</u> and is a <u>world of pleasure</u>.

"We have planted some peas and I've gathered 1/2 bu. of beans and have that many more that must be gathered. . . I call Jackie every time he gets out of my sight and he always answers. He said tell you he'd been out and got you some eggs. Sure enough - he brought in <u>5</u> and put them in a carton. . . We will go to Westminster today or tomorrow. I'm going to get a straw hat [for him] if there is any down there."

That summer Mother began to sort and save old letters (most helpful to this manuscript), and commented about what she was reading when Cena Griffin called:

"I told them I found the one Stewart wrote Jack about his coming wedding and in it he said he was so busy he couldn't possibly go with them on their honeymoon, then said, 'Is Mrs. Gibson going?' "

Grandma sent cookies to the grandchildren. Jean wrote soon thereafter, "Richard [two years+] got in our bed before we were up. I looked over and he had already gotten a cookie and was eating it."

Family photographs document recreational activities in 1959: a few days at Meridian State Park, a trip to Bryan and a fall visit in Kingsville. Throughout the year, photographs were taken at Sedalia including Jackie's June visit and Beth's July attendance at Vacation Bible School with Grandma Blanche at Westminster. We all attended Beth's September piano recital.

A Second Family-Professional Decision

Max Houtchins called from Central Office Thursday, September 17, 1959: "Sharm will be moving to a hospital – we will need an Area Chief in St. Louis - need you very badly - Think in terms of draft - keep close to belt - Get 57 in to us."

Here we go again! It had been only two months since the Columbus, Ohio request was rejected. Why St. Louis, an Area Office that covered twelve states? Why was Dr. Phillips leaving?

I wrote Dr. Houtchens four days later, and gave a tentative agreement to travel to St. Louis and talk with the Director, and added: "For the past two months I have been undergoing a barrage of verbal aggression, and am anxious to get out from under it. Everyone, the Manager, the Medical School, hospital staff, etc., expect me to stabilize and give indirect leadership without any real authority. I would want to make sure I'm not getting out of the frying pan into the fire."

The "verbal aggression" reference was to the hospital psychiatrist's organizational and treatment decisions accompanied by his often used metaphor, "cut with a sharp knife." A Form 57 was submitted for evaluation by the Director of Professional Service, Dr. Earl B. Ross. I gave Dr. Houtchens permission to begin the first protocol step, a telephone call to the Manager, Dr. Buckholts. 4

Dr. Houtchins gave answers to all questions in a two page letter on September 24, and praised the new Area Psychiatrist, Dr. William E. Olson. Max Houtchens was correct, Dr. Olson proved to be a very good choice.

Sharm Phillips Communicates

An uncomfortable unknown: Was Area Medical Director Dr. Charles H. Beasley trying to remove Sharm? Dr. Phillips was a good friend - my post doctoral mentor. Dr. Phillips and I conferred by telephone, and on October 2 wrote him: "I have agreed to come to St. Louis to discuss the Area position . . . after much thought, and per your counsel."

Sharm wrote an undated letter, and am uncertain whether it arrived before or after the letter of October 2.

"Dear Jack (at end, get out match and burn. I feel I must write this but shouldn't.) This note should be in confidence between us absolutely. I don't feel officially I should communicate with you and you haven't written any inquiry. I judge you'll be invited up for a visit (VA funds 'ed. travel') but since that halfway commits you (to accept an invite- should even you expect to take area job).

"The facts are, once again this status of a psychology job in Area is threatened. A decision which Max [Houtchens] was not let in on was made (prior to APA) to eliminate job. Neither he nor

I knew this at APA, [in Cincinnati] but were both told on return. [I attended the Cincinnati APA to recruit a staff psychologist.]

"In finally getting funds restored, it was opined by CO a fresh face [Psychologist] was needed for our new psychiatrist. (W. C. Olson, from K. City). The fact of my being fired for the 2nd or third time, behind Max or Hal's [Hildreth] (old chief at one time), etc. should not deter you if your are comfortable in working in a role where psychology (in area) is a definite level below physicians and where, with my leaving, psychology will probably be back under area psychiatrist. Keep in mind I survived."

Ever the old work horse, Area Chief, Sharm Phillips added a P.S. 'I dug up and read your projected program. Looks fine! Dallas.'"

One of the family variables considered was our need to give support to Mother. She responded positively to the announcement of a possible move to St. Louis. Following are excerpts from a letter to her in early October.

"A move such as this has so many complexities that it requires much prayer and thought . . . St. Louis is 625 miles away and can be driven in 12 or 14 hours. This makes a long weekend trip possible."

The Area Medical Director requested an immediate visit.

I flew to St. Louis October 6, and was pleasantly surprised when Sharm Phillips met the plane on a chilly October evening. He drove me to the Pick-Mark Twain Hotel, and was a most gracious host during off duty hours. We visited his home so I could get a feel for St. Louis housing, and drove through school neighborhoods appropriate to the age of our children.

Excerpts from my letter to Max Houtchens dated October 13, 1959:

"It has been five days since the return from St. Louis. After much thought and consideration, I believe it is unwise for me to accept a transfer to Area Office when the Chief Psychologist position becomes vacant.

". . . I received a warm reception from everyone in St. Louis, yet the trip had a negative effect on the decision. The review of the position with Dr. Beasley and Dr. Westman for approximately three hours brought more clearly into focus the requirements of the position . . . field trips are on a two weeks basis. Absence from home is a type of sacrifice to me and my family to which I could never adjust.

". . . I know Central Office and Area Office are doing everything possible to develop an assignment which will be attractive and rewarding to Dr. Phillips. His desire for a change after years of dedicated service will be honored, and the reassignment cannot be accelerated. This is as it should be."

". . . I would not be happy taking a tour of duty in Area Office, and if my perception is accurate, then I don't feel I am the man for the job."

I did not express the antipathy for the manner in which, according to Sharm, he was being fired for "political reasons."

The Manager wrote to Dr. Charles H. Beasley, Area Medical Director withdrawing my name as a candidate for the Area Chief Psychologist position. The cover memo from Dr. Buckholts stated:

"When you originally contacted me concerning Dr. Jernigan, I felt there was a possibility he might be interested in the position of Area Chief Psychologist. From a selfish point of view I am indeed happy to retain Dr. Jernigan at this station."

In the mail came a hand written letter from Sharm telling of other VA position offers from Central Office, all of which he rejected. He felt he was "Starting out, after 55, on my own and build a career, etc." I conveyed to Sharm before leaving St. Louis that the area job was unattractive because of the way he was being treated. He concluded the letter with, "If you have changed mind, the job needs you."

Dr. Houtchins wrote October 16, 1959 that he appreciated the ". . . candid letter, regretted the decision, and read between the lines" that the job as outlined by Dr. Beasley was the source of my decision, and they had been concerned about his "rigidity." He continued, ". . . talked to Beasley yesterday and he was very disappointed in your decision since he was highly impressed with you and said he would have liked nothing better than to have had you on his staff."

Max was gracious in his remarks and encouraged me to continue working on the problems at Dallas VAH. It was a relief to have survived another offer.

Sharm wrote an official letter in December, as Area Chief, and included a personal letter that was more positive in tone. He appreciated my support, and perhaps my decision gave him some extra time. He later found an administrative position with the state hospital system in one of the Dakotas.

Ben Goodwin left to enter fulltime private practice. The ward was open for a few months, then closed. Management returned to its recruiting pattern of "looking for a Psychiatrist."

The 1959 Annual Meeting of the Texas Psychological Association was held at the Texas Hotel, Fort Worth, Texas, December 11 and 12, 1959. I served on a panel, "Should Universities Teach Clinical Skills" led by Austin E. Grigg, University of Texas. Other participants were: Irwin J. Knopf, Southwestern Medical School, James L. McCary, University of

Houston, J. R. Kinser, V. A. Regional Training Secretary and Carl Hereford, Austin Community Guidance Center.

That Christmas all the Jernigan sons and their families met at Sedalia. Blanche sat for a photo with her seven grandchildren in front of the 1959 Christmas tree.

Chapter 5 - 1960 - 1962

Dallas Psychological Association

Dr. Joseph Siegel, a psychologist in private practice encouraged Dallas psychologists to form a local professional association in May 1956. Psychology faculty members of Southern Methodist University (SMU) were key participants and many of the interested persons were or had been students in the SMU Psychology Masters program. I was invited to attend a meeting of the group in October 1956. The first officers of the Dallas Psychological Association (DPA), 1957-1958, were: President, John Geers; Vice-President, Robert Stoltz; Secretary, Genette Burrus; and Treasurer, Kal Lifson.

I served as Program Chairman the second year, 1958-1959, with Harold Crasilneck, President, Jack Strange, Vice-Chairman, Marguerite Topper, Secretary, and Kal Lifson Treasurer. Dr. Robert C. Topper served as Master of Ceremonies for Dr. Crasilneck's Presidential address at Sammy's Restaurant, 3900 Oak Lawn on Tuesday, May 5, 1959 (dinner $2.50 per person). 1

I was elected President of DPA for 1959 - 1960. Other officers were: Vice-President, Jack Strange, Ph. D., Chairman Department of Psychology, SMU; Secretary, Virginia Chancey, M.S., member of SMU Psychology staff; and Treasurer, Bill Garretson, M.S., psychologist with a private Psychiatric Hospital.

The Dallas VA Psychology staff supported DPA, served on many committees, panels, and as members of the Executive Committee. Earl Wilkinson was Treasurer in 1960-1961 and Vice-President in 1961-1962. The Treasurer in 1961-1962 was Dr. Don Giller, our first Clinical Psychology Intern.

Social Security

In 1958 I began accepting an occasional private practice referral from Grady Niblo, and used Dr. Niblo's office on Saturdays. Later Sales Aptitude Testing of New York invited me to serve as their representative in Dallas, and assess salesmen applicants for companies such as Cheeseboro-Pond and Kimberly-Clark.

Sales Aptitude gave a modest $20 fee, but that income combined with fees from the few private practice referrals made it possible to meet Social Security's minimum $400 annual income requirement. The goal: Acquire ten quarters (two and one-half years) of tax payments to Social Security and qualify our young family for many benefits in case of my death. It was (is) an excellent, inexpensive family insurance plan. The Veterans Administration's superior Federal Retirement Act did not cover children until age eighteen upon death of parent.

Educational Exchange

The Director of Clinical Training in Psychology at the University of Texas, Austin E. Grigg, Ph.D., wrote in January 1960 to inquire about my interest in a possible educational leave that Dr. Bob Morton, Chief of Houston VA Psychology had considered. Dr. Grigg proposed I spend a semester on their campus, he in turn would spend a semester at the VA Hospital as a lecturer-practicing Psychologist.

Dr. Grigg once worked with Dr. Ed Harris in Virginia and knew of our association together in the Air Force and at University of Kentucky. Dr. Grigg was impressed with the Rorschach training Ed and I received under Dr. Graham B. Dimmick at Kentucky. He wrote, "I think you would enjoy teaching our testing courses such as I teach now and also Ira [Iscoe] teaches." Dr. Grigg believed his semester as a clinician at the VA Hospital would enhance the University's Clinical Training program.

Neither the Personnel Officer nor the Area Chief Psychologist (visiting at the time) was familiar with an exchange plan. I expressed interest in teaching a course for clinical psychology graduate students, but distance from the University precluded such a possibility. Dr. Grigg dropped the idea, but continued his consultation pattern to review progress of UT-VA Trainees at Dallas VAH.

A Sad Story

Frank Davis, one of Mother's former pupils at Sedalia, came from a respected family of many children, son of Sedalia Baptist Church's prominent lay leaders. Frank entered Dallas VA Hospital soon after the Psychiatric Ward opened in October 1959. I examined him through our group assessment program, did not participate in his treatment beyond that, but followed his progress through staff conferences. 2

Following are excerpts from an article in Section 4, Dallas Morning News, Friday March 25, 1960: "Foreman Fatally Shot By Ex-Mental Patient."

"A recently discharged mental patient who jovially played dominoes with fellow employees Wednesday came to work with a pistol Thursday and killed his foreman with two shots.

". . . The shooting occurred about 7:30 a.m., minutes after 28-year-old Frank James Davis, a fork lift operator, was admitted to the warehouse of the United Motors Service, 6303 Cedar Springs. Davis walked straight to the office of warehouse foreman Vernon Cecil Norman, 53, who was sitting at his desk.

"Office Mgr. E. C. Casey, 47, sprang from his desk in a nearby office when he heard two shots, ran to Norman's office and found Davis standing at the doorway, holding a snub-nosed pistol.

Norman lay crumpled behind his desk. The bullets had hit the foreman in the right shoulder about an inch apart.

"Casey said Davis obeyed him when he ordered him to put the pistol on the desk. 'He never said a word- just stood there shaking,' Casey told newsmen. I said several times, 'Frank, what has happened? And he never would answer me.'

"Davis remained mute hours later as detectives plied him with questions.

". . . A bachelor, Davis took a voluntary sick leave in October to undergo treatment at the Lisbon Veterans Administration Hospital for what a company official described as a 'persecution complex.' Davis returned to work two weeks ago after the hospital pronounced him physically and mentally fit, a company official said.

". . . Casey described Davis as a 'model employee' who took an active part in the firm's recreational program until he was overcome with 'a sense other people were after him.' Norman several times had talked with Davis about his problems, Casey said. Their conversations were on a friendly basis.

"Davis joined the auto parts firm, a division of General Motors, in 1951 and returned in 1957 after military service."

Frank Davis' trial was pending in Dallas County. His Dad, Mr. Joe Davis, searched for help for his son, and asked Weldon Lane to contact Mother to see if I would visit Frank. Mother mailed a "Special Delivery" letter to the VA Hospital office May 11, 1960 with a note from Mr. Davis.

Excerpts from the "enclosed note" from Mr. Joe Davis, father of Frank Davis, the subject of this good family's concern:

"If going to see Frank or going to court conflicts with your position at hospital we understand . . . Visiting day is Tuesday, visiting hours are 8 AM till 11 AM.

"Dick Davis will go with you. Thanks Joe"

Mr. Davis did not indicate the purpose for the visit. I contacted Lawyer Dick Davis about his cousin and we decided there was no professional reason for me to interview Frank or participate in the pending legal review.

The court committed Frank to the State Hospital for Criminals at Rusk, Texas. Mother kept in contact with Frank through his parents and sent him home-made candy from time to time. It is a sad story.

A Silent Year

The story of Frank Davis is my only extant documentation of the Psychiatric Ward for 1960. The Ward remained open a few months after Dr. Ben Goodwin left the VA to enter private practice. A correspondence file indicates a staff psychologist was recruited for the Ward in September 1959, following-up a lead from the Cincinnati APA annual meeting. Responses to letters of inquiry during 1960 indicate funds were unavailable for hiring, and were probably withdrawn because of the dormant Psychiatric Service.

I attended a workshop at the University of Texas, Austin, April 21, 1960 titled, "Behavior From Viewpoints of Social Learning, Small Groups and Cultural-Sociological Concepts" sponsored by the Veterans Administration in cooperation with the Department of Psychology, University of Texas. Served as chairman one afternoon for a series of presentations made by Dr. Julian Rotter, University of Ohio, Dr. Sidney E. Cleveland, Assistant Chief of Psychology, VA Hospital, Houston, Dr. Robert Blake, Professor of Psychology, University of Texas and Dr.

Max Houtchens, Chief Clinical Psychologist, VA Central Office, Washington, D. C.

On May 24, 1960 I wrote a detailed (two page) evaluation of a University of Texas Clinical Psychology trainee applicant, John Kregarman. Dr. Austin Grigg, Director of Clinical Training at UT discussed the applicant with our Training Committee during a consultant visit.

We accepted Mr. Kregarman, but there is no documentation of his Dallas VAH training. John, very academically bright, made an effort to comply with our training outline, but did not complete the internship year at Dallas. We encouraged a second try at Waco VAH.

In December I responded to a request for ". . . a description and projection of my future interests" from Dr. Jerry Carter, Chief Clinical Psychologist, Community Service Branch of the National Institute of Mental Health, Bethesda, Maryland. The letter indicated we visited December 5, 1960, probably at the annual meeting of the Texas Psychological Association. A Form 57 was enclosed in the letter.

Some positive interests expressed in the cover letter: ". . . to be in a setting where I can participate . . . in the basic practice of clinical psychology . . . work with people who work with people . . . the consulting role . . . would like working with people in the general area of Mental Health . . . to serve as a group leader on community projects which fostered research, education, and the application of mental health principles at a practical level."

Negative interests: ". . . a community mental health position which required frequent lectures to inspire and stimulate interest in mental health . . . not interested in extensive traveling . . . do not wish to make frequent moves. . . to the extent I know my feelings, want to be frank with you."

The restrictions made me an unlikely candidate for Dr. Carter's section at NIMH. There is no other extant correspondence with Dr. Carter.

Family Happenings - 1960

Letters and a few still photos document 1960 family events. Also, approximately thirty minutes of silent movie film of birthdays, vacations, and Christmas celebration gave a synopsis of family proceedings. Jean was greeted in bed by her family with many presents and kisses the morning of her 34th birthday. The next month was Richard's turn to be surrounded by family, a cake with three candles, and many gifts.

Grandmas Jernigan and Younger traveled together to Bryan in May to attend their mutual grandson's high school graduation. David Jernigan was their first grandchild to graduate from high school.

The area behind our house on Swansee Street was vacant, and amounted to an undeveloped park with a creek and trees for the children of the neighborhood. In the center of this open area was a large excavated spot identified by the children as "the hole," ideal for riding bicycles, wagons, and other such vehicles up and down the sloping hill into the hole. The three Tilton cousins, Bobby, Kathy and Jim, the three Jernigans, Beth, Jackie and Richard, along with many children in the neighborhood were filmed one afternoon riding up and down "the hole."

The JCJ's spent Easter at Sedalia and the five grandchildren had an Easter Egg hunt in the front yard. A few weeks later there was a large family gathering of Gibson children and grandchildren. In June we drove to Kingsville, stopped at the Aquarena in San Marcos, and took the glass bottom boat ride. At Kingsville the two families took an afternoon outing on the shores of Padre Island building castles, wading in the gulf, and ate a picnic supper from the back of Jamie's Rambler Station Wagon at dusk.

Stewart wrote an "official" letter on July 1, and began with his, ". . . displeasure over your failing to visit us, but now a professional matter has arisen and I have to ask your help. So much for personal pique!" In the "official" section of his letter, Stewart said Mr. Kerley, Director of Texas A&M College's recently established Counseling and Testing Center was in search of a Clinical Psychologist and asked Stewart to inquire if I knew of a possible qualified candidate for the position. I didn't.

The children of the neighborhood celebrated Jackie's sixth birthday with all kinds of food including birthday cake, ice cream, hot dogs, etc. Jackie kissed Leria Lewis during the party. The next day he dictated a letter to his grandmother and Rover, the dog.

"August 22, 1960

Dearest Grandma Blanche,

"I got a knife, and I am very proud of it.

"We have read both the books several times. They are very nice. I also have a new ball glove and a pencil box. I put 6 pennies in the Sunday School bank.

"Yesterday afternoon we had the Malloys, Terrells and Leria down for hot dogs and ice cream and cake. It rained, so we ate in the kitchen at 4 o'clock. Bridget [Malloy] gave me a belt; Robbie [Terrill], a log cabin and cowboy set, and Leria a dollar. I now have $7.46. I am really rich! Also Jimbo and Laura sent me a tile set. I am building a ship with it now. I have just written them a letter to thank them for it.

"Rover, I am sorry I couldn't play with you on my birthday. Maybe I can next time.

Love to Grandma and Rover,

J A C K I E"

"[P.S.] These past few years I want to know if you are all right. Write this down in a letter if you have or have not been all right. Next birthday maybe I can come and hunt with Rover and my new knife that I got for my birthday.

"As dictated! Excuse the writing. Love, Jean"

The Arnold Krugmans, former University of Kentucky graduate school classmate, visited one afternoon in the fall of 1960. They brought pictures of their children, and updated life since leaving Lexington.

Beth's 9th birthday was celebrated September 26 with much fanfare and many guests. She rapidly opened a variety of gifts while all the little girls watched with anticipation.

Beth began the fourth grade and Jackie enrolled in the first grade at Carpenter Elementary School in the fall of 1960. Beth attended Williamson Private School her first year as she missed eligibility by 26 days for public school because of the State's rule of September 1 as the birthday cut-off date. Jackie attended a kindergarten sponsored by Wynnewood Presbyterian Church prior to his first public school year.

Cousin Natalie Murray invited us to place the children in her Lamplighter School in north Dallas on Churchill Way. It was a gracious offer, but the extensive transportation prohibited acceptance. And Jean and I were of the opinion the children needed to learn to live with the people in their neighborhood. Jean and I were pleased with the training they were receiving when we visited Beth and Jackie in their classrooms for a half day two months after school started.

In November I came in possession of a good used bicycle and began refurbishing it as a possible Christmas gift for Jackie. He had outgrown the previous year's purchase of an excellent

Huffy bike that Hubert (Peanut) Page's son had outgrown. (Hubert was a fellow VA employee, formerly from the Cannon community north of Sedalia.)

Our garage on Swansee had a small enclosed workshop with a locked door. It was there I worked on the bicycle and also a large doll house for Beth. Jean decorated the several rooms of the doll house. We were able to keep the gifts a secret. An 8mm movie film recorded the two "stealth" gifts under the 1960 Christmas tree, along with many other "store bought" gifts.

We traded the 1950 Plymouth for a new 1960 Ford Falcon Station Wagon in December. The 1954 Plymouth became our "second" car. We attended the NAIA football game in Dallas as guests of Dean J. C. Jernigan and watched his Texas A&I team win the National Championship. I wrote Mother on December 30 mentioning the two events, and the marriage of high school friend Boyd Newman, who at one time was County Attorney for Grayson County.

"Boyd Newman called last week inviting us to his wedding last Saturday afternoon (the day of the A&I game here). We would have gone if it hadn't been for that. He married a widow of a Baptist minister at Carrolton. I sure hope this works out well for both of them. . . We are liking our new station wagon. It is about due for the 1,000 mile check and I'll have to get that arranged next week."

The marriage did "work out" for my good friend. He was able to conquer his addiction to alcohol, and later retired from his Lewisville law practice to live in Rusk, Texas.

The final 1960 movie scene came early morning, January 1, 1961, with Jimbo helping raise the American flag at our home. Nearby, Jamie's Rambler exhaust puffed white smoke, as we all gathered in the driveway to say goodbye just before the JCJ's left on their long journey to Kingsville. The black Rambler, with white mist drifting from its exhaust was parked to the side of the new white Falcon.

A Ready Made Psychiatric Service

There are no available extant data that tell when the Dallas VA Psychiatric Service closed in 1960. It is my recollection the bed service was inactive for several months, then:

In its desperation to activate the Psychiatric Service, the Veterans Administration's Central Office ordered transfer of 60 patients from the Waco VAH to Dallas VAH in March of 1961, and shortly thereafter transferred an additional 23 patients. Housekeeping quickly prepared the dormant 8th floor facilities for patient care as well as offices for staff. Therapeutic services were alerted. Dr. Buckholts issued Bulletin 11-18, Dated March 17, 1961, "Hereafter Wards 8-A and 8-C, will be referred to as Ward 8-C, and Wards 7-A and 7-C will be referred to as Ward 7-C. The Director, Professional Services will be the Administrative Chief of these Wards."

Psychiatric Charge Nurse Elmore and the Nursing Service prepared for the admission of 83 patients. Dr. E. Garrett Sills, general physician with the Outpatient Service was assigned to cover the medical needs of the patients, and according to Bulletin 11-18, ". . .spend each morning in professional activities with those patients transferred from Waco."

Psychology Service prepared to assess the population and assist in the development of treatment plans. A questionnaire designed to elicit a patient's perception of the transfer and therapy expectations was added to the group psychological assessment battery. Patients were brought to the ninth floor conference room in groups of ten, and the entire population was assessed within a week. Most patients carried a chronic psychiatric diagnosis in remission, and Waco Psychiatrists evaluated all the patients unable to function outside a hospital. I knew many of the men during 1951-1956 when on the Waco VA Hospital staff.

John Geers surveyed all hospital departments and developed Industrial Therapy assignments for the patients. John's Vocational Counseling contacts made it possible on short notice to locate Industrial Therapy (IT) positions for the patients. This IT program became a benchmark for other Psychologists to follow. As soon as the test data were collected, John and I discussed the findings and together suggested tentative IT assignments. The days were hectic but rewarding as we successfully responded to an enormous challenge.

The Area Chief Psychiatrist (Dr. Olson, see Chapter 4) came from St. Louis the second week of the "exodus" to lead an afternoon staff meeting. All relevant services were present, Nursing, Social Work, Psychology, Physical Medicine, etc. By the time of the meeting, I had scored all tests, summarized the data, had not dictated reports, but was able to give global demographic and mental status reviews of the patient population. The group assessment approach was invaluable for it enabled the staff to become knowledgeable and comfortable with the population, some of whom had never worked with psychiatric patients.

The transfer and assimilation of the 83 psychiatric patients was perceived as a positive experience by the patients and the hard-working, dedicated staff. Since many of the patients had lived on closed wards for years at the Waco VAH, the new hospital environment gave them new hope. 3

A month before the "exodus" Phil Roos, Supervisor of Psychological Services with the Board of Texas State Hospital and Special Schools, invited me to become a consultant with the State Adult Mental Health Clinic as he was encouraging the Dallas Clinic to develop a group psychotherapy program. Grady Niblo was also a consultant to the Clinic and encouraged the proposal. However, the director of the Clinic was not immediately responsive to the recommendation. The sudden reopening of the Psychiatric Service at Dallas VA postponed the project, never to be revived.

Recruitment - To and Fro

Prior to the exodus, Hospital Management promised to place another psychologist position in the 1962 budget (effective October), and to that end a February letter to the recently appointed St. Louis Area Chief Psychologist, Dr. W. K. Rigby asked him to be on the alert for a qualified Clinical-Counseling candidate. Immediate authority was given by Management to recruit a psychologist.

At the April meeting of the Southwestern Psychological Association in Little Rock, Will Rigby introduced me to Frank Horner, scheduled to graduate from the University of Tennessee in June. A letter to Max Houtchens in Central Office informed him of Dr. Horner's interest and our urgent need, explaining that John Geers and I were devoting full time to the Psychiatric Service, and ". . . our other activities in the hospital were running on the momentum of the organization of the past, being coordinated by our secretary."

Former Waco Trainee, Pat Kuekes again became interested in Dallas, but wanted a grade advancement as well as opportunity to conduct research. Margaret Chetham expressed interest, but decided to take a position at Waco VAH. However, soon thereafter, Ruth Hubbard graciously endorsed Ralph Robinowitz's request to transfer to Dallas. Dr. Robinowitz became a member of the Dallas VAH Staff on June 5, 1961.

Dr. Frank Horner also joined the staff in June 1961. Two excellent psychologists went on duty in an active Psychology Service: Ralph assigned to the Psychiatric Service and Frank to share Clinical and Vocational Counseling referrals through the Consultation Service for GM&S patients.

Recruiting requests arrived in October from two Kentucky friends, Dudley Roberts, Chief Psychologist at Lexington, and classmate Dick Thomas with Systems Development Corporation in Santa Monica, California. Both letters were answered October 16, 1961. Dick was searching for employees with "Master and above," and my response, ". . . 60 to 70 psychologists in the metropolitan area . . . might well find a sample who would be interested in making a move." Jean and I were excited that Dick might be a guest; however he did not make the visit.

The response to Dudley Roberts: "We are now established as a Psychology Service and have a staff of five psychologists . . . hope no one is interested in leaving, but will inform everyone of the opportunity you outline in your letter." The October 16, 1961 letters carried the earliest extant official title, "Chief, Psychology Service - 5140/183."

State Board Advisory Committee

Charter Number 170414 was granted December 2, 1960 to "The Texas Board of Psychological Examiners Under the laws of Texas", as a non-statutory provision for the certification of psychologists. The board met in Austin October 29, 1961 with the following members present: Gladys Brown, Raymond Fletcher, Harold Goolishian, James Kinser, John MacNaughton, Carson McGuire, Harry Martin, Glenn Ramsey, Philip Roos, and Jack Wheeler. Austin Foster and Saul Sells were absent. A decision summarized in the minutes stated: "The Board agreed to request approval of the Advisory Committee to send out the revised bylaws . . . so that all psychologists will have a copy available before the TPA meeting in Dallas on 7, 8, and 9, December 1961."

The invitation to become a member of the Advisory Committee has been destroyed, but Ruth Hubbard's thoughtful letter to Dr. John I. Wheeler, Jr. on February 28, 1961, with copies sent to "A. Foster, H. Goolishian, I. J. Knopf, C. Hereford, A. J. Jernigan, and R. Fletcher," were to those asked to be Advisory

Committee members. Dr. Hubbard presented some early decisions to be met in the establishment of certification-licensure in the State of Texas.

I participated in 1957 and 1959 in affirmative votes for self-certification at TPA annual meetings, and also attended a meeting to discuss certification issues led by Dr. Saul Sells in his Fort Worth home.

Dr. Jack Wheeler clarified issues raised by Ruth Hubbard. As member of the Advisory Committee, I wrote Jack November 21, 1961: ". . . congratulate you and members of your committee on the work you have done in bringing about a revision in the by-laws. . . approve the circulation of the by-laws to the psychologists in Texas as soon as possible." 4

Another Central Office Call

Max Houtchens or Cecil Peck called from Central Office November 16, 1961, "to talk informally about a couple of matters." Bob Morton was retiring or vacating the position as Chief Psychologist at Houston VA. It was a Central Office policy (preference) to bring in a new chief from the outside and not promote from within, thus their request of my "availability to go to Houston VAH - a nice promotion, a more sizeable program, etc."

Houston's Assistant Chief, Sid Cleveland was highly respected as a psychologist and I inquired why he wasn't the natural selection for the Chief's position. The response was that Sid would be offered the Chief's position at Dallas VA. Central Office wanted us to swap locations.

Again as in 1959, the dilemma was multifold: Did not want to interrupt the school and church environment for our family; Dallas VA Psychology had a staff of five (John Geers, Ralph Robinowitz, Frank Horner, Earl Wilkinson and myself) and was at the point of demonstrating the many contributions of psychology to an expanding VAH Hospital. It was my belief Houston had the correct Chief candidate in Sid Cleveland. CO insisted a trip be made to Houston VA Hospital to evaluate the possibility.

A TWX followed: "Desire to determine interest and candidacy of Dr. A. J. Jernigan, Chief Psychology Service for position of Chief Psychology Service VAH Houston. Also desire to determine interest of Dr. S. E. Cleveland, Asst. Chief Psychologist VAH Houston for position of Chief Psychology Service Dallas. Stations concerned establish contact and explore possibility for station visit."

The Travel Voucher covered the period November 29-30, 1961. Excerpts from the December 6, 1961 letter to Dr. Cecil Peck summarized the visit to Houston and the decision:

". . . I was told at Houston that a packet of material had been forwarded to Central Office with a number of people, including the Dean of the Medical School, the Manager, Dr. Pokorney [Chief, Psychiatry], and perhaps others, who are recommending Sid Cleveland for the job. You recall in our telephone conversation I emphasized I would be influenced by the attitude of the members of the Psychology staff and those directly related to Psychology at Houston concerning an outsider being sent down as a candidate.

"I was very cordially received at Houston. People were frank in expressing their amazement that Central Office would consider anyone but Sid for the job. Sid expressed some anger that he had not been informed of Central Office's plan to recommend someone else and that he had recently been told by Central Office that he would be the Chief when Bob left. Dr. Boyd [Asst. Chief, Psychiatry]. . . stated the hospital had great respect for Sid and his ability, and had always considered he would be the Chief should Morton leave, and predicted that if he were not the Chief, it would greatly disrupt Psychology and indirectly affect Psychiatry. She also predicted a number of the staff would leave should someone new be brought in.

"I realize there are a number of ways of interpreting their reactions . . . the hospital had not been prepared for my visit. . . With the attitudes I found it would be unwise for the profession, or for me professionally to continue as a candidate.

"Cec, I sincerely appreciate your considering me for this spot. . .I have given you most of the details, but if you like, I will be glad to review it more fully this next month at Wadsworth [Kansas]."

Sid Cleveland was appointed Chief of Psychology. He and I had many, many professional contacts over the ensuing years, and don't recall we ever again discussed the December 1961 visit. As would be expected, after three position turn-downs (Columbus, Ohio; St. Louis, Missouri; and Houston, Texas), there were no further job offers from Central Office.

However another opportunity came when Dr. Bob Stubblefield recommended that Timberlawn Psychiatric Hospital recruit me to direct their Psychology Section. Dr. Stubblefield, familiar with my work with his residents encouraged me to explore the possibility. I visited the hospital, but became disinterested upon evaluating their perception of psychology, for example, a psychologist would not be permitted to participate in ownership, a privilege given to psychiatrists.

Family Happenings - 1961

Richard inherited Jackie's small Huffy bicycle and was filmed riding the bike with training wheels. Richard, Jackie and Beth were filmed celebrating their birthday parties in the backyard at ages four, seven and ten.

Beth Jernigan had a "Mid-Term Recital at Wadley Piano and Organ Company February 4, 1961 at 7:00 o'clock P.M." Music teacher, Mrs. Jack Williams selected "Two on a Tandom" by Hazel Cobb for Beth's performance.

Easter Sunday

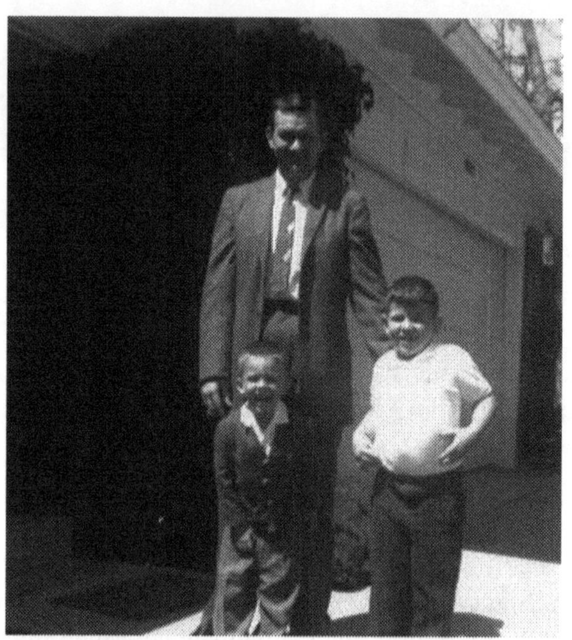

A backyard Easter Egg hunt came in the spring, and later I served as the only male parent among many mothers who accompanied Beth's Brownie Troop on a downtown Dallas trip that included a view from top of Southland Life Building.

A huge "Pelt & Foley Builders" sign felled by time and/or wind lay in the grass along Highway 67 not far from our house.

Easter Sunday

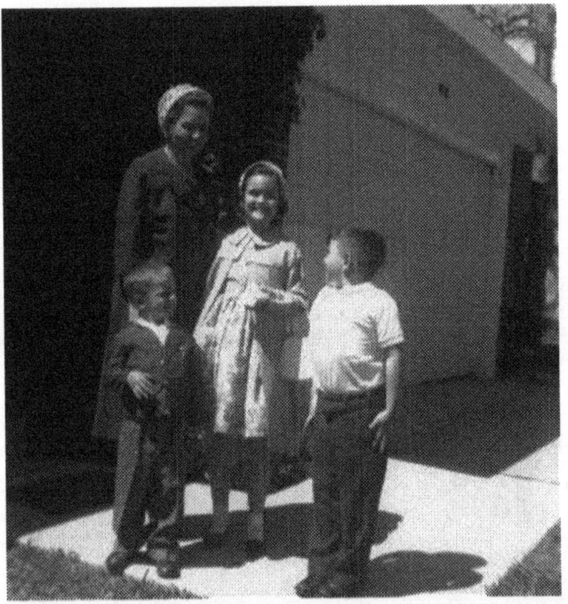

The sign was constructed of 4x8 sheets of plywood on a frame of 4x4 posts connected with heavy bolts. With permission (hopefully), I dismantled the flattened, discarded sign, and carted the pieces on the children's red wagon to our backyard. We constructed a jungle-gym type platform out of the material with slide, a chinning bar, etc. A playhouse was built from the plywood sheets. Our children and their guests had many hours of pleasure with the two home-made items.

Our summer vacation trip included a tour of the Texas State Capitol with 8mm scenes of the children standing with a group of Pakistan soldiers in the U. S. for specialized training. From Austin we drove to Padre Island, rented a cabin, and frolicked in the Gulf. From Padre we drove to Kingsville and a side-trip to Laredo, Mexico with Frances Jernigan as guide and our collective five children, Richard, Jackie, Beth, Laura and Jimbo.

Our return trip home took us through Junction where Stewart taught at A&M College's summer school. There is a movie scene of Uncle Stewart preparing a piece of edible cactus for his nephews and niece - pricking his finger in the process. The trip ended with a backyard patio view of the children surveying their Gulf sea shell collection.

Gibson Fiftieth Wedding Anniversary

Mr. and Mrs. Gibson celebrated their 50th Wedding Anniversary the weekend of July 5, 1961 and were filmed welcoming all their children, grandchildren, and a host of other relatives and friends to their Melissa home.

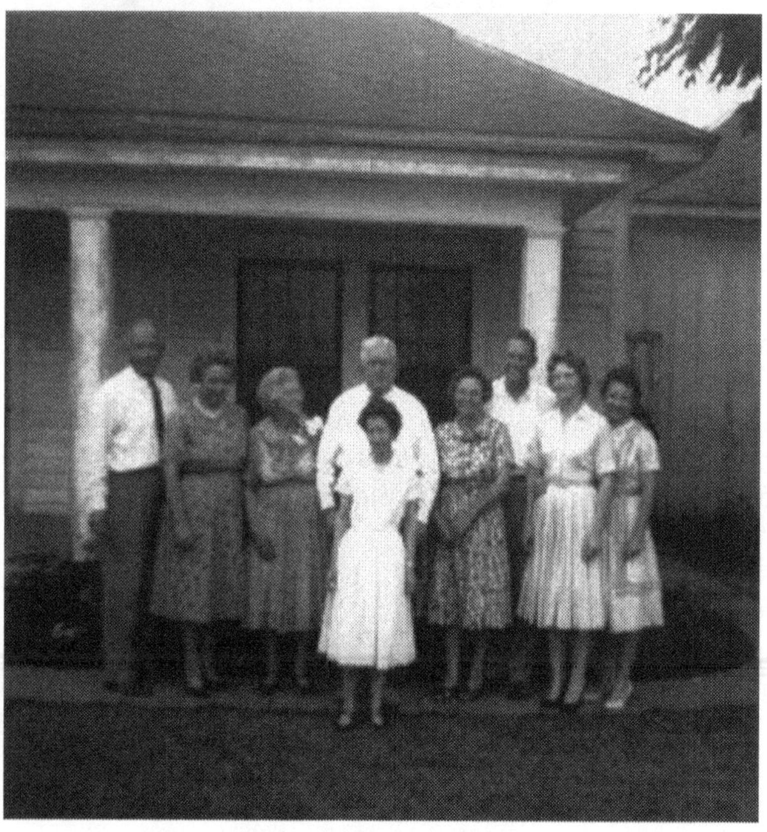

John – Frances – Mary and W. M. (Jake) Gibson - Doris (in front) Marian – Bill – Margaret - Jean

Red Skelton came to Dallas in August. An unforgettable memory of that hilarious evening was Jackie literally rolling in the aisle with laughter when Red by mistake picked up the "wrong" speech and began delivering his little son's school paper, the A-B-C's.

In late August we visited "Six Flags Over Texas", spending "$15.90." Labor Day weekend, the Niblos invited us to their Lake Texoma cabin for a full day of boating and picnicking. Grady patiently gave each child an opportunity to participate in a water activity, e. g. pulled on a sled or water ski.

Mother wrote a note of encouragement to Speaker Sam Rayburn, ill at his home in Bonham. The dying Mr. Sam's office responded September 25, 1961: "Thanks for your kind letter of September 22nd. I appreciate it very much.

"I am doing fine here at home with my own doctor. I have a pretty bad case of lumbago but he claims he is going to take care of it.

"With every good wish, I am Sincerely yours, Sam Rayburn."

Sam Rayburn died of cancer in the fall of 1961 and we drove to Bonham where his body lay in state at the Sam Rayburn Library. The day of his funeral the five of us and Grandma Blanche became a part of the silent crowd outside the Baptist Church where inside were four living presidents, Truman, Eisenhower, Kennedy, Johnson (to be). Home movie scenes documented the retreat of the hearse carrying Speaker Rayburn's remains to the cemetery and Grandma Blanche and Beth rapidly entering the church sanctuary to sit in the pew that President Kennedy and the past presidents had just vacated.

Halloween found Richard dressed as a Pirate, Jackie as a Devil, and Beth wearing an adult-like dress, hat, shoes and face rouged for exaggeration.

We attended Grandma Blanche's 75th birthday at Sedalia December 6. Jean took a cake with candles to celebrate the event. Aunt Ella was also present for the party.

Christmas concluded the year with rounds of family events and a tree loaded with presents that included a bicycle for Beth, a Civil War set for Jackie and a boat with wind-up motor for Richard. The warm holiday weather brought forth many outdoor movie scenes at Sedalia and Melissa.

As in January 1961, snow again covered the landscape in January 1962, but Richard, with swollen cheeks, sat by the window watching the neighborhood children romp in the snow. His mother sat with him. He had the mumps!

Jean wrote her mother-in-law January 18, 1962 that Richard was ". . . still a little peaked . . . none of the rest have symptoms." She continued with:

"The teachers at school are having an in-service training course and asked 5 mothers (including me) to be on a panel - 'What the School should do for the Child.' It was an informal discussion, and I really did enjoy it - just wish every parent could have such a wonderful opportunity. Was also glad the children are doing well, so I could be complimentary of the teachers! They said our school community is unusual in the amount of interest the parents show in the children's work - that it is not that way in many parts of town.

"Jack's sec'y. is leaving and they are having coffee for her today. I made brownies and Bea Geers is making nut bread. I surely hope they get a new one who suits. This lady was very good."

One other member of the family came down with the mumps: Jean! Neighbors and church family brought food and Dr. Buckholts came one afternoon with a huge pot of soup that lasted most of the week. Jean struggled through the uncomfortable episode with her usual pattern of few complaints, expressing more concern for family than self.

Because of their illness, I did not attend the Regional Chiefs of Psychology Services Meeting held in Wadsworth, Kansas. Cecil Peck, Chief Consulting Psychologist, VACO, Washington referred to Richard and Jean's illness in a letter dated February 2, 1962.

"I am sorry to have missed you at the Wadsworth meeting. Although I managed to have the mumps some years ago I did not feel tempted to trust my luck to visit your family during such episode. I hope that you have survived the ordeal. I expect Jean was really very sick to have acquired the mumps at her age, and probably a lot sicker than the kids.

"We had a very good meeting at Wadsworth and I am sure that you will find the minutes of the meeting interesting and helpful to you. I am sorry that the opportunity was not available to clarify with you the recent position regarding the Houston hospital, but I hope that this opportunity will avail itself at the APA meeting in St. Louis this fall. I had a good opportunity to talk with Sid Cleveland and I think things will work out quite nicely. My best personal regards to you, Jean, and the family.

Cordially,
Cec"

The Psychology staff selected Mrs. Mary Ingram to replace Mrs. Helen Dennis as Secretary, Psychology Service. These ladies were key participants in scheduling and recording the work of consultants for the Consultation Service. Dr. Dave Fuller and Mrs. Ingram became good friends and he soon appropriately gave her the nickname "Mary Sunshine" because of her cheerful and friendly attitude.

Pig-Lot Orchard

John Geers and I planted a fruit orchard in an abandoned hog-lot at the Sedalia farm on a warm Saturday that winter. John was a horticulturist with a green thumb. He loved the soil, and consulting others on plant growth.

As Mother watched the growth of the trees during the years, our most pleasure from the orchard came in anticipation of the fruit to be harvested. We received a few peaches but the Allred Plum was the most productive and the last of the eighteen trees to survive. 5

Chapter 6 - 1962 - 1963

A Swapping Story

Dr. Joe Rickard, Chief Psychology Service, Temple, Texas and I attended a VA sponsored professional meeting in St. Louis in April 1962. Joe discovered his car keys were missing from the raincoat pocket when he arrived at Love Field.

"Dear Joe: (April 11, 1962) The story of "The Keys." Last night. . . I reached in my raincoat pocket and discovered a set of keys. I was delighted because last December Jean lost a set. . . She informed me these were not her keys. I decided they must be yours. I assume our rain coats were hanging on the same coat rack last Thursday, and you slipped them in my pocket instead of yours. . . I am happy to return yours. I enjoyed being with you . . . wish you the best . . . on recruitment."

"Dear Joe: (April 12, 1962) "The Raincoat," a sequel to the story of "The Keys." As I was driving home from work yesterday afternoon it suddenly dawned on me that my raincoat had a button missing from the bottom of the row rather than the second button from the top. . . I took off the coat and didn't find my name. . . I'll trade 'even Stephen.' It is made by the same company, the same color, and the coat I now have is cleaner."

"Unless there are new developments, don't look for a letter from me tomorrow."

Good fellow Joe forgave me for swapping raincoats.

A Summer Vacation

In May 1962 we prepared for a vacation trip to Tennessee and Kentucky by purchasing books for the children to read, travel checks for the trip, clothes, a water jug, rented a Car Top Carrier for the Falcon Station Wagon, and distributed trip allowances to each child. We invited Mother to go along and visit Daddy's cousin, Nannie Wright, a widow living in Orlinda, Tennessee. Mother and Nannie corresponded, but had never met.

We left early June 3, traveled through Arkansas where someone in the car spotted a dead pig at the side of the road and commented, "See the dead pig." Richard cried out, "I didn't see the dead pig. I want to see the dead pig!" In retrospect, "Why didn't we turn around, locate the poor dead animal and satisfy Richard?" However, we didn't, and ever so often during the day we heard, "I wanted to see the dead pig."

But it was a happy day. That night we stayed at a Memphis motel. Beth and Grandma Blanche occupied one room and the four of us an adjacent room. The next day we drove on toward Cross Plains, visited Ft. Donelson, a Civil War Battle site that Jean and I drove by each year we lived in Kentucky, but never had the time to visit. The three adults wondered if Grandpa Jack Jernigan might have fought at Ft. Donelson.

Two years later the research to establish a Civil War marker at Grandpa's Sedalia gravesite led to the discovery that Sgt. Andrew J. Jernigan was captured at Ft. Donelson in February 1862. We visited the battlefield on the 100th anniversary of Grandpa's capture.

Grandfather Jack enlisted in the Confederate Army in 1861 with a host of other relatives from Robertson County, Tennessee. Men from Sumner, Smith and Davidson Counties joined those of Robertson County to form the Thirtieth Tennessee Infantry. In November 1861 the 975 men of the Thirtieth Tennessee were ordered to Fort Donelson on the Cumberland River, 87 miles northwest of Nashville, and participated in the construction of the fort. They were captured by Ulysses S. Grant and imprisoned February 16, 1862.

We took poignant home movie scenes at Ft. Donaleson of Jackie and Richard wearing their Centennial Year Civil War caps "charging" up the hill to recapture the huge, silent cannons along the embankment. And there was Mother reading the Historical Plaques that described significant events in the life of her beloved father-in-law. Little did we know these great-grandsons and great-great-nephews were playing war on the site where so many ancestors were captured on that snow storm day in February 1862. Grandma Laura Stewart Jernigan's baby brother, Billy Stewart contracted measles at Fort Donelson and died. 1

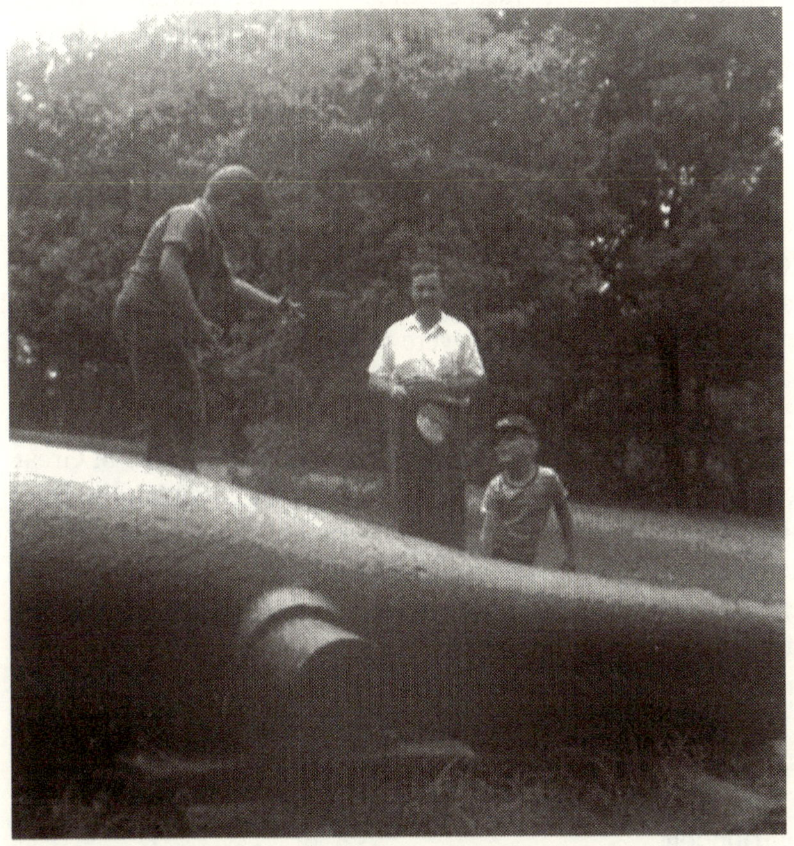

Jackie – Jack – Richard at Fort Donelson

From Donelson we drove on toward Nannie Wright's home in Orlinda where Blanche and Nannie came face to face for the first time. Soon these two Baptist Sunday School teachers were chatting as if they saw each other every day. We left them talking, and drove to Bowling Green, Kentucky for the night.

The next day we visited Abraham Lincoln's birth place at Hodgenville, Ketucky and later made a brief stop at Mammoth Cave. We pointed out to the children Kentucky scenes along the Bowling Green to Lexington roads their parents traveled in 1947-1951. The children saw the race horses at Calumet Farm in Lexington, and later at a race track site watched harness racers practice their beautiful racing skills. We visited familiar University places, the houses where we once lived, and ended the day in the swimming pool at Holiday Inn.

The following day we drove south by west to Cumberland Falls State Park to spend a day and night before retracing our travels toward Orlinda to pick up Grandma Blanche. At White House, Tennessee, we visited the two-story house built in 1870 by James P. ("Colonel") Jernigan, youngest brother of Albert and Jack Jernigan. Many of his barns were still in use and the spring house was intact.

On a hill above the spring house were the graves of Great-grandparents, James A. Jernigan and Deborah Strickland Jernigan, their son, James P. Jernigan and his wife Mollie, and son Ralph and members of the Strickland family. The farm bell that sat serenely on its tower at the side of the James P. Jernigan house would some day stand beside our Texas home. That is a later story.

We arrived back at Sedalia, Texas late Saturday afternoon June 9, 1962. Our account book recorded we spent $168. True to her nature, Grandma Blanche made a generous money contribution.

Summer 1962

Beth returned to Sedalia ten days later to attend Vacation Bible School at Westminster. She mailed three letters on Jun. 20, 1962, one to her parents and one to each brother. In the brothers' letters she added some personal cartoons describing her farm experience. Excerpts from the letter to parents follow:

"Dear Mother and Daddy,

"I miss you terribly. I got your cards today. In V. B. S. we are making pictures out of cloth.

"Did you see the 'Andy Griffith Show' last night? It was the Officer Friendly one (Ha-Ha-Ha).

". . . There are more boys - bratty boys - than girls in V. B. S. Grandma asked who denied Christ 3 times before the cock crowed. None of her Intermediates knew. But of course I knew; Peter.

"I miss you and love you,

Beth"

Beth told the brothers she loved them and in a postscript to Jackie added, "I love and miss you. Isn't Uncle Jamie's news grand." Jamie announced to his family he was to be appointed the next President of Texas A&I College.

As she did each summer, Jean took the three children to Vacation Bible School at Cliff Temple Baptist, swimming in the public pools, clothed, fed, and entertained them. The family visited Six Flags that August. Although the children had their "spats," they were very fond of each other and became close friends for life. Jean was/is a very good teacher.

Professional

The VA Psychology Training Committee assigned four Psychology Trainees to Dallas VA for the summer of 1962. The four graduate students from the University of Texas at Austin were: David Hardt, Level III Counseling; Wayne Carroll, Level II, Clinical; Gerald Clore and Don Nelson, Level I, Clinical.

Three of the four trainees were assigned for only three months. It was a challenge to develop a program for graduate students with no previous hospital experience for such a brief period. The psychology staff created an innovative clinical and research training means for this influx of summer trainees. Each student was asked to design a time limited research study to blend with his clinical assignment - thereby collecting research data as new clinical skills evolved. The trainee was required to complete a written summary of his research findings.

A Second Chief of Psychiatry

There are no extant documents to identify the date in 1961 when Dr. Jack Sandt was appointed Chief, Psychiatry Service at Dallas VAH, nor the date of his departure in 1963. After the dramatic influx of Waco VA patients to the 8th floor Psychiatric Ward, medical and psychiatric needs of patients were covered by Dr. Garrett Sills, Internal Medicine, assisted by Psychiatric Consultants from the Medical School. Dr. Ralph Robinowitz remembered that when he came in June 1961 there was "a very nice working arrangement with Dr. Bob Leon from the Medical School who consulted one afternoon a week to cover the ward." 2

Jack Sandt, a bright, young, Psychiatric Resident graduate from a New York Medical School was more interested in research than service. He requested and was generously given sophisticated recording equipment for the sound room adjacent to the conference room across from our offices on the 9th floor. When Dr. Sandt departed, Psychology became caretakers of the equipment that required frequent servicing, and was never adequately used. Dr. Sandt, whom I personally liked, made intolerable requests that Staff Psychologist Ralph Robinowitz give him the raw psychological assessment data.

Temporary resolution of the Sandt conflict was referred to in an October 25, 1962 letter to Dr. A. Earl Wilkinson. Earl resigned his position at the Dallas Mental Hygiene Clinic in August 1962 to accept a staff position at the North Little Rock VA Hospital. Following are excerpts from the letter that began with a word of sympathy to his wife, Kathy, in the death of her mother.

". . . We have some changes in our staffing here. Because of the disparity in the perception of Psychiatry and Psychology's perception of the role of the psychologist on a ward, we have removed direct psychological service from the psychiatric ward. Ralph is now assigned to the Clinic on a temporary basis and is working also a day and a half on the Neurology Ward. This may ultimately become a permanent assignment and perhaps a permanent distribution of service time. I thought we had recruited a psychologist at the APA for your old position, but he informed us the first of the month he could not accept the position. We now have a vacant position on the psychiatric ward, but are not at this time actively recruiting.

"I am continuing your psychotherapy group on Thursday morning and added a couple of men from the individual cases to this group. I am enjoying the work."

The outpatient psychotherapy group referred to was composed of WWII schizophrenic patients, in remission. Some traveled many miles each week to attend. One Bonham resident with an interest in politics visited occasionally with U. S. Senator Ralph Yarborough in his Austin office and told the group of their discussions. A former Japanese POW from East Texas told of lying on his back in a POW camp and watching B-29's coming in to bomb Japan. A black member of the group frequently discussed conflict with his extravagant-living Dallas minister. One member attended garage sales and once brought the therapist the gift of a pair of coveralls purchased at one of the sales. Federal employees are prohibited from accepting gifts, but the Chief of Staff and I concluded it might be perceived as rejection by the patient not to accept his gift.

The "APA" meeting mentioned in the Earl Wilkinson letter was held in St. Louis in 1962. Mother retained a picture postcard of the "Statue of St. Louis and City Art Museum" mailed to her on September 2, 1962.

"Dear Mother:

"I enjoyed walking through the old World's Fair grounds today. I have had a very pleasant and busy stay here. I have seen a number of old friends. I return home tomorrow night and I'm looking forward to seeing the family again.

Love, Jack"

I wrote Mother on September 6, 1962:

". . . back from St. Louis and it is good to be home. . . I know you would have enjoyed going through Forest Park in St. Louis as I did. One can visualize what the [St. Louis World's] Fair was like and I kept imagining the way Daddy must have viewed it in 1904.

"The family is well and school got off to a good start yesterday. Beth and Jackie like their teachers. . . I sent Jamie a Telegram Saturday morning being as that was his first official day in office [September 1, 1962].

The September Announcement

The Board of Directors of
Texas College Of Arts and Industries

are pleased to announce the appointment of

James Coffey Jernigan
as the seventh President

and

Robert David Rhode
as Dean of the College

Texas College Of Arts And Industries
September 1, 1962

Clinical Psychology Training - Academic and/or Medical

Dr. Jay Knopf, Chairman Psychology Section at the Medical School, proposed a training consortium with the University of Texas Department of Psychology at Austin. The proposal was discussed with Cecil Peck at the St. Louis APA convention.

After Cecil returned to Washington, he wrote a PERSONAL - OFFICIAL - DO NOT OPEN IN MAIL ROOM letter on September 10, 1962 to ". . . keep us informed on developments pertaining to the Ph.D. Degree program in Clinical Psychology in the Medical School." Cec went ahead to mention:

"I had an occasion to briefly discuss it with Dr. [Starke] Hathaway from the University of Minnesota Medical School. He expressed interest in developments of this type and agreed with me that some type of understanding and communication would exist with the Evaluation and Training Board of the American Psychological Association. I am sure it is clear to you that a major VA policy decision will hinge on the outcome of the deliberations which are underway with the University of Texas."

Cecil signed the letter "Chief, Psychology Section, Psychiatry, Neurology and Psychology Service." I wrote September 19, 1962 stating what a pleasure it was to see his official title that he had privately shared would be forthcoming. Following are excerpts from my response to Cecil's request to be kept informed, a summary of contacts with Drs. Donne Byrne and Jay Knopf:

"Donne Byrne. . . University of Texas . . . expressed some reservation about the projected program for the Medical School. . . a trend toward moving Clinical Psychology under the academic direction of Psychiatry. . . recognizes that unless the University takes more positive action in training graduate students in the area of Clinical Psychology that the University could lose this privilege in time by default. . . Donne is ambivalent about the concept.

". . . Jay Knopf states the Medical School plan follows successful completion of the qualifying examinations. University of Texas would give the first year academic study . . . second year the student takes the qualifying examination. The University then expects the student to take the clinical courses following successful completion of the qualifying examination . . . at this point the student can elect to take either the Medical School route or the University route.

"Dr. Knopf believed that if the University held to its pattern of training, the student could not elect alternative route until the third year. And in answer to the question of what was his plan if unable to reach a satisfactory agreement with the University of Texas, replied, '. . . we intend to go ahead with the program, regardless. . . selecting students from acceptable Master Level programs within this area, e.g., TCU, SMU.' He recognizes that this route would not have APA approval. I will keep you informed of further developments.

"Best wishes to you and Jo. Cordially yours, Jack"

Cecil responded October 10, 1962. He addressed the letter to 1808 Swansee and said in part:

"Your last letter concerning the Psychology Training Program and the University of Texas and the Texas Medical School was appreciated. . . we are making a complete study of the VA Psychology Training Program and will no doubt by early January plan to have some major revisions in operational procedures, etc. . . It is always a pleasure to hear from you and if any interesting aspects of the realignment for psychology training in Texas develops, please keep us informed.

Cordially, Cec"

The Medical School did follow its plan of action, and in time developed a program independent of official ties with the University of Texas. We subsequently hired one of its first Ph. D. graduates.

Breaking the Cigarette Habit

In the fall of 1962 I was asked to consult with a patient with Burger's Disease who had lost one leg and was subject to lose the other if he didn't quit smoking. My smoking habit was slightly less than a pack a day. How could a therapist addicted to nicotine help a patient quit smoking?

There is a vivid memory of the 1962 effort to quit smoking. Richard had outgrown his small Huffy bike and Jackie's rebuilt bike needed to be replaced. A "pre-Christmas Special" bike-advertisement encouraged parents to come in and make a down payment that would "hold the gift until Christmas." I had been off nicotine long enough in November 1962 to be experiencing withdrawal when we stopped by the bicycle store to select two bikes and make a down payment. The clerk said to make the down payment check out for "x% of the total cost." A very simple calculation became a very difficult problem.

This temporary cognitive loss was so impressive that I wrote a detailed description of the withdrawal symptoms (no longer extant). The paper included teenage recollections of lighting a cigarette while plowing with the F-12 Farmall Tractor on the backside of the farm (where not likely to be discovered smoking), and experiencing the distinct increase in the motor's pitch with the first inhalation of the nicotine. The diary-paper recorded those two memories along with other recollections, and the conclusion reached that smoking was more than a psychological habit: It is a physiological addiction.

To conclude: regression took place, smoking resumed by becoming dependent on a pipe. It was equally addictive; cigars, the same. Chewing tobacco, more so, for membranes of the mouth quickly absorb nicotine into the blood stream. After shifting to chewing tobacco, I began to experience the desire to chew at the office. Chewing was not the answer.

It would be approximately seven years before "cold turkey" brought the experience of freedom, pride of self control, and renewed taste buds. A compulsive smoker, I recalled the smoking-time schedule, and had a fantasy of how good a cigarette would taste. At that moment, money was put in a jar for the cigarettes that would have been bought. The "reward-jar" produced a prize of more than $60 (cigarettes were much cheaper then) before it was no longer felt necessary to use the reward technique.

I do not recall asking for Divine help in conquering the smoking habit. It was years later that the Alcoholics Anonymous 12 Step Program expanded to other addictions including nicotine. However, Jean used prayer to help her husband break another irritating habit.

Breaking the Towel Habit

After hurriedly dressing in the mornings to get to work, I would throw the towel toward the bathroom towel rack. It was usually left in a rumpled or wadded mess on the sink. Jean, patiently (usually) asked that the towel be folded and placed on the towel rack, but I rarely complied. She became really "put out."

Then, Jean read Theologian Emmett Fox's recommendation on forgiveness through prayer. When Jean saw the "thrown" towel instead of a neatly folded towel on the rack, she quietly prayed, "Bless Jack." She no longer complained about the towel, but when she saw the disarray, prayed, "Bless Jack." 3

Then, she noticed a neatly folded towel hanging on the rack each day. I was unaware a change was taking place until she pointed out the new behavior. We were pleased and thankful for answered prayer. I have used this personal example with patients in therapy who have difficulty in forgiving an offending spouse, parent or family member.

A Christmas Scene

Back to the purchase of two bicycles for our sons' Christmas gifts. The 1962 home movies documented two shiny red Huffy Bicycles under the tree, but Jackie's being the larger, was toward the back of the tree, partly concealed, and Richard's was out in front of the pile of presents. When the children ran in Christmas morning to look at their presents, all three immediately saw Richard's bike. Jackie was so sweet, helping his little brother mount his bike. After congratulating Richard, Jackie began to look at some of the smaller packages that had his name. One of us asked, "Jackie did you see <u>your</u> bike?"

And for the first time, this brother who rode an old (rebuilt) bike, so glad his younger brother received a new bicycle, saw his shiny new Huffy Bicycle, and said, "Did I get one too?" It is one of my precious Christmas memories of a son's happiness for his brother, and did not express disappointment if he felt it.

1963

Nineteen hundred and sixty three was a signal year for the United States and also the Jernigan Family. John Connally was inaugurated Governor of Texas in January, and seriously wounded November 22, 1963 during the assassination of President John F. Kennedy in Dallas, Texas. Governor George Wallace tried to block the enrollment of two black students at the door of the University of Alabama. The Southern Baptist Convention adopted "The Baptist Faith and Message."

Susan Jernigan became the first AWJ grandchild to marry. Jamie was inaugurated as the seventh President of Texas College of Arts and Industries.

Jean and I attended the 1963 New Years Day Cotton Bowl game. The children spent the day with Grandma Blanche.

The five of us and Grandma Blanche drove to Bryan for the wedding of Susan Jernigan and Ray Gibbs on February 10, 1963. Jamie and Frances and children came from Kingsville to attend Susan's wedding. Our cousin, Natalie Murray was also present to witness the ceremony.

Seventh President - Texas A&I

Approximately four weeks later our family and Grandma Blanche drove to Kingsville to witness Jamie's inauguration as President of Texas College of Arts and Industries Monday morning, March 25, 1963. Governor Connally was the principal speaker and following the ceremonies was a guest at the reception at the President's Home. Jimbo and Jackie saved the Governor's empty Coca Cola bottle as a souvenir and deliberated how to share it. One consideration was to break it into two pieces, but they rejected the thought.

Jackie – Governor – Jim –Beth - Jamie
Gov. Connally and Coca Cola bottle

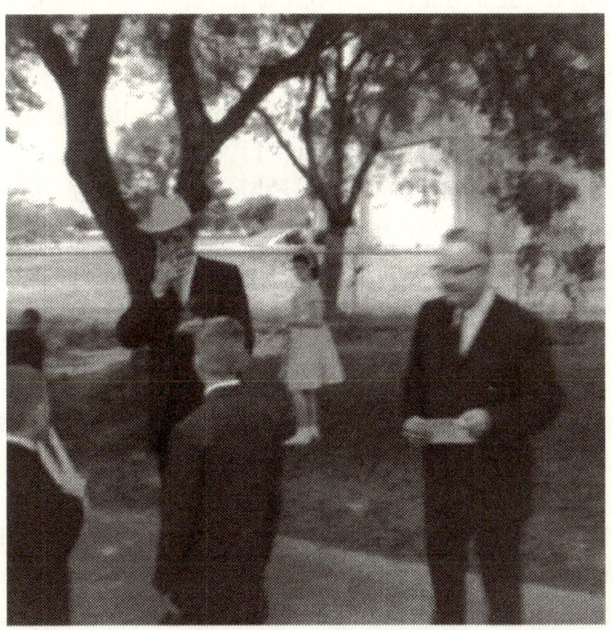

I took home movies of the gala event including the "marching in" of the A&I faculty, invited faculty and administrators from other colleges and universities wearing their caps and gowns along with the Governor of Texas wearing his University of Texas regalia, with Jamie bringing up the rear wearing the colors of the University of Chicago. Jamie and the Governor spoke and we, the unbiased family, believed Jamie was the better speaker. Florence Reagin, Frances' sister and Natalie Murray flew down for the ceremony. Stewart and Mary were unable to attend.

The inauguration activities concluded at 2:30 p.m. with a public reception at the Student Union Building.

The Corpus Christi Caller, for Tuesday, March 26, 1963 reported the event. 4

Brief TPA Assignment

While on the staff at Waco VA Hospital, and then a member of the TPA Ethics Committee, Dr Mitchell, a VA Hospital Psychiatrist, requested a review of the psychological activity of a person in Waco whose ethical behavior was questioned by Dr. Mitchell. In 1963 an Amarillo member of the Texas Psychological Association in private practice in that city was charged with unethical behavior. I was one of two TPA members asked to fly to Amarillo and investigate, either as Ethics Committee Members or as an ad hoc committee to investigate a specific charge.

Ethic Committee's had no legal teeth for there was no state law that regulated the behavior of people calling themselves psychologists, trained or untrained. Thus, our standards could be maintained only by diplomacy, peer pressure, and exclusion from membership in psychological associations.

The name of the Amarillo Psychologist is not recalled, and would not be given if known, but I do remember he was a very gracious and charming individual. The documented trip occurred May 5-6, 1963.

Open House

Arthur Giles, one of Mother's 1907 pupils at Westminster, Texas initiated the plan that all of "Miss Blanche's former pupils surprise and honor her with an open house at her home in Sedalia." Many people from Westminster, Sedalia, and surrounding communities as well as her sons participated in the "surprise" plans. When Grace Shields and Nannie Smoot of Sedalia began to encourage her to do some house interior redecorating as well as furniture restoration, she knew something was afoot. She was informed a week or so before the big day.

Excerpts from the Van Alstyne Leader for Friday, September 6, 1963:

MANY ADD TO PLEASURE OF OPEN HOUSE FOR MRS. A. W. JERNIGAN SUNDAY

"Friends from far and near were at the home of Mrs. A. W. Jernigan of Sedalia Sunday, when friends honored her with a 'surprise' open house in her home. The guiding genius of the event was Mrs. U. L. Downey who taught school with Mrs. Jernigan for 19 years.

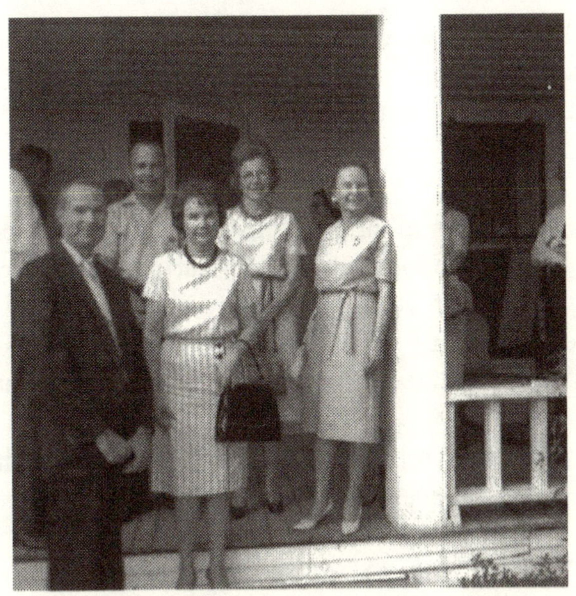

Five of Twelve Alfred Hill Children

Former Students

". . . Congressman Ray Roberts of McKinney was among the well wishers. Other guests were there from Sedalia, Westminster, Anna, Van Alstyne, Sherman, Oklahoma, Nobility, Forney, Dallas, Ft. Worth, Richardson, Plano, McKinney, Blue Ridge, Greenville, Bryan, Houston, Kingsville, Celina, Pilot Point, Whitewright, Arlington, Leonard, Wichita Falls, Tom Bean, Red Oak, Allen, Elmont and Gainesville. Among the many guests were her three sons, all of whom have Ph.D. degrees.

". . . Mrs. Jernigan taught her first school at Pike, Texas in 1904-05. She taught at Westminster, 1905-06 and 1907-08 and at Sedalia in the old school building in Shirley's pasture in 1908-1909-10. She did not teach any more until 1923, when she resumed at Sedalia and continued until the school was closed in 1946--they were pleasant and fruitful years in Mrs. Jernigan's memory."

Mother's only regret: It kept her family from attending Sunday School and church.

Following are excerpts from her letter two days later:

"I know this is a busy day for all your family. My youngest grand child [Richard] starts to school today bless his heart.

". . . I hated for all of us to miss S.S. and church because of something being done for me but after hearing Jack's prayer with all of us together I felt we had not missed church after all. . . Jack - I appreciate <u>Jean</u> having you write down the gifts and all as I called them out. I didn't realize how very important that was until later.*

"Must get to work. Think I'll start my washer right now. Still can scarcely believe I have had such a day. Love Mother"

Richard did indeed begin the first grade on September 6, 1963. He was ready to begin a new direction for in February one of us closed the car door on a finger, his tonsils were removed in May, and that summer he pestered Beth, she ran him out of her room, and slammed the door. However, one foot was still in the door. Richard's cast was removed from his fractured ankle shortly before school began.

New Trainees

Walter Penk was assigned as a Level II Clinical Psychology Trainee from the University of Houston in February 1963. Walter was promoted to Level III, and began his internship in 1963.

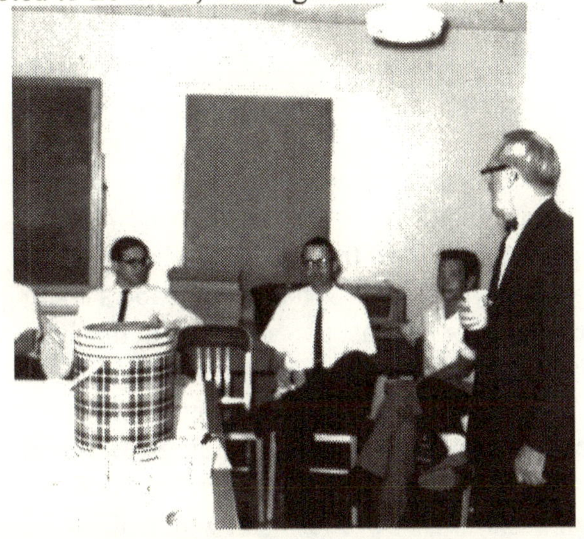

Penk – Hardt – Lee- Gaubert -9th Floor

David Andres, appointed as a Level I Trainee from the University of Texas, began a summer assignment in June 1963. Dave was asked to design a time limited research study to blend with his clinical assignment, continuing the 1962 pattern.

We received a Level IV Trainee in the fall of 1963, Charles E. Bounds, an accomplished musician, and former Texas A&I faculty member. Charles, at age forty, entered graduate school at University of Texas to pursue a doctorate in clinical psychology.

Mother wrote October 12, 1963 and stated she hoped our staff party would be all "it is hoped to be." (She also commented how happy she was that Beth was in the Church Choir and was pleased with her music teacher.) The late afternoon staff backyard hamburger supper was documented on 8 mm movie film. Among those photographed were Charlie Bounds and wife with their two children, and Frank and Marie Horner.

A November 19, 1963 memo to the Chief of Staff recognized the successful completion of the trainee's assignments and requested funds to attend the annual meeting of TPA to present a symposium.

Subject: Student Research Symposium

1. The Texas Psychological Association meets at the Driskell Hotel in Austin on December 5, 6, and 7. On Saturday morning, December 7, at 10:00 a.m., the Dallas VA Hospital is sponsoring a student research symposium. Papers coming out of research projects over the past two summers at this hospital will be presented by VA psychology trainees Don Nelson, Gerald Clore, and David Andres. Wayne Carroll is currently out of the State and will be unable to present his research findings. Dr. Frank Horner, who worked with Mr. Carroll, will present for Mr. Carroll at the research symposium. Dr. A. J. Jernigan will be the moderator and discussion leader.

2. Travel and per diem are requested for Drs. Jernigan and Horner to attend this symposium. VA Forms 10-1053 are enclosed.

A. J. Jernigan, Ph.D. 5

Dallas - November 22, 1963

There was excitement at our house on November 22, 1963 - the President of the United States, John F. Kennedy was coming to town! The next day I wrote a seven page summary of personal decisions and observations that fateful day in Dallas. Following are highlights:

"I was a sideline eye-witness to history on Friday, November 22, 1963. Friday broke with a heavy overcast. We seriously considered taking the children from school so they could attend the parade honoring the President of the United States. Because of the inclement weather, we decided against taking the children to the parade, and concluded I would not go unless the weather changed by 10:30 a.m. 'Just in case' I placed the movie camera in the car. The streets leading to the Veterans Hospital at 7:40 a.m. that morning were damp and slick.

"Psychology Intern, Walter Penk inquired if I was going to the parade, and I responded the decision depended on the weather, suggested Main and Lamar would be a good viewing site. Walter said he would go to Love Field if he went. We intended to take annual leave, unaware that 2 hours of official leave had been granted employees.

"On leaving the office for an appointment at 9:10, conveyed to Psychology's Secretary, Mrs. Ingram that should I attend the parade would return by way of Sears on Lamar and pick up an ordered item, "In that way I can kill two birds with one stone." John Geers laughingly remarked he would forget the statement if something should happen at the parade.

*"T*he patient I was to interview on the 4th Floor of Building 1 was watching T.V. as the President was being introduced at the Ft. Worth breakfast. The patient and I listened to seven or eight minutes of the President's speech. President Kennedy made reference to his dead brother, Joseph and that the brother had flown a Ft. Worth built plane in World War II.

*"A*t 10:35, the sky was overcast, but dry. Walter Penk and I agreed to leave immediately for Love Field where he was to meet his wife and son at Ramada Inn. Called Jean and said Jamie and Frances were in town to attend the luncheon for the President at the Trade Mart. They were to leave Dallas at 2:30 to fly to Austin and attend the scheduled dinner for the President at Austin Friday night. I was extremely proud to learn a member of our family was to receive such an honor.

"As Walter and I drove to Love Field the sky began to clear and Walter remarked that God seemed to be on Kennedy's side.

We also discussed the recent political events and our hope that a great turnout would appear to honor the President. We had some misgivings in this regard for we noted a poverty of traffic at the Love Field entrance, it then being about 11:00 a.m.

"After parking the car, I took a position on the west side of the extreme right lane of the Love Field exit to wait for Walter and his family. The four of us decided to await the President at that position rather than risk having a poor view-point at his debarking site. Approximately six other people clustered with us as we waited for the President's arrival. Vice-President Johnson's plane landed, followed 5 minutes later by Air Force 1.

"From our position, approximately 1/2 mile away, we witnessed Mrs. Kennedy and the President alight from the plane. The caravan began to form approximately 15 minutes later. Ahead of the caravan, an old pick up truck went by with "Yarborough Exterminators" painted on the side. A very charming lady standing by smiled, and the two of us commented on the irony of the event. Senator Ralph Yarborough and Vice-President Johnson were on speaking terms again for the first time in months, and were riding together in the VP's automobile

"My goal was to obtain a good "shot" of the President but as the Secret Service car approached, felt a moment of concern less they misperceive the 8mm Kodak camera as a weapon.

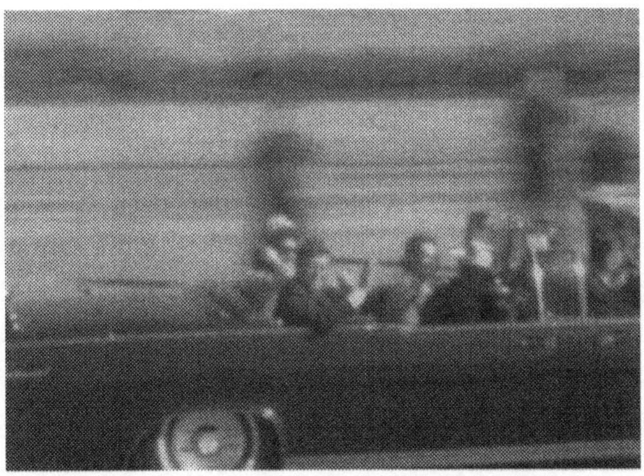

JFK as he leaves Love Field for Dallas

"For I stood alone on a circular, concrete platform, approximately 3 feet high, and the only person at that location taking movie film. The President waved and I had the distinct impression he was aware of my presence and waved for the camera. The entire caravan was by in an instant.

"Walter and I walked across the two Love Field roadways to the car in the improvised parking lot east of the Love Field entrance. The traffic was heavy and moved slowly on Mockingbird Lane to the Stemmons Freeway entrance from where we drove toward the Mart. By then the caravan was going down Main. It was approximately 12:30 p.m.

"One of the Press Buses was pulling in at the Trade Mart and we assumed the caravan had already arrived. Approximately 5 feet of film remained in the camera and I asked Walter to get a shot of the Mart as we drove by, decided to pull off at Harry Hines, and hopefully film the President entering the Mart.

"As Walter took the wheel in the slow moving traffic I ran through the underpass, saw a huge crowd on the corner waiting the caravan's arrival, and asked a man if the President had gone in. He said the President was inside and told his tale of woe of how he had missed by just a moment witnessing the whole procedure. I took a brief shot of the marquee welcoming President and Mrs. Kennedy, then a few frames of the crowd, ran back through the underpass and caught the car.

"I drove on to the expressway and began moving in the direction of the V. A. Hospital. As we turned the bend looking south along the Expressway adjacent to the Triple Underpass, we entered a traffic jam in our out-bound south lanes and the north bound lanes were also dead still. As far as the eye could see, all Dallas traffic was at a standstill, with motorcycle policemen driving frantically along the banks and across the expressways, some standing beside their vehicles holding back the traffic. Dallas traffic stood frozen.

"Since approximately 11:50 when we got in the car at Love Field, we had been listening to the radio. Just as the jammed traffic began to move the announcer stated there was an unconfirmed report that the President had been shot.

"We could not accept this, knew it was a false rumor. More and more as we drove down the expressway we began to say it might be true, having just experienced the unusual Expressway scene. It was difficult to concentrate on driving. A car flashed by and the man driving looked like a former patient, and the thought occurred, "Could he be the assailant?" Two men were in the car, a two-tone blue 1957 or 1958 Chrysler or Ford product. Could we have seen the assassinator?

"When we arrived at the hospital at 12:55, I went immediately to the Recreation Hall. A stunned group of hospital employees and patients listened as the news came at about 1:15 that President Kennedy had been assassinated."

*M*emory is that the TV was tuned to CBS and I heard and saw Walter Cronkite hold back the sob as he removed his glasses, looked at the clock and gave the time of the President's death.

The afternoon of November 22 was devoted to working with hospital staff to prepare special attention for patients on the psychiatric ward and coverage for the coming weekend. We were shocked and sad!

As I left the hospital grounds, the remaining movie film was used to capture a late afternoon scene of the Veterans Hospital with flag at half-mast. The film became a collector's item, and a special story to be told later. 6

As the Psychiatry Service was without a chief, it was covered by Ward Physician, Dr. Edward Arman. Dr. Arman sent the following memo to the Chief of Staff on November 29, 1963, with copies to "Chiefs of Services, T. W. Wade (PM&R), A. J. Jernigan (Psychology), D. E. Torrie (Social Work) and Mary F. Friedman (Nursing Service)."

"It was most gratifying to have received the sincere and unselfish support from the Physical Medicine and Rehabilitation Service, Psychology Service, Social Work Service, and Nursing Service during the period November 23rd, 24th, and 25th, when the tragic events caused us to cancel all patients' passes. With the generous voluntary help of these Services, I feel that the patients on the Psychiatry Service received extraordinarily good care and that the entire service operated more smoothly because of their efforts.

Edward W. Arman, M.D."

Jernigan-Coffey Family Reunion

During the week of the President's death, Mother was preoccupied with preparation for a Jernigan - Coffey family reunion scheduled November 30, 1963. The reunion was a great success as recorded by the December 6, 1963 issue of the Van Alstyne Leader.

"Saturday, Nov. 30th, was an ideal autumn day for the Jernigan-Coffey family reunion at the home of Mrs. A. W. Jernigan of Sedalia. There was an abundance of delicious food as everyone brought a variety of delectable dishes."

The Leader listed forty-five guests present for the reunion. Our family was present but neither Stewart nor Jamie came. Frances would later write they were too distressed after November 22 to return to Dallas the next week.

Jackie wrote his grandmother, "We are looking forward in coming to your house for Christmas. I hope we will have a good time.

"Richard is going to be an angel at school on the Christmas program.

"We are studying about Alaska inside the Arctic Circle. Friday we went on a whale hunt and yesterday we went to a movie."

Jackie received his wish. Mother informed the Van Alstyne Leader and editor, Mr. D. H. Reeves published the following on January 10, 1964: "Mrs. A. W. Jernigan of Sedalia enjoyed having all her family with her on Christmas Eve except one granddaughter [Susan Gibbs], for a Christmas tree. Christmas carols and old songs were sung. Jack Jernigan, Jr. read the Christmas story from the second chapter of Luke. The six grandchildren sang Silent Night for their grandmother."

Chapter 7 - 1964 - 1965

Veterans Administration Friendships

A fraternity of Veterans Administration Psychology Chiefs evolved over the years composed of former Kentucky classmates, psychology trainees and postdoctoral friends. Many of us joined ranks each year at state, regional and national psychological meetings, or at a VA Central Office meeting.

Kentucky classmate Cecil Peck, Chief Psychologist, VACO came to Dallas for an official visit February 10, and spent the night in our home. Beth's hamster escaped from its cage. Suddenly Cecil's quiet voice shifted tone, "Jean, I believe you have a rat in the house, I just saw it run under the couch!" With help from each of us, Beth corralled her hamster, returned him to its cage, and there remained for Beth's Science Fair project until he tripped a rat trap under the kitchen sink and died.

Cecil sent a thank you note:

"Although my stay in Dallas was very brief, it was most pleasant. It was certainly wonderful seeing you and Jean again and to meet your children. I wish to thank you for everything that you did for me while I was in Dallas.

Cordially, Cec"

Life Member

The Texas Congress of Parents and Teachers certified Mrs. A. J. Jernigan a "Life Member of the Texas Congress of Parents and Teachers" February 11, 1964. The recognition came as a result of Jean's leadership in the PTA organizations of Daniel Webster and Carpenter Elementary Schools.

A VA Central Office meeting for Chiefs of Psychology scheduled for March 1964 brought a letter from Verner Baugh requesting, ". . . put in a good word to Cecil Peck concerning my application as Chief, Psychology Service at Knoxville VA Hospital, Knoxville, Iowa."

Dr. Verner Baugh, my post doctoral year supervisor at Waco VA Hospital was Acting Chief at Knoxville VAH. His staff members included wife, Counseling Psychologist Annie Baugh, and former Baylor faculty member, Clinical Psychologist Kenneth Bean.

The reply, ". . . the Manager at Iowa is to be commended for recommending you for the Chief's position. . . I will be glad to speak to Cecil about you and, if he so wishes, put it in writing. I suppose you want me to emphasize what a good farmer and horse trader you are, but in addition, will also tell him about your good qualifications as a psychologist and that I think most highly of you." 1

Former Kentucky classmate Jack Griffiths, Psychology Chief at Ft. Lyon, Colorado wrote in February that he and wife, Betty would be attending the New Orleans conference, would drive through Dallas, and invited us to ride with them to New Orleans. However, Jean could not go so I flew to New Orleans and visited there with the Griffiths.

Promotions came to two former VA Psychology Trainees. A letter of congratulations went to Phil Roos February 13, 1964 following Phil's announcement in the State Hospitals' "Psychology Newsletter" that Phil had transferred from the position, "Chief of Clinical Psychology Services to Superintendent, Austin State School." The same Newsletter announced that, "Dr. Don Giller, Chief Clinical Psychologist at Terrell State Hospital since March 1960 transferred to the Dallas Outpatient Clinic September 1963."

I wrote Phil, "The State of Texas is fortunate to have had an individual who was willing and able to give such fine leadership. The Austin State School will profit from your being designated as Superintendent."

Visiting Scientist Program

In a letter, dated Friday, January 24, 1964, Mother asked, "Isn't it Monday or Tuesday when you go somewhere for a talk, Jack?" Her reference was to an invitation from a Texas High School to visit and share information with the students and faculty about psychology. The program, sponsored by the Texas Academy of Science ". . .Designed to improve science and mathematics education in Texas for junior and senior high schools" was supported and funded by the National Science Foundation and various industrial organizations.

Dr. Wayne Holtzman of the Hogg Foundation submitted my name to the Texas Academy of Science in 1961. The first request came in October 1962 from a small school south of Cedar Creek Lake. Driving back to Dallas, I listened with intense interest the radio's minute by minute discussion of the National Cuban Missile Crisis.

The "Visiting Scientist Program File" documented a speaking engagement at Jacksonville High School January 27, 1964. The title of the talk was "The Scientific Measurement of Human Behavior" explaining the expanding role of psychology in a medical setting. I informed the students there were very few clinical psychologists prior to WWII, and at war's conclusion there was an immediate need for psychologists to respond to possible rehabilitation requests from sixteen million WWII veterans. The students were told about the VA Psychology Training Program as a possible future vocational goal.

The students participated in a sample slide presentation of copying forms, and listened to how psychologists' evaluate a person's response. The demonstration stimulated much student discussion. The Visiting Scientist requests were rare opportunities to go into a classroom, and interact with students.

New Orleans - 1964

The Area Psychology Conference - Saint Louis Medical Area met March 19-20, 1964 in New Orleans, Louisiana. I stayed at the Buel Hotel in New Orleans. Dr. Irwin A. Berg, Chairman, Department of Psychology, Louisiana State University gave the opening address, titled, "The Task of Psychology." Special Reports on "Domiciliary" and "Administrative Matters" were presented by Central Office personnel. And there were "Contributed Papers" and Panel Discussions." My paper was titled, "Summer Romance or the Research Project as an Introductory Training Technique."

Jackie requested information about the Battle of New Orleans. I caught a bus and rode out to the National Cemetery Area, Chalmette National Park to photograph an 8mm movie of the historic 1812 Battle site. Chalmette is the name of the battlefield where the Battle of New Orleans was fought, and a local brush fire added reality to the movie scene.

Civil War Centennial & Genealogy

The Civil War Centennial Years brought many questions about ancestors and their participation in the war. We discovered members of the Chambers, Coffey, Gibson, Griffin, Jernigan, and Stewart families who fought on the Southern side. The post Civil War first generation children of veterans retained only a few memories about their parent's role in the war. Documents were lost that told who did what, with whom, where and when during the four year national tragedy. By 1961-1965, the surviving older generation knew little more than that a father or grandfather was a Civil War Veteran.

The initial research began with Jean's maternal grandfather, Elijah Windsor Chambers and my paternal grandfather, Andrew Jackson Jernigan, two who were known to have fought in the Civil War. Information about Grandpa Chambers' service history came alive with the transcription of his Civil War Diary. The diary was preserved by Mary Chambers Gibson, and passed on to us. 2

The search for Grandpa Jernigan's Civil War history began when Grayson County announced its drive to place a Civil War Marker at the grave of every Civil War Veteran. Mother wrote, "Where did Grandpa Jernigan serve during the Civil War? We need to put up a marker?"

Grandpa Chambers' Diary gave background information about his Civil War service at Mansfield, Louisiana when the five of us traveled to Mansfield, La. to participate in the "Texas Muster" at the Centennial Commemoration of the Battle of Mansfield - Red River Campaign, April 4, 1864. All descendants of those who fought at Mansfield were invited to witness a reenactment of the battle. Jean's mother Mary Gibson canceled her invitation to accompany us when Doris became ill.

Stewart and I requested photocopies of Andrew Jackson Jernigan's service record from the National Archives and Records Service, and received records for two Andrew Jackson Jernigans from Tennessee. Our grandfather's service record was verified a year later. 3

Civil War research increased an interest in family genealogy. The search for ancestor information began by reading old family letters, a review of books from family libraries, and other related documents. Also we began reading books about the fascinating and tragic saga, the Civil War.

Professional Meeting

The week after the "Battle of Mansfield" festivities, an April 8, 1964 letter to Mother told of a projected trip to San Antonio where I was to be a participant "on a program" at the Southwest Psychological Annual meeting.

A Historical Note

Jack Ruby's trial was headline news in the spring of 1964. Jack Ruby murdered Lee Harvey Oswald before Oswald could be investigated for the assassination of President Kennedy. Psychologist Roy Shafer was invited to evaluate Jack Ruby, and Dallas Psychologists followed Dr. Shafer's media reported testimony. Dr. Shafer was author of a key internship text used at Kentucky, titled, Clinical Application of Psychological Tests.

An artist's sketch of Dr. Shafer as he testified was published in a local paper. After Dr. Shafer returned to New Haven, Connecticut, I sent him a copy of the sketch and wrote April 17, 1964, "Dallas Psychologists followed with interest your testimony. You are to be congratulated on the professional manner in which you represented the field of Psychology."

Dr. Shafer responded, "Thank you for the clipping and for your words of appreciation. It was a difficult situation and it is gratifying to know of the favorable response of colleagues.

Sincerely yours,

Roy Shafer."

A New Home

Jean began a search for larger living quarters in the spring. She located an attractive house built by Clifford E. Yeldell in

Kimball Estates near Browne Junior High School, Kimball High School, convenient to Carpenter Elementary.

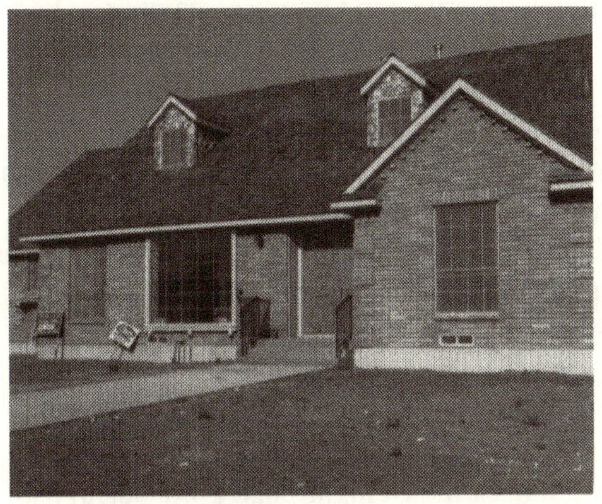

Mr. Yeldell agreed to apply our Club Oaks Home to the sale price of $24,000 for the new house, and negotiate a new $18,000 loan. Jean initiated a great trade. The monthly loan payment of $110 began August 1964. Check stubs indicate a total cost of $508 to make the trade including $45 paid Oak Cliff Transfer to move the "heavy" household objects. We carried the rest of our belongings in the Kentucky trailer in many round trips from 1808 Swansee to 4012 Fountainhead on July 4, 1964.

Vacation

We left home on a vacation a few days later, and spent the first night and day at Lake of the Pines in East Texas. We rented a barge and the children enjoyed taking turns at the pilot wheel of a rented barge on Lake of the Pines. The next day we drove to Arkansas and searched for War sites identified by Grandpa Chamber's in his Civil War Diary. Pvt. Chambers wrote:

"May 1864, I went to Princeton, Dallas, Co. ark with some wounded wounded (sic) . . . I was tending to the wounded, in the Courthouse. . . I bought a side knife for $5, confederate. . . Joseph [brother] is able to take a little exercise."

A crumbling red brick wall was identified as part of the hospital building described in Grandpa Chambers' Diary. We retrieved a fallen brick from the Civil War Hospital that the mason inserted in the chimney in our Chambersville home in 1984.

Movies of the trip included a brief stop in Hot Springs where Richard and Jackie tested the water's temperature. A scene of Jean and Beth walking toward one of the springs documented Beth had grown to the same height as her Mother.

The vacation was reviewed in a letter to Mother, July 26, 1964.

"We got back in last night - had a wonderful trip. We stayed a day at the Lake of the Pines - then to Camden, Arkansas - visited two battlefield sites where Grandpa Chambers was stationed and reported in his diary. We visited a Bauxite Mine - looks like a small scale Grande Canyon - then to Hot Springs - down to Arkadelphia to spend the night. We ate in the cafeteria, where we ate on the last day of our trip back from Tennessee. Yesterday we came through the diamond mines and the children thoroughly enjoyed collecting rocks (no diamonds).

"We have you a small box of the salt water taffy like that you bought on our trip [to Tennessee]. You were remembered and thought of many times by all five."

Trainees – Staff - Research

Charles Bounds completed his internship and academic requirements in early 1964, qualified for staff at the GS-11 level. He accepted a Dallas VA Hospital staff position on March 9, 1964 and assigned to the Psychiatric Service.

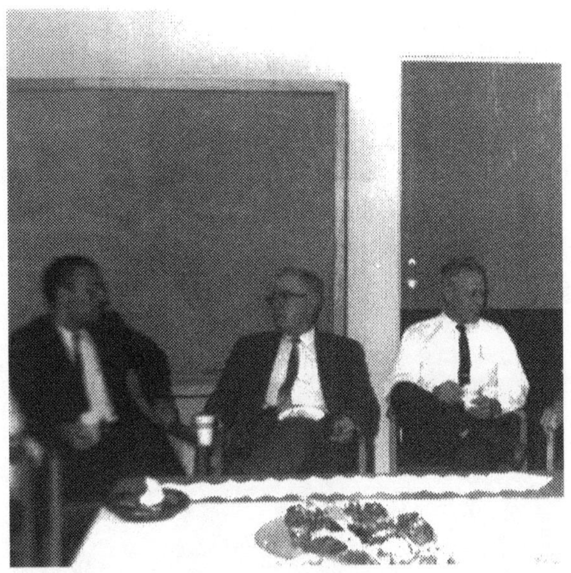

R. Robinowitz, Dr. Buckholts, C. Bounds

Mrs. Anna J. Campbell, Level III Psychology Trainee transferred to the Dallas VAH from VA Hospital Phoenix April 6, 1964. Anna was assigned to the Consulting Service, participated in a weekly teaching conference held by the Chief of Neurology, and presented psychological test findings at monthly teaching conferences for medical residents led by Dr. Stubblefield, Chairman, Department of Psychiatry, Southwestern Medical School. She also conducted a time limited research project.

Mark Schwartz, University of Texas, Level I Trainee was assigned to Dallas from June 15 to August 28, 1964, and supervised by Dr. Geers, Assistant Chief Psychology Service. As the trainee had not received academic training in clinical testing, John Geers taught Mark the Wechsler Adult Intelligence Test and assigned forty patients for supervised assessment with the WAIS.

I wrote Area Chief, Bill Rigby in August requesting 600 hours of additional training for Anna Campbell effective October 1, 1964, and added she and Walter Penk would soon be eligible for a VA staff appointment. Anna accepted a continuation of internship in Child Psychology at Southwestern Medical School, but we successfully recruited Walter Penk for a staff position at Dallas VAH.

Frank Horner transferred to the Tuscaloosa Alabama VAH. His wife, Marie, a native of Alabama, encouraged the transfer. We received a Tuscaloosa postmarked letter of appreciation from Dr. Horner August 12, 1964 signed by each family member.

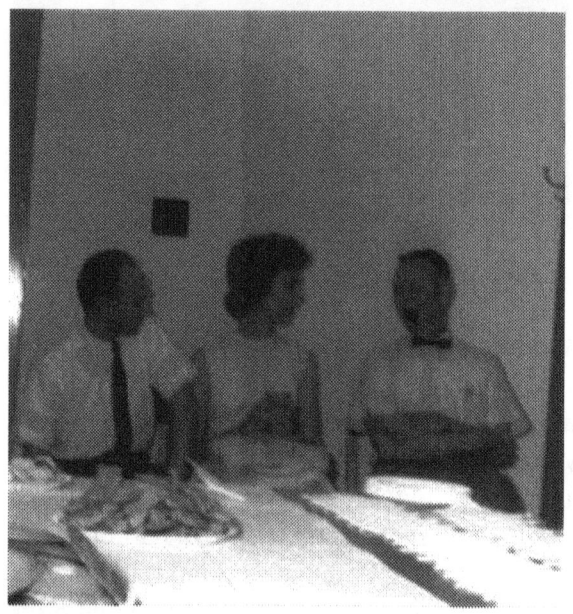

Frank & Marie Horner – John Geers

Review of Psychiatric Consultation

Psychology Service initiated a demographic study of the seven year Psychiatric Consultation Referral Program. Mrs. Mary Ingram, Secretary, Psychology Service collected the data for the review of 297 referrals completed in 1963 by four psychiatrists and eight psychiatric residents. Dr. Dave Fuller, Coordinator of Psychiatric Residents, served as a consultant to the study, suggested areas for review, and among other contributions designed the breakdown for the classification of the variety of drugs recommended by the consultants.

The nine page review submitted November 24, 1964 brought together a number of demographic and clinical facts about the referral program, and concluded: "No two identical cases were found, emphasizing the highly individualized nature of the consultation process. . . The findings may be found helpful to those who make referrals, to those who respond and to those who teach."

A copy of the report was routed June 29, 1966 to Dr. James Uloth, Chief Psychiatry Service. The routing slip was the earliest extant document to identify James Uloth as Chief of Service at Dallas VAH.

Family Activities

Jackie celebrated his tenth birthday at the Grady Niblo Farm. Beth visited Grandma Blanche on the Sedalia farm and rode the Continental bus back to Dallas.

Doris Gibson's chronic heart continued to cause much concern. We visited her, and Jean reported Doris seemed to be feeling well. I took Mr. Gibson to get some cantaloupes at Chambersville.

Jean invited her mother-in-law for a visit in October. She added, "Richard told me yesterday he is the best reader in his class - don't know whether he is or the teacher decided that, but they are all pleased about their schools."

Mother made the visit and afterwards sent this report for publication in the Van Alstyne Leader for Friday, October 23, 1964:

"Mrs. A. W. Jernigan of Sedalia visited in Dallas last week with her son, Jack Jernigan, and his family. Dr. and Mrs. Jernigan and children recently moved into their new home on Fountainhead Drive. During Mrs. Jernigan's visit, they gave a luncheon for her and their uncle and aunts. Present were Mr. and Mrs. G. A. Coffey, Mrs. J. M. Hoyle, Mrs. R. L. Johnsey, Mrs. Pansy McDougal, and two cousins, Mrs. Swain Tidwell and Mrs. Dezslo Kolozsy, all of Dallas. Mrs. Jernigan was accompanied home by her sister, Mrs. R. L. Johnsey, for a short visit."

Beth was a member of the Bell Choir at Cliff Temple. I wrote Mother November 1 that it seemed like we had been in church all day, "The children and Jean went to Training Union and then Beth stayed for fellowship and I am going down at 9 p.m. to pick her up. I took her at 8:30 this morning so she could practice playing the bells at the morning service, and it was worth the effort. Dr. Bassett always seems to enjoy the girls' performance so much."

Beth invited a host of friends from Browne Junior High School to a boy and girl party at our house that fall. Many of the guests were children who had been classmates throughout the years. Home movies captured some delightful scenes.

Cliff Temple Baptist Church committee schedule for 1964-1965 listed Dr. and Mrs. A. J. Jernigan as members of the Hospitality Committee. I was also a member of the Stewardship Committee and Family Counseling Committee.

We celebrated Thanksgiving with the JCJ's in Kingsville. One side trip was a tour of the King Ranch. Mother returned with us to Dallas. We stopped in San Antonio to visit the Alamo and later drove by the LBJ ranch.

We bought a living Christmas tree for our first Christmas at 4012 Fountainhead. The potted fir tree, planted in the front yard survived only one year.

The boys received an elaborate motorized roadway set for Christmas with cars, bridges, and other gadgets they laid out in the upstairs playroom. A 1964 movie scene recorded Uncle Stewart and his two nephews on the floor racing the small cars.

1965

I drove the 1960 Falcon to Gene Hays Motors in McKinney the second day of January 1965 and traded it for a 1965 Plymouth for $2400. The new, white Plymouth with blue interior was our first automobile to have factory installed air conditioning

Mother gave Jean a renewal subscription to the Reader's Digest as a birthday gift. Excerpts from Jean's March letter of thanks:

"Dearest Mother J.,

"The Reader's Digest came today, and it was really welcomed . . . Richard had such a good time on his birthday. He bought an outfit for "GI Joe" with his $3.00. . .I didn't get to go to Week of Prayer as much as I wanted. Our Circle had the program Tuesday, as I helped that day. Our revival is next week. The Young People visited last Saturday. I enjoyed going with them but it really threw me behind.

"Thank you so much for the Reader's Digest. I am looking forward to having it again.

Love,
Jean"

In mid-March we hired Globe Fence Co. to enclose our backyard with a combination wood panel and chain-link fence. Globe installed a double gate at the alley driveway entrance leading to the two-car garage. The boys and I built a basketball goal along side the driveway between the alley gate and garage.

A Bit of 1965 History

Feature writer, Larry Powell selected samples from the Dallas Morning News, for his Thursday, April 15, 1965 article. Excerpts:

"President Lyndon Johnson toured areas of the Midwest struck by tornadoes and violent weather. . . The Dallas school board OK'd a Project Head Start program for underprivileged children . . . the teachers would make only 90 cents an hour. . . Washington rejected a North Vietnamese peace plan because the State Department said it would result in a Communist takeover of the south.

"At Woolworth's, seamless nylon stocking cost 98 cents a pair. . .Sears sold men's tropical slacks in "Iridescent hues" for $4.77 . . . At A&P a pound of Eight O' Clock coffee cost 69 cents and an 18 ounce box of Cheerios was 35 cents. Beginning female secretaries with college degrees, $365 a month. . . Volkswagon bugs, $1495. . . in North Dallas, tri-level four-bedroom home, $35,000. At the movies: The 'Sound of Music' with Julie Andrews at the Inwood. The U. S. Post Office Department declared the ZIP Code --Zip Improvement Plan, if you wondered -- to be a help in pushing forward the goal of overnight delivery by 1967 of a letter mailed anywhere in the United States."

Professional Meetings & Visits

I attended the Southwestern Psychological Association Annual Meeting in Oklahoma City April 19, 1965. Mother's life long friend, former 1904 classmate at Westminster Baptist Academy, Mrs. Elizabeth Hollums lived in Oklahoma City. Mother rode with me to Oklahoma, I dropped her off at 3335 N. W. 19, Oklahoma City, and drove on to the meetings at the Skirvin Hotel. The two friends had a half century of "catching up" to do

The VA Central Office planned a Chief of Psychology Services meeting in Washington, D. C. in late April 1965. Notes on back of Lafayette Hotel stationery identified some of the men attending the conference: "Len Krasner, Palo Alto; Less Oseas, Cincinnati; Phil Carman, Wadsworth; Sid Cleveland, Houston; Lou Sherman, Boston; John Brownfain, Dearborn; Bill Rigby, Area Chief, St. Louis; Dick Filer, Research VACO. The topics discussed were not identified.

I took annual leave after the meeting to sight see and do personal research. Following are excerpts from four picture postcards mailed to family April 27-29:

"I had a fine trip up. Lunch was served over Texarkana; finished past Memphis. The Dulles Airport is quite a place - was cloudy, but no rain - around 60 degrees. Beautiful view coming into the city. Saw the monument 1st as we drove up the Potomac. The Trees are as beautiful as 'they' say. I will share a room with one of the participants (has not yet arrived). It is still light out, and I'm going walking. Wish each of you were here. Love, Daddy

"Dearest Jean: Had dinner with the Pecks Wed. night. They doubly insisted I remain with them on Thurs. & Fri., and I will. Weather is reported to be mild & sunny for the weekend. I am very pleased with the visit. Just wish you were with me to share the next two days. I love you, Jack."

"Dear Jackie: My hotel is the one nearest the White House. (I am about as close as we live to Brown Jr. Hi.) I am having a good visit. I will see you Saturday. I love you. Daddy"

"Dear Richard: I can't get this close to the White House. But I will go inside tomorrow morning. I am having a good time. I wish you, Jackie and Beth and Mother could see this with me. I love you, Daddy."

Tuesday and Wednesday nights were spent at the "Hotel Lafayette Overlooking the White House" (check stub, $16.64). Thursday and Friday nights were spent with the Pecks at their home on Honey Bee Lane.

The office of Congressman Earle Cabell of the 5th District (Dallas) scheduled a Congressional White House Tour for Friday, April 30, 1965. Passes were also included for the House and Senate.

At breakfast the morning of April 30, 1965, I read in the Washington Post Lady Bird Johnson would be planting a tree a few blocks from the White House at 9:30 that morning. I began an early D. C., self guided tour carrying along the 8mm movie camera, hopeful the long anticipated White House tour would be completed in time to attend the tree planting. Personal photographs were not permitted during the White House tour, but a few movie frames were taken outside the White House. The "Arbor Day in the Nation's Capital" site was reached in time to get a second row seat. Photographs were permitted.

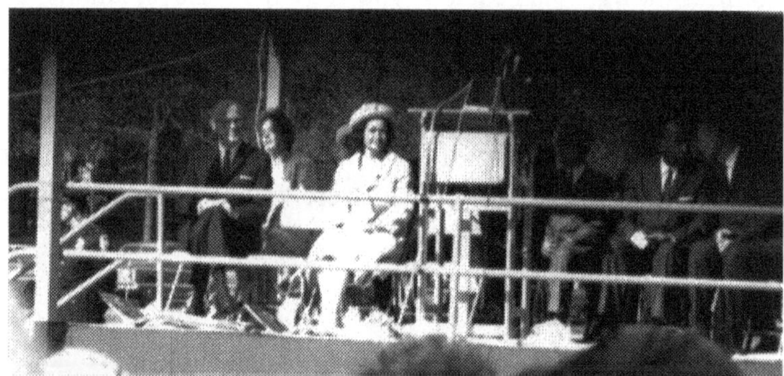

The "Arbor Day" brochure listed Walter N. Tobriner, President Board of Commissioner D. C. as Master of Ceremonies. Music was by the United States Army Band, Lt. Col. Samuel Loboda Leader. Mrs. Johnson sat front and center on the platform. Following the playing of the National Anthem, The Rev. William M. Baxter, St. Marks Episcopal Church gave the Invocation. Brigadier General C. M. Duke, Engineer Commissioner, D.C., read an Arbor Day Proclamation, followed by an introduction of distinguished guests. Mrs. Johnson made a few remarks as did Rep. George H. Fallon of the U. S. House of Representatives.

Mrs. Johnson turned the first spade at the tree planting. I took some decent movie frames of the entire ceremony including the arrival of Mrs. Johnson's limousine to return her to the White House.

As I packed the cameras, a uniformed black man tapped me on the shoulder and remarked he observed the filming and wondered if he could purchase a copy. There was a cautious response to the African American's request because of the increased racial tensions in D. C. at that time.

I soon learned that Mr. Harvey Lewis was the Tour Guide Driver for Sightseeing Tours, 4428 Ponds Street, N. E. Mr. Lewis explained he had lived in Washington all his life, had never been that close an observer of such an historic event, and wanted to own a copy of the movie film. I asked for his name and address, took a few movie frames of Mr. Lewis at the Arbor Day site to prove he had been present at the ceremony, and promised to mail him a copy of the film. In gratitude, Mr. Lewis said he would take me anywhere in Washington I might wish to visit. He drove me to the steps of Congress.

During the visit to the Senate Chamber, I listened to Senator Ted Kennedy give a brief speech. Later that same morning, April 30, 1965, I visited Senator Robert F. Kennedy's Office and spoke with a member of his staff about donating a copy of the 8 mm movie film of President Kennedy taken at Love Field November 22, 1963. The staff member suggested a copy be forwarded to Senator Kennedy for his review.

A description of the 1963 filming and copy of the film were mailed to Senator Robert F. Kennedy, May 15, 1965, with these added remarks:

"Several months ago a group of local people collected similar film and compiled a brief documentary for commercial purposes. I did not think this was appropriate and said so. However, I do wish to share a copy of the film with those who loved our President. I believe you or a member of your family can best determine the proper method for sharing these scenes."

Senator Kennedy's framed letter of acceptance and four scenes from the film grace our living room wall. The JFK Film story will be continued in another book.

National Archives

Another exciting opportunity came that afternoon: A "Card of Admission to Search Rooms at the National Archives and Records Service" dated 30 April 1965, valid until 3 May 1965. The card gave permission to enter the Search Room area for original Civil War documents and review of the Muster Rolls of the 30th Tennessee Regiment. Ten of twenty Muster Rolls for 30th Tennessee were delivered to the desk, but I had time to copy data from only four Muster Rolls.

The third Muster Roll included the Company's Pay Roll. "A. J. Jernigan, listed # 6" on the payroll, signed for his pay, "signature witnessed by J. H. Burney." Archives Mission accomplished. The distinct signature identified the 30th Tennessee Regiment Andrew Jackson Jernigan was our Grandpa A. J. Jernigan.

But I continued to read the one hundred year old Muster Rolls, each signed by "Jas L Jones, Capt," Grandma Laura Stewart Jernigan's cousin. After his surrender at Ft. Donelson, Capt. Jones wrote Laura Stewart's mother, Elizabeth Young Stewart from prison. The Captain told her of his effort to send her son home when Billy Stewart first contracted measles. Billy began to walk toward home just before the 30th Tennessee surrendered.

The fourth Muster Roll listed A. J. Jernigan as # 5 on the list of 31 names and signed by "C. Armstrong 2 Lt." Three men of the 30th were "killed at Chickamauga 19th of September, 1963. Jones, J. L. Capt" headed the list!

A shock of sadness came as I copied the 4th Muster Roll and read the notation of Capt. Jones' death. I felt the death of a loved one at the Archives. Also copied: "William C. Stewart - Age 19, enlisted Oct 22, Red Sp., Died at Springfield Tenn Feb 1862." A great-uncle died at the Archives that day.

Archives closing time neared. I pushed to read and copy a Muster Roll of Pvt. Elijah Chambers of "Company K, 16th Regiment Texas Calvary." 5

One final effort made while at the Archives: Identify the service record of James M. Griffin, Mother's maternal grandfather, born November 22, 1813 - died January 6, 1880.

The search was unsuccessful, but a "downstairs" Archives resource gave the Texas death record of J. M. Griffin. 6

Excerpts from the May 6, 1965 joint-letter to Stewart and Jamie:

". . . I feel confident that the A. J. Jernigan of the 30th Reg. was our grandfather. On one of the ten muster rolls of this particular regiment, all the men signed the payroll. The A. J. Jernigan signature is definitely the same as those we have for Grandpa Jernigan. . . I am having all the muster rolls micro-filmed. Each carries a log of the battles, and there are many notations after the names of individual soldiers (none after Grandpa's name). . . I copied the one muster roll, attached, and then inquired if I could get copies on microfilm. For $2.50, one can get 50 pictures. So I asked for the 20 from Grandpa's group, and the rest of Grandpa Chambers."

The National Archives did not send photocopies of Muster Rolls, but forwarded photocopies of copyist's recording of very limited data. Had I known that was the policy, I would have remained in Washington another day, returned to the Archives the next morning and copied the remaining Muster Rolls. I am very thankful for what was copied on April 30.

Significant Letter

Mr. Lewis wrote June 10, 1965, and enclosed a money order for $6.00.

"Dear Mr. Jernigan,

"Thank you very much for the film. I showed them to my church members last week.

"Best regards,

Harvey."

It was a nice experience for both of us.

Request for Leave

Before leaving for Washington, I received a memo from Dr. Geers asking for leave for a period of six months, ". . . effective April 26, 1965" to use all his accrued annual leave and the balance in leave without pay. The purpose: "This leave is requested in order that I can have time to resolve some personal problems."

That is the only extant document, and do not recall the circumstance for the request. John's "Memo" was forwarded to Dr. A. H. Hinshaw, Chief of Staff with this statement, "This request is forwarded for your review and consideration." John canceled his request and served with distinction that summer in supervising new trainees.

Psychology Trainees - 1965

Two Psychology Trainees from the University of Texas at Austin were assigned to Dallas VA Hospital in June 1965: Joyzelle Herod, Level I Psychology Trainee (Counseling), June 1, 1965 and Alan R. Brown, Level III (Clinical), June 7, 1965. Joy Herod was a "joy" as was Alan Brown. Joy was a "first" - a second generation psychologist in training: Her father, Dr. Tom Herod, was a Counseling Psychologist with the Temple VA Hospital.

Joy Herod came with little formal training in test administration and interpretation. She was introduced to such techniques as the Wechsler Adult Intelligence Test and the Strong Vocational Inventory. Her primary assignment centered on a study of youth volunteers and young people employed by the hospital in cooperation with the Educational Opportunities Act. Miss Herod sought to evaluate changes in attitude that might be related to the work experience. Tests and a questionnaire were administered at the beginning of the youth's work experience and repeated near the close of summer. Joy evidenced a great deal of initiative in completing the project with help and assistance from members of the staff, especially Dr. John Geers. Before Joy was able to analyze the data she returned to the University (September 17, 1965), but promised to complete the study in the summer of 1966. And she did.

Alan R. Brown entered the VA training program in June of 1964 as a Level II trainee at Waco VA Hospital and promoted to Level III in March 1965. The evaluation of Alan's 1965 summer experience was not retained, and do not recall his psychology unit assignment or the staff person who supervised his training. However, the report of his subsequent training will be presented in the next chapter. Alan was married and the Browns' daughter, Lisa, became one of Beth's first baby sitting experiences.

Crede, Colorado

We left home Saturday, June 26, 1965 for a vacation week at Antlers Guest Ranch, Crede, Colorado. We stopped at Love Field to visit with Jamie and family flying en route to Thailand on an Education Mission for the U. S. Department of Education and then around the world on return trip. As both families were to be "out of the country" in our Mother's perception, each family made extra efforts to keep her informed. She wrote June 29:

"I was extra lonesome Saturday and Sunday knowing 2/3 of my family were away. I was surely glad I wasn't at Love Field Saturday. Jamie called and said they'd just seen you all off in your car and they surely appreciated your being there when they got there and I did too. It was so thoughtful of you and Jean. . . I talked to all four of them but when I hung up after hearing Jamie say "Goodbye Mama" I had me a nice little cry [WW II flashback?]. We never know what may happen but as I told him we know the Lord is every where and he watches over us. . . There was a piece in <u>Sherman Democrat</u> (Sunday) about Dr. Jernigan and family going over seas. A. V. [mailman] told me he'd seen it."

At destination, June 28, 1965, mailed Mother a picture postcard of Crede's main street: "Crede, Colo. Colorful Pioneer Mining Town - Still active as a mining center. Very active as a hunting, fishing and resort area. Elevation 8,854 Feet."

"We had a very nice trip up. Our cabin is very warm (was in the upper <u>20's</u> this morning). We brought heavy clothes. I have never seen more breath-taking scenery. All of us are well and looking forward to a pleasant week. I hope you are well.

Love, Jack"

One day later a picture postcard of: "ANTLER'S PARK A beautiful home-like resort between Crede and Lake City on the banks of the Rio Grande River. Surrounded by the Rio Grande

National Forest. Fishing and hunting. A typical place for the whole family. 5 1/4 miles above Crede, Colorado."

"Won't write every day, but found this card showing our cabins. I marked ours with an X. Dr. Buckholts wrote urging us to come over this Sunday (they are about 150 miles away). We may do that. No one has caught any fish, but Jackie fished from 8 to 1 today. The Mgr. said he never saw a boy with so much patience. All the children have found things to keep them happy. We plan to go to a near bye silver mine this afternoon.

Love Jack "

"Thursday, July 1, 1965

Dear Mother:

"The boys have had some cold but are about over it. Beth is begging to stay over Monday AM so you know she's having a good time. We haven't caught any fish but the Sears fishing kit the children gave me for Fathers Day has been a boon. We visited an old silver mine yesterday. . . A Methodist minister, the couple who manage the lodge and the rest of us sat up to 10 last night singing. These are wonderful people here and wholesome for the children. Hope you are well. Love, Jack"

Jean wrote the following note to Beth one morning:

"Beth----

Cereal in box
apple pie in oven
We are in Meadow on other
side of rec. room. I wore
your Jacket --"

It was cold at Crede, Colorado during the early morning hours. Crede was a once in a lifetime vacation - never repeated. Wish we had.

Dr. and Mrs. Walter Buckholts moved to their "vacation retreat" in Colorado when he retired as Manager of Dallas VAH in 1965. We visited and had lunch with them on our return to Dallas. Dr. Buckholts took Jackie fishing as recorded on movie film.

Back at the Office

Many items awaited my response upon return to work from the refreshing vacation. The Civil Service Commission asked our new Hospital Director, Dr. J. B. Chandler, to encourage staff to participate in a guest-lecturer program, ". . . to strengthen the relationships between Federal agencies and our major personnel source, the colleges and universities." The Regional Commission Director, Louis S. Lyon asked for a reply by August 2, 1965. Dr. Chandler requested a response from each Service Chief.

The form asked for the usual demographic information: education, memberships, honors, research, etc. and "Suggested Titles of Special Talks and Lectures." My titles for possible "Special Talks and Lectures" were:

"The Role of the Psychologist in a General Medical Hospital"
"The Scientific Measurement of Human Behavior"
"Research as a Training Technique"

Past experiences with presentations to high school students were rewarding, though I am not a gifted public speaker. The Veterans Administration granted official leave to give talks during daytime working hours of 8:00 to 4:30.

Dr. Will Rigby wrote he had ". . .transferred from Jefferson Barracks to NIMH in early October 1965 and I am now located in the Regional Office of the Public Health Service at Kansas City,

Missouri." I thanked him for his letter, and invited suggestions for a job description request that would justify a GS-14 rating.

He pointed out that Houston VA with its large Psychology staff was the only GM&S Hospital of the St. Louis Region with a Chief at grade level GS-14. It would be four years before the GS-14 pay grade came to Dallas.

Family Happenings - 1965

Richard and I participated in Indian Guides and the fathers and sons of several "Oak Cliff Tribes" took an overnight outing to Possum Kingdom Lake. Mother mentioned the trip in her late September 1965 letter.

I became bored with Sunday School in 1965 and after dropping off Jean and the children at Church, drove on to the nearby Cliff Towers Nursing Home for a visit with Aunt Claude, who was blind. However, Aunt Claude always asked, "What is today's lesson?" and I was prepared to give a summary. It is a happy memory.

I wrote I was scheduled to talk on Stewardship at a Cliff Temple Baptist Church morning service.

Grady Niblo and I went to Sedalia and Melissa to cut firewood. On the return trip to Dallas the Kentucky trailer had a flat, and thankfully discovered the 1965 Plymouth spare fit the trailer's 1942 Dodge wheel hub.

Jean became a substitute teacher in Dallas Schools. She wrote her mother-in-law on Monday, November 8, 1965 about teaching and other happenings.

"Dearest Mother J.,

"I am teaching LATIN [in Duncanville] today and tomorrow. It has not been too hard so far. They know enough to correct each other.

"We all had a good time at the carnival. I was a Slimy-Hand Ghost and Jack took tickets.

"Beth said Jack did "OK" yesterday, which probably means his talk was a good one. . . Jack has gone to a funeral for one of the doctor's wife. We went to see them last Monday night and knew it could not be long. She was unconscious after a brain tumor and he was caring for her at home [wife of Dr. Ludlow Pence].

"I have an off period, so thought I'd get some use from it by writing a while. Take care of yourself. We are so proud of you for all you do. Please don't wait to call if and when we can help out."

Mother commended Jean in a return letter: "I've wondered how many days you taught Jean. I've always thought a substitute teacher the smartest kind. I could never have done that I'm sure - not in a big school, anyway."

A Sister's Death

Marian Wysong made Social Security payments for Doris Gibson's baby-sitting Ann, Marian's daughter, but Doris was declared not eligible for Social Security Disability because she baby sat in her home. However it was possible for Doris to receive a heart operation through the Texas Rehabilitation Act.

The operation carried a great risk. This brave, sweet person elected to take the operation at St Paul's Hospital on Harry Hines in Dallas, stating if she lived or died she would have a new heart. She did not survive the December 1965 surgery, but she received a "new heart."

We bought an artificial "White Christmas Tree" for our living room in early December 1965. Mrs. Gibson slept on the couch in the living room the night after Doris' operation. We woke her early in the morning to tell her of Doris' death. For Jean, "White Christmas Tree" symbolized Doris' death, and she gave it to Goodwill Industries. From that time onward we always had a "Green Christmas Tree."

Doris was buried December 17, 1965. Jean spoke to Doris' death in a letter December 20, 1965.

"Dearest Mother J.,

"I am teaching today at Crozier Tech and have an off period. Am glad the students don't know what a poor typist I am; this is a new style keyboard and all the keys are blank. In addition, there is an extra row on the right hand, and I keep getting my fingers mixed up.

"Beth had a very lovely Christmas program last night at the church. Jack and I went to two open houses and to Sunday School and church yesterday morning, then all of us back last night, so it was a busy day. Aunt Claudya has been walking around the block. We plan to go to see her at Anita's during Christmas. It does seem impossible that she could be that much better.

"Jackie made an "A" on a report he worked on last weekend, and is doing much better in his school work. Richard is slacking off but he will pick back up I'm sure. His music teacher will have a party for his group Wednesday and his Cub Scouts are going caroling tomorrow. So he will be busy. He simply cannot wait to see if he is going to get a bicycle [with a Banana seat]. Surely hope he does!

"Jamie and Frances called Saturday night. They had sent Daddy and Mother a [condolence] telegram. Everyone has been so nice to us. They wanted to know about Christmas, and we suggested we all come up Friday [December 24] to your house. If this does not suit, we will change, as we have no other plans. Other than visiting, I am sure there will be no other plans at Melissa.

"We will always be grateful to the Murphy's for bringing you Friday [December 17 to the funeral], and tell the others how much we appreciated their coming to the funeral. Jack thought it was a little short, but Doris had said she didn't want a long service. We miss her, but can't wish for her any more of the kind of suffering she had to live with.

Love, Jean"

All three Jernigan families were at Sedalia during the Christmas holidays. It was a quiet Christmas at Grandpa and Grandma Gibson's home.

Chapter 8 - 1966

1966 - Quite a Year

Family Happenings

Jackie and Richard begin 1966 with a bang after they received permission to light small firecrackers New Years Day at Sedalia! Later, I drove Mr. Gibson to Highland Cemetery on a cold Saturday afternoon because he, ". . . wanted to see that the dirt had been spread correctly at Doris' grave."

It snowed twice in January, and Jean especially enjoyed the new clothes dryer. I wrote Mother January 24, 1966 that, "We had a very pleasant weekend in the snow. The children all played out Saturday and no one got a cold. We burned lots of wood."

The Department of Psychology, University of Texas sponsored a clinical training workshop January 28, 1966 at Lakeway Resort north of Austin. Wives were invited, but Jean did not wish to attend.

I wrote Mother the good news of Richard's conversion experience on Sunday the 23rd of February: His acceptance of Jesus Christ as Lord.

". . . it was a most moving scene. . . the 'feeding of the five thousand.' The role of the boy had been emphasized. . . Dr. Bassett asked them to sing one more verse (there had been no response). Richard pulled my sleeve and said he wanted to go down. I told him to go right ahead and followed . . . have no doubt about his understanding."

It was Dr. Bassett's last baptism before retirement. All three of our children were baptized by Dr. Wallace Bassett. I wrote him a note February 24, 1966:

"I was quite moved by the penetrating interpretation you gave Sunday of John's description of the 'feeding of the five thousand.' I was even more moved when I realized your words had reached the mind and heart of our 8 year old son, Richard. To me, this eight year old boy coming forward symbolized the message of the miracle.

"You will be receiving countless statements of appreciation in the next few weeks. This note is not to thank you for the past (although I do), but to thank you for your on-going creative work of the present."

Aunt Sis Coffey died February 23, 1966. The following was abstracted from a McKinney Examiner article titled, "Smile Her Trademark."

"ANNA - A friendly hand, a cheery word, an almost [un]erasable smile were the trademark of Miss Cynthia McKinney Coffey, of Anna, who was more than 100 years old when she died at 6:30 p.m. Wednesday in a McKinney hospital after an illness of several weeks.

"Miss Coffey was the last of a large family of Mr. and Mrs. Jess Coffey, Collin pioneers. All of the children lived to be more than 80 years of age. Miss Coffey was born on Oct. 8, 1865. She was a member of the Christian Church in which she was active until infirmity slowed her steps."

In March the children watched their cat, Petula have kittens. We built a cedar-wood screen on the south side of our patio in May for privacy and to mask air compressor noise.

Dr. Bassett retired, Cliff Temple called Dr. Darold Morgan to be pastor. Jean became a member of the Long Range Planning Committee, and she and I were members of the Hospitality Committee. I was also Vice-Chairman of the Family Counseling Committee, and a member of the Stewardship Committee.

A Challenging Request

Sid Cleveland, Chief Psychologist Houston VAH wrote May 10, 1966:

"I am trying to gather some information on experience of psychologists regarding the usefulness of group testing of psychiatric patients. You may have heard that a psychiatric work-up is being planned on a sample of Texas State Hospital patients, including psychological testing. It seems to me that in terms of the numbers to be examined (1800) individual testing is out of the question.

"I would appreciate from you any of your experiences with group testing, including the types of tests used, which are more useful and which not appropriate. Also, any comments regarding testing conditions, size of subject group, etc. I would be interested in the kind of information you feel can be gained from group testing and what sort of information can only be gained in individual sessions."

Excerpts from my response to Sid's May 10, 1966 letter:

". . . Four years ago we developed a standardized approach enabling us to collect norms for our hospital population, using the following tests: Kent E-G-Y, Scale D; Memory for Meaningful Stories (Taken from Wechsler Memory Scale, Form 2); Grayson Perceptualizaton Test; Bender Gestalt Test; Human Figure Drawings; Rotter Sentence Completion Test; Illness Description Test.

"From time to time, additional tests are included. . . For example, we experimented with The Roos Time Reference Inventory. . . Last year, Walter Penk included the Ravens Progressive Matrices.

"I am convinced group testing has considerable merit as an assessment procedure. . . The battery takes approximately 90 minutes. I limit the size of the group to ten, unless I have an assistant. A number of behavioral observations can be made . . . we are developing a check list for recording such observations. A large group reduces the opportunity for gaining subtle clinical cues; however, this can be overcome to some extent by having trained observers present.

"The idea of testing 1800 patients intrigues me. This certainly offers an opportunity to test out many variables in group testing . . . examiner differences, varieties of tests, order of tests, etc."

Texas Department of Mental Health
Mental Retardation

The 59th Texas Legislature passed the "Texas Mental Health and Mental Retardation Act" designed to strengthen the Texas Mental Health Program. The Act created an Operations Research Division within the Texas Department of Mental Health and Mental Retardation. Governor Connally appointed Shervert Frazier, M.D., to be Commissioner of Mental Health and Mental Retardation effective December 1, 1965. Dr. Frazier's first act was to recommend a study that came to be the 1966 Administrative Survey of Texas State Mental Hospitals.

The Commissioner held his first planning session in Austin February 2, 1966. Representative leaders from the National Institute of Mental Health (NIMH), the Department of Health, Education and Welfare, from University of Texas, Austin; University of Texas Southwestern Medical School, Dallas; and the Texas Department of Mental Health and Mental Retardation attended the meeting.

A NIMH grant application evolved from the second planning session that named Dr. Shervert Frazier, Director, and Dr.

Alex Pokorny, Co-Director of the survey. The design: 1. Complete a State Hospital patient census; 2. Survey behavioral characteristics and nursing care needs of patients; 3. Do an intensive examination of a 10% sample of the entire hospital system; 4. An evaluation of each of the seven mental hospital's programs, assets, problems, etc.

"Intensive examinations" were to be conducted at San Antonio, Austin, and Terrell Hospitals that included examinations by a psychiatrist, psychologist, neurologist (selected cases), social worker, 9 laboratory tests and x-ray examinations, physical examination by physician, review of each case record, and contacts with relatives and friends. Four group panels assembled in May to outline the project consisting of: Sociologist/Social Workers, Psychiatrists, Medical Examiners and Neurologists, and Psychologists. The Sociologist/Social Worker Panel met in Austin; all other panels met in Houston.

The Psychologist Panel that met in Houston May 25-26, 1966 established the general outline and selected key leaders for the survey. Members of the assembled panel were: James Bieri, Ph.D, Maurice Korman, Ph.D., Harold Goolishian, Ph.D, Sidney Cleveland, Ph.D., Wayne Holtzman, Ph.D., Paul Baer, Ph.D., David Wright, Ph.D., Sanford Goldstone, Ph.D., Shervert Frazier, M.D., Alex Pokorny, M.D., Fred Crawford, Ph.D., Hubert Reese, George McBee, and Carl Taube.

The panel made these general recommendations: 1. Group psychological testing should be used wherever possible; 2. as many as possible of the remaining patients should be given individual psychological testing; 3. all of the remaining patients in the sample should be seen by a senior psychologist; 4. a well qualified psychologist should take charge of the entire psychology testing program; 5. teams of testers should be organized, so that all of the testing within one hospital could be completed within a few days; and 6. a behavior rating scale to describe each patient's participation in the testing should be developed and employed. 1

An Invitation

The Houston Psychological Panel designated Dr. David Wright to contact me by telephone, Thursday May 26, 1966 and ask that I consider the position of Coordinator of Psychological Testing for the 1966 Administrative Survey of Texas State Mental Hospitals. Later that day I talked with Sid Cleveland who explained: "The survey design called for an examination of 1700 patients, 1/3 from each of 3 state hospitals. Teams of graduate students would go to each hospital; follow-up testing to be done by Ph.D.s later; survey to begin July 9."

Diary

I began a "State Survey Diary" that day and recorded all contacts and decisions. The diary was later transcribed by Mrs. Mary Ingram, Secretary to Psychology Service, a forty-page, single spaced document titled, "Notes on Administrative Survey." Within the diary rest the names of many of the leaders of Texas Psychology as well as a host of graduate students, many of whom became future leaders. It seemed the entire Association of Texas Psychologists became invested in seeing that the project succeeded. Their collective cooperation made it possible to achieve a monumental testing goal in the span of two weeks in July 1966. Highlights as recorded in the Diary follow.

Excerpts from Diary

"A quick review of the Panel's request was made with the psychology staff and the Chief of Staff. The following day, Friday, May 27 Maurice Korman, a member of the Houston Panel, gave a detailed summary of the committee actions and decisions. . . pointed out that the decisions were guide lines and not hard and fast rules of procedure. Returned call to Sid Cleveland, and gave provisional agreement to serve as Coordinator.

"5-30-66 (Monday) Met with Psychology Staff, began to make proposals regarding battery, e.g. that Ph.D.s serve as group examiners.

"5-31-66 (Tuesday) Met with Dr. Frazier at Executive Inn, Austin; reviewed Dallas' tentative recommendations.

"6-1-66 (Wednesday) Dr. Pokorny called. His areas of interest: Intelligence, organicity, psychoses, personality assessment; reviewed Dr. Pokorny's telephone call with Dr. Hinshaw, Chief of Staff, VAH."

On June 1, 1966 the Texas Commissioner of Mental Health informed the Director of Dallas VAH of the Advisory Panel's recommendation that the Chief Psychologist of Dallas VAH be asked to help coordinate the psychological examinations. The Director granted the request.

"6-2-66 (Thursday) Called Cecil Peck. He suggested Cornell and Shipley Tests.

"6-3-66 (Friday) Flew Braniff to Houston to confer with Dr. Pokorny. He suggested Stanford-Binet front sheet for rating of patients.

"6-6-66 (Monday) Talked with Hubert Reese of Operations Research Division for first time. Reviewed week's contacts with Psychology Staff."

Hubert Reese, Chief, Field Data Systems, Operations Research Division, Texas Department of Mental Health and Mental Retardation became the key liaison person in Austin. Hubert was a bright, affable person with a "can do" attitude.

The following memo was submitted to the Chief of Staff, Dallas VAH June 7, 1966 to document previously approved verbal decisions by Hospital Administration:

"Subject: Coordination of Psychological Examinations of the 10% Sample of State Psychiatric Patients.

"1. The services of the Chief Psychologist have been requested by the Commissioner of Mental Health and Mental Retardation, Dr. Shervert Frazier, Jr., to participate in a state-wide examination of psychiatric patients. The general plan is that beginning July 9, 1966, approximately 1700 psychiatric patients will be administered group psychological screening tests at the following State Hospitals: Austin, Terrell, and San Antonio. It is anticipated, five teams of three psychologists each, will examine, on a group basis, a total of 200 patients a day. Thus, group testing will go on at each of these three hospitals for approximately three days each during the month of July.

"2. As coordinator of this phase of the project, I will be working directly with the Chief of Psychiatry, Dr. Alex Pokorny, of the Houston VAH. Dr. Pokorny is responsible for the coordination of the psychiatric examinations; also, he will give general supervision to the entire project.

"3. It is estimated that my services will be needed for approximately thirty working days. As much as possible, time devoted to this project will be confined to week-ends and evenings. However, it will be necessary to be on leave from my position for probably 10 to 15 working days. Rate of compensation is $100 a day for each full consulting workday, with some additional funds being made available for travel expenses.

"4. Plans have not yet completely crystallized concerning the over-all details of this project. The general outline has been approved by the National Institute of Mental Health and the State of Texas is matching the funds granted by the National Institute of Mental Health. It is my understanding that, in addition, the state has additional funds available for implementing this project. The consulting fee paid to any federal employee will come from the state fund. If permitted to participate in this project, I plan to request annual leave on those days where I will be away from my full-time duty assignment. I will attempt to use no more leave than would ordinarily be used during regular summer vacation. It is felt this is a most worthwhile project, and that each person invited to participate should make an effort to contribute.

A. J. Jernigan, Ph.D."

Support Groups

The hospital administration was most supportive, and gave blanket permission to use Psychological Service Staff and facilities in the development of the group test battery, to recruit personnel by telephone and letter, and blend all necessary background work with regular duties as Chief Psychologist. Except for general guidelines from the Houston Panel, we started from scratch. The project became one of the most challenging and rewarding experiences of my professional career.

Dallas VAH Psychology staff: John Geers, Ralph Robinowitz, Walter Penk, Psychology Trainees Joy Herod and Alan Brown were enthusiastic contributors and supporters of the project. Dr. William M. Hales, Program Director of the Dallas Office of Mental Health Services of the Department of Health, Education and Welfare joined our staff. Bill was a participant in the February 2, 1966 Houston planning meeting. He became a key advisor-contributor to the project.

Bill Hales neared retirement and wanted to lighten his duties after a long and responsible Federal Service career. Dr. Hales applied for and accepted a vacant Psychology position at Dallas VA as a Ward Psychologist. His many past accomplishments included participating with Starke Hathaway at Minnesota in the development of the MMPI. It was Dr. Hale's strong, convincing recommendation that the Cornell Medical Index became a part of the test battery instead of a modified version of the MMPI suggested by others.

Dr. Wayne Holtzman became the central consultant to the project, in part because his Holtzman Ink Blot Test (HIT) was included in the battery, but primarily because of his strong state and national leadership as a psychologist in the field of mental health. Our relationship went back to the early days at Waco when he served as consultant to Waco VA Psychology staff.

Wayne and I spent several hours Sunday June 12, 1966, reviewing the June 11 field trip observations made at Terrell State Hospital with Dr. Pokorny, Hubert Reese, Bob Humble and Dr. Metzger. Wayne agreed with the decision that a standard Ph.D. team be recruited for test administration at all three hospitals.

We discussed several possible tests to be used in the survey. Wayne suggested we look into Reitan's work which led to a call to former Kentucky classmate Dick Thomas who stated the Reitan Test was not applicable as a group test. Wayne also suggested former Waco mentor, Dr. Don Gorham be contacted and review his method for presenting HIT slides to groups. Dr. Holtzman and I drafted a tentative group battery and the estimated time to administer.

At the conclusion of the meeting, I returned to the Austin Chariot Inn to visit with the family. Jean and the three children accompanied me to Austin the previous afternoon for an overnight stay at Chariot Inn. The days had become so busy that it was difficult to have time with Jean and the children. The Austin trip was one of those few times the family received special pleasure from the State Survey.

Pilot Study

Walter Penk and I conducted our first pilot study Friday, June 17, 1966. Walter selected a group of patients from the

Psychiatric Ward and we attempted to create the anticipated State Hospital test environment. Walter served as observer. We devoted the entire day to the pilot, recorded the test session, and reviewed the experiment the following afternoon (Saturday). He and I drafted a tentative observation scale, subsequently refined by Walter, and identified as the BOR (Behavior Observation Rating).

Sunday afternoon, June 19, I outlined the coming week's agenda: "(1) order following tests: Kent; Widerange Achievement; HIT; W. M. Form I; Bender Gestalt; Sentence Completion; Cornell Medical Index; Adjective Check List. (2) Write letters to 10 psychologists. (3) Call 4 psychologists locally. (4) Write instructions for all tests. (5) Draft and pursue procedure for development of test booklet. (6) Work on procedure for administering individual tests."

Sid Cleveland, Joe Rickard and Reese Kinser were helpful in supplying names of psychologists and trainees willing to take annual leave and serve. By Monday, June 20, 1966, we confirmed acceptance from five test examiners: Ralph Robinowitz (Dallas), Joe Rickard (Temple), Clarence Miller (Houston), Reese Kinser (San Antonio) and Wayne Gill (San Antonio). Wayne communicated in Spanish, a necessary requirement for the San Antonio State Hospital.

Following are excerpts from a June 21, 1966 letter to Dr. James Bieri, Director of Clinical Training at University of Texas:

"Enclosed is a draft of a rating form Walter Penk and I constructed this past Saturday. The items listed were empirically derived based on a testing experience of 6-17-66 with seven schizophrenic patients . . . would appreciate your review and criticism of the rating schedule . . . appreciate very much the counsel and advice you gave during your recent consultant visit . . . am tentatively scheduling Sunday, July 10, as an orientation day in Austin, with the plan that testing will begin July 11."

"Diary: 6-23-66 (Thursday) Second pilot. Tested 20 patients. Reviewed tape recording of procedure that evening. First draft of BOR. Ralph Robinowitz and Bob Brown, Southwest Medical School Psychologist were observer-critics. Tests: Kent, Logical Memory, HIT, Memory for Designs, Word Association [Moran], Bender Gestalt, Human Figure Drawings, Sentence Completion, Cornell Index, Arithmetic (Wide Range), Illness Description, Adjective Check List. Total time for slowest patient: 3 hours and 8 minutes. Refreshments served at midpoint by Nursing Service. Notes from tape review: Reduce HIT instructions (6 minutes). Is calling blot number an acceptable procedure? Make certain projector table is stable. Jean Jernigan suggested instructions for Memory for Design: "Look - Draw." Word Association: Allow time for confusion; should one give examples? Rules on smoking should be established. Each record must be scored, select tests that can be scored. Don't push patient to limit on the final tests. Medical School supplied ACL (Adjective Check List). Used Form A and B of HIT.

"Feedback from Reese, Pokorny, Brown, Bieri, Holtzman, Rickard and Kinser: Reese recommended Mrs. Ingram be paid her overtime Federal pay rate. Pokorny gave tentative breakdown of 600 patients from Austin, 470 from Terrell and 470 from San Antonio to be stratified into 72 cells proportionate to entire hospital system.

"Bill Hales and I began a draft of the Manual of Instructions on Saturday June 25, 1966. Bill suggested we give the rationale for each test and its contribution toward the testing goal. Walter Penk worked on BOR."

Sunday afternoon June 26, 1966, outlined procedure for ordering test forms; worked on Manual. Developed agenda for week: "(1) Letters and calls to Bieri, Gill, Stanley Blumberg, Balbona, Reinehr; (2) write final instructions for all tests; (3) refute, or move forward on test booklet; (4) procedure for individual tests; (5) order tests; (6) order equipment, e.g. tablets, pencils, etc.; (7) check with W. Holtzman on projectors; (8) complete Manual."

The preparation pitch reached crescendo level on Monday, worked until 11:30 pm. Consultants polled for their special test entries during the day. Wayne Holtzman supported dropping Adjective Check List and limit HIT to 30 slides. Made calls throughout day requesting rush orders for test forms, then sent confirming letters to each Test Company. VA Medical Illustration agreed to make slides for Form C of Benton.

Bill Hales and I tested 4 patients Tuesday. Worked from 6:30 pm to 12:30 am on Instructions to Examiners. We conducted the third and final pilot with 18 subjects Wednesday morning (June 29, 1966). Joy Herod and Alan Brown were proctor-observers, John Geers and Walter Penk observer-critics and Ralph Robinowitz dropping in. Was the first complete run using final test battery; completed in 2 hours, 32 minutes for slowest patient.

That afternoon entire staff scored tests, reviewed rating scale and manual. John Geers made especially relevant suggestions: "Collect patients and bring to test room as a group; make sure all patients have glasses; identify hard of hearing; arrange room so observer can walk among patients; cut off projector at end of HIT demonstration; have one of three psychologists responsible for changing a bulb in projector; give more time on Benton, improve instructions; enunciate WA [Word Association] more clearly; have a nursing aide present in room; set up test material in 2 packets for ease of distribution."

Hubert Reese called Thursday, asked me to fly to Austin Saturday and on to San Antonio to meet with Nursing Staff and review test rooms. Talked with Dr. Arthur Benton, he recommended Form E of Benton, contracted with Walter Sullivan of Medical Illustration to produce five sets of Benton slides. Mrs. Ingram and I verifaxed and assembled 15 copies of Manual.

Flew to Austin Saturday July 2, 1966 and met with Dr. Pokorny, State Hospital staff, Hubert Reese, Bob Humble. At their Central Office (CO) drafted a mock-up of test booklet - scheduled reproduction of 2,000 copies of each Form - BOR, WA, DOC. Learned the sample size from each hospital: 638 Austin; 480 Terrell; 419 San Antonio, total 1537 patients. From 11:00 to 12:30 met with Wayne and Jon Swartz, and also Bob Humble and Hubert Reese at Wayne Holtzman's office. Opened and checked all tests received from Test Companies. Hubert Reese agreed to mail HIT manuals to all examiners. Drove to San Antonio with Bob Humble and Hubert Reese to meet Hospital personnel and check out testing rooms. Flew home.

Sunday to church and some rest. Consolidated notes from Saturday and read Bob Brown's observation-critique of Pilot # 2. Bob wrote at length about purpose of study and the need to establish scoring and interpretation procedures before we began testing the 1500+ patients. He offered complete backing of Southwestern Medical School psychologists.

The final week of preparation arrived Monday, July 4, 1966; outlined thirteen steps to be completed. (All were checked off except #11: "Method and Procedures for Scoring Tests.") Each day of the week's Diary is filled with mind-boggling details: telephone calls, letters, assuring all test material, booklets, manuals, testing equipment were available and in place; confirmed personnel and located replacements for one individual; and smoothed a few "hurt feelings" of some who felt overlooked in the decision making. John Geers drafted a rating scale for "un-testable" patients. Contracted with a "Dr. Kleen" to translate test instructions into Spanish. By telephone with Hubert Reese: discussed test booklet page by page, decided on number of M and F forms, Spanish forms, and front of booklet. Joy Herod completed observer work sheet form.

Friday, July 8, 1966 filled with last minute details, locating and packing spare equipment. Called Phil Roos, Lou Moran and others, asked them to be present at the Sunday orientation-demonstration test session. Searched for additional Female forms of Cornell; wrote letters of invitation to two Houston students, letter to George Parker explaining why Adjective Check list excluded, etc. Left home by car drove to Austin at 7:00 pm.

Saturday, July 9, 1966. Oriented by Hubert Reese and others on procedure for recording data. Psychiatrists were oriented by Dr. Pokorny. Worked with Hubert Reese and his Central Office staff on the assembly of the 2,000 booklets. Conferred with Wayne Holtzman and his staff on scoring; reviewed brief scoring suggestions accumulated at Dallas. Surveyed test rooms at State Hospital with Mrs. Eidelbach and Bob Reinehr. Explained why state psychologists were not participating in the survey. From 4:00 to 6:00 pm Hubert and I checked all equipment. Met in evening with Phil Roos - reviewed survey. Later, completed outline of Sunday's orientation.

Orientation of testing staff and consultants began at 9:00 am Sunday, July 10, 1966. Ph.D.s present: Robinowitz, Gill, Miller, Kinser and Rickard. Trainees: Laird, Hooks, Klein, Brown, Mandell, Lyles, Witzke, Sachs, Yale, Jackson, and Haywood. Consultants: Holtzman, Roos, Moran. Administrative: Reese and Humble. Dr. Pokorny gave brief summary of plans, purpose, and some results from psychiatrist's interviews on Saturday.

I reviewed the Houston Panel's recommendations and gave summary of development of group battery. Identified the individuals who participated in the June preparation: Ingram, Penk, Hales, Robinowitz, Geers, Brown, Herod, Korman, Bob Brown, Bieri, Holtzman, Cleveland, Iscoe, Bounds, Art Benton, Parker, Cecil Peck, Dr. Kleen, Pokorny, Thomas, Gorham, Kinser and Rickard.

Three Dallas Pilot studies involving 45 patients summarized. Named tests explored and not included in final battery: Rotter S.C.; A.C.L.; Wide Range Achievement; Wechsler Memory (Design); MMPI; Mid-Town Manhatten Scale; Cornell N-

2; and Benton Form C. The test battery and manual were presented to the panel.

Wayne Holtzman discussed the HIT - gave brief history - its potential contribution - and the method of adapting the procedure to group testing. In a similar way Lou Moran discussed the Word Association. Phil Roos made pertinent observations about the procedure and shared his experience and knowledge of the State Hospital System.

A group of 12 hospitalized patients were brought to the conference room after lunch and administered pertinent sections of the battery. Kept the patients for approximately an hour - took break and the staff returned to critique the procedure. Mandell and Jackson as volunteer observer-proctors reported problems they encountered: some forgot glasses, not all could hear well, compulsive patients required more time, need for clarity of instructions, etc. The group discussed minor recommendations: Put all B.G. Designs on one page, rejected requiring HFD be placed on 2 pages, tear out last page of HIT, etc. Decided patients would be told to smoke only at the break.

Nurse Eidelbach gave general orientation to hospital and nursing procedures. Team assignments were announced: (1) Ralph Robinowitz - Don Laird U. of T. and Walter Hooks VA Houston; (2) Wayne Gill - Dan Klein U. of T. and Alen Brown VA Dallas; (3) Clarence Miller - David Mandell U. of T. and Dick Lyles VA Houston; (4) Reese Kinser - Don Witzke U. of T. and Stan Sacks VA Houston; (5) Joe Rickard - Pat Yale VA Houston and Joe Jackson VA Temple.

Each team loaded a carousel, checked out equipment in its assigned room, and made ready for first day's testing.

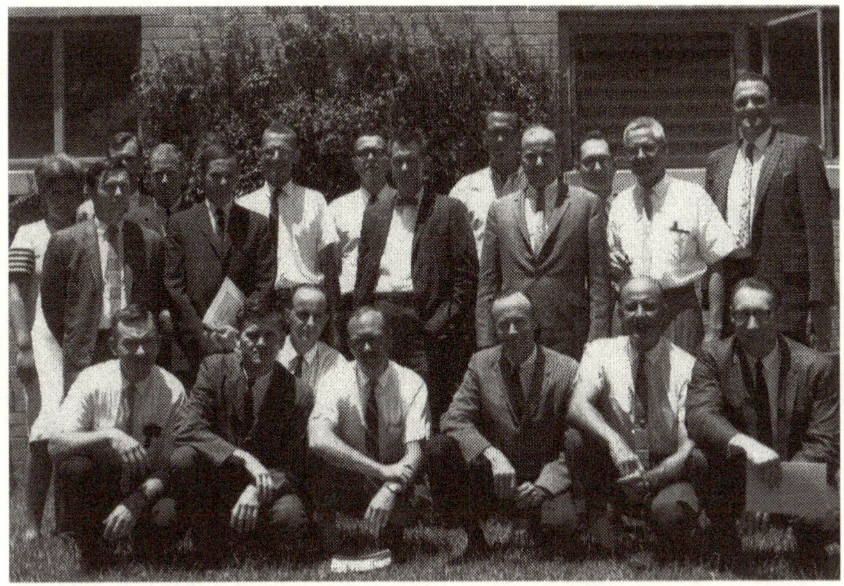

Standing: Yale, Haywood, Lyles, Brown, Sacks, Robinowitz, Hooks, Rickard, Jackson, Gill, Laird, Moran, Klein
Front row: Jernigan, Miller, Mandell, Witzke, Kinser, Holtzman, Roos

I met with all examiners Monday, July 11, 1966 for final instructions. At 10:00 am made a tour of the groups and happily discovered everything going well, all examinations on schedule. The five teams of examiners-proctors (with exception of Mandell) ate together at noon and discussed problems, and did some fine tuning. Five teams tested 94 patients. All were quite pleased with the results. I was reminded of the similarity of the experience and WWII days as Chief Examiner in Miami and Coordinator of experimental testing at Randolph Field.

Nurse Eidelbach and I discussed the testing of the 67 patients of the sample living at the Confederate Home in Austin. Forty five patients were rated by psychiatrists as un-testable. Three children were included in the 10% sample and arrangement made for Graduate Student Haywood to examine those three. Mrs. Eidelbach and I visited the Confederate Home on West Sixth Street (beyond Albert Jernigan's historical home) at 1:45 pm Monday afternoon, and determined there was a space for group testing and sufficient offices for individual exams.

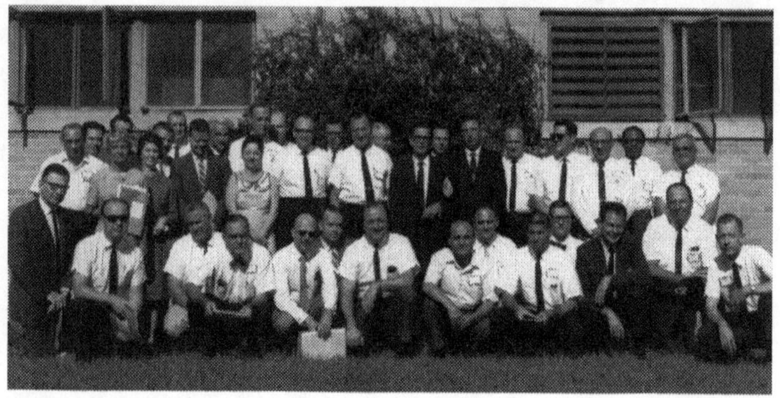

Psychiatrists – Austin: Alex Pokorny, front row center, Isham Kimball, next to last on front row, right.

The Monday afternoon group of patients was somewhat more regressed, three tested individually, one hard of hearing, two Spanish-speaking. We assessed 191 patients that first day. In the evening, Ralph Robinowitz and I attended a party at Wayne Holtzman's home where the project was discussed with a number of psychologists, and recruited some individual examiners from those present.

We tested 95 patients Tuesday morning, July 12, 1966. In the afternoon three teams remained at the Hospital while the Rickard and Miller teams moved to the Confederate Home. U. of T. Graduate Student Haywood and I went along to assist. We found 45 patients seated on benches in the Chapel. All psychologists rapidly reorganized the room, moved benches brought in tables, set up screen to project slides, etc. The appointed examiner, Joe Rickard asked for a show of hands of those unable to write. Pat Yale and I took the six individuals that required individual examinations to an adjacent building. It soon became evident that most of the patients required individual attention. Back at the Hospital Wayne Gill recruited the assistance of Spanish-speaking aides to help in the examination of his afternoon group. Even with so many complications, we examined 100 patients individually and in groups on Tuesday afternoon.

Tuesday evening Clarence Miller, Alan Brown and I spent three hours reading psychiatric reports in preparation for Wednesday's psychological assessment. We developed the following breakdown: marginal, 15; some possible data, 36; glasses-hearing-language, 21; un-testable estimate, 136.

We used a reduced staff on Wednesday, July 13, 1966, finding very few patients testable in groups. Experienced psychologists paid dividends in that we were able to examine 45 patients. That afternoon Bob Humble, Hubert Reese and I met with Wayne Holtzman to discuss scoring and data processing. Accounted for equipment and prepared to rent equipment for Terrell and San Antonio testing. Left for Dallas at 6:00 pm, having examined 433 patients in two and one half days.

At Home

Jean was taking care of the home front those busy days. Beth left by plane to Galveston with some of her friends. She wrote postcards to each brother, postmarked July 14, 1966.

"Dear Jack,

"The plane ride down was bumpy and I got right sick. It's real hot and we've been swimming twice already. There are thousands of seagulls and you can feel the sea in the air. The air conditioner in our old room sounded like it would explode any minute and leaked all over the floor.

See ya, Beth"

"Dear Richard,

"On the plane from Beaumont there was a Green Beret. I guess going to Viet Nam. Later this after [noon] we're going to the

"Pleasure Pier" (there's a hotel on it out in the middle of the water) get souvenirs and there on a train ride. One hotel pool is much like the one in Austin Chariot. Beth."

On to Terrell

A number of issues awaited my arrival back at the office Thursday morning: correspondence to be answered; locating proctors and psychologists to assist in individual testing at Terrell before Monday, July 18, 1966; responded to administrative problems at San Antonio; conferred with Dr. Pokorny; streamline test procedures for un-testable patients; outline plan for residual Austin testing. Dr. Bob Brown began recruiting staff for Terrell. Sid Cleveland and Reese Kinser were contacted about staff for Austin and San Antonio. State Social Workers discovered 15 Germans, 1 Chinese and 1 Greek non-English speaking patient in San Antonio sample.

On Friday, July 15, 1966, Joy Herod checked all test material for Monday's testing at Terrell. Borrowed some test items from SWM, a spare projector bulb from VA Medical Illustration. Summarized Austin testing and wrote addendum for individual instructions. Alan Brown developed a deaf version for administration of Kent and ran 50 copies. To SWM in afternoon to orient five proctors: Adams, Lovitt, Sullivan, Lowry and Hannum; gave each proctor his Monday assignment. Returned to VAH and packed all equipment and material for Terrell testing.

I arrived in Terrell at 8:30 Saturday morning to attend Dr. Pokorny's orientation of psychiatrists. (Some Waco VA psychiatrists were present.) I agreed to arrive early Sunday morning to photograph the psychiatric staff as was done the previous Sunday morning for the Austin psychiatric staff. During the day: coordinated with the State C.O. staff from Austin; conferred with Mrs. Ballard, Terrell Director of Nursing Service and her Assistant, Mrs. Jackson; examined the testing rooms - devoted most of day rearranging the rooms, moving equipment, insisting there be 20 chairs for each room, etc. I left at 3:00 pm for Dallas to attempt to locate a projector lens replacement, dowels to be used as pointers, etc.

Sunday morning, July 17, 1966, took group photo of the psychiatrists, and began setting up and checking equipment with Mrs. Jackson. Received call from Bob Humble at San Antonio who related a number of problems to be resolved at San Antonio. About mid-morning, Dr. Gordon Shaw, Sociologist at SWM (arrived at 8:20 am, left at 6:00 pm), announced regret he had just been informed of the Administrative Survey and wanted to be oriented. Mike Woods of C. O. discovered the Nursing Staff had incorrectly scheduled the patients for Monday and Tuesday testing. The nurses quickly recovered from shock and spent the afternoon revising schedules based on psychiatric reports. Dr. Shaw attempted to help them. Called Hubert Reese when we discovered shortage of forms - he placed forms on bus for Terrell to arrive at 1:00 am Tuesday. Left Terrell at 6:00 pm drove by VAH to pick up additional forms. Called Bob Brown to discuss Dr. Shaw's presence and called Walter Penk to locate more BOR forms.

All psychologists were present at 7:30 am, Monday July 17, 1966. Mrs. Bales of O.T. had coffee waiting for psychologists. Examiners and the assigned graduate student proctors by teams were: (1) Ralph Robinowitz - Walter Hooks, Roger Adams SWM Intern (Vanderbilt U.); (2) Wayne Gill - Alan Brown, Tom Lowry, U.T. SWM; (3) Clarence Miller - Dick Lyles, Bob Lovitt, SWM Intern (LSU); (4) Reese Kinser - Stan Sacks, Joy Herod; (5) Joe Rickard - Pat Yale, Jerry Sullivan, U.T. SWM. Jon Hannum, a University of Oklahoma, post-doctoral intern at SWM was assigned individual testing. Teams advised to make an all-out effort to exam patients in groups; reviewed some of the Austin procedural adjustments; scheduled group picture at noon. All groups moved smoothly and simultaneously paced test administration sequence. Five patients were removed from groups and assigned to Jon Hannum and Jon was utilized equally as effective in afternoon.

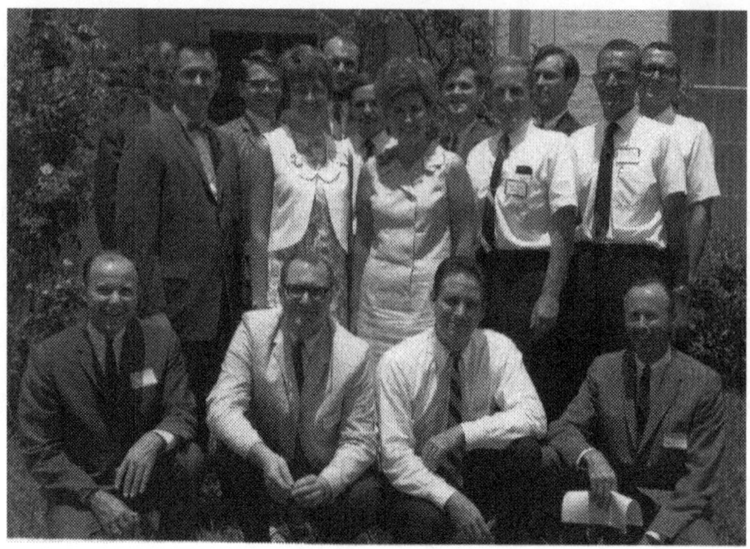

Terrell Psychology Team

Standing, left to right: Adams, Rickard, Sullivan, Herod, Lowry, Sacks, Yale, Miller, Brown, Lyles, Robinowitz, Hooks.
Front: Gill, Lovitt, Hannum, Kinser.

I telephoned Hubert Reese on missing forms and discussed Dr. Shaw's unscheduled presence. Received a call from Medical School requesting Dr. Shaw be given opportunity to observe provided he did not invalidate procedure. Official count for day was 194 patients, 97 in am and pm.

Tuesday July 19, 1966, drove the forty-one miles to Terrell, arrived at 7:00 am. Mrs. Bales had coffee for all psychologists. Plan for the day was to test 100 patients in the am and attempt average of 5 patients for each psychologist in pm. The morning group was more regressed than those of Monday, approximately half could read, but we were able to test 95 patients. We took group photograph at noon. Nursing staff provided sixty patients for afternoon, and we closed down two teams, Kinser and Rickard, to examine patients individually on the wards. The two efficient psychologists examined 91 patients in pm, a day's total of 186. Dr. Shaw visited, sat in on Dr. Gill's group. Dr. Tom Herod, Temple VAH called at 9:30 pm that he could help in the coming Saturday's "clean-up" testing at Austin State Hospital. His was the fifth commitment and two psychologists on standby.

Soon to be fifteen year old daughter, Beth accompanied me July 20, 1966 to Terrell for the final day of testing. She assisted Joy Herod in preparation of material for San Antonio testing, as well as collected the necessary supplies to test the remaining Austin patient sample on Saturday and Sunday. Dr. Jack Black of Dallas, five Medical School Interns, and three from Dallas VAH assessed 59 Terrell State Hospital patients by 2:00 pm. Jerry Sullivan received a shocking experience. The patient Jerry evaluated died immediately after the interview.

We examined 439 patients in 2 and 3/4th days. Logistically it was a highly successful week.

The next two days at the VAH were filled with a multitude of calls, clarifying staff needs for the Austin and San Antonio projects, each with its unique demands. Brought on duty some new personnel, Dr. Don Johns of Kerrville VAH and Virginia Chancey of SMU to assist in the assessment of San Antonio's Spanish patients. Mrs. Eidelbach sent a roster of 220 patients yet to be tested in Austin. Even with the greatest of care in clearing Terrell, we came up missing test slides, Manuals, etc. that needed to be located or replaced. Joy Herod was approved as an Administrative Assistant for Austin testing. Left Dallas at 7:00 pm Friday night, arrived in Austin at 10:00 pm and conferred with Don Johns until midnight, reviewing his role in the Austin testing schedule.

The following psychologists were present in Austin at 8:00 am Saturday July 23, 1966: Don Johns; Tom Herod, Temple VAH; George Fabish and Bob Bates, Houston VAH; Pat Kuekes, San Antonio, VA MHC, Clarence Miller, Ralph Robinowitz and Joy Herod. Psychiatrists predicted that most of the 220 patients would require individual assessment. However, we outlined a method of reporting group testable patients, and those located, to be examined by either Miller or Robinowitz. I was interviewed by one of the local T. V. Stations later in the morning, and left at noon for San Antonio leaving Dr. Robinowitz in charge, assisted by Joy Herod.

San Antonio State Hospital

After registering at the Menger Hotel, drove out to State Hospital and met at 2:30 pm with Mrs. Pollard, Director of Nursing, her staff Mrs. Spain, Mrs. Robinson and LVN, Mrs. Trzesmick. We toured the assigned test rooms and requested an additional room. Checked test equipment and found all items present. I brought Dr. Pokorny up to date on psychological assessment at Terrell and the ongoing Austin State Hospital testing.

Sunday morning, July 24, 1966: Arrived at San Antonio State Hospital at 8:00 am, took photographs of psychiatrists and nurse groups. (All Administrative Survey photographs were black and white, using the Rolliflex Camera.)

Bill Little assisted in helping move test equipment and supplies to test rooms. Mid-morning sat in on conference led by Dr. Pokorny and C. O. staff, reviewed immediate and long term report needs. Sixteen areas of information were covered including some discussion of coding and classification of psychological data.

From 3:30 to 7:30 pm prepared for 1st day's testing. We selected the groups with the help of nurses and C.O. representatives. We drew up lists of patients for 8 and 1/2 groups, one of which was Spanish speaking. Discovered there was a shortage of Herod's Proctor Work Sheet.

I called Ralph Robinowitz and Joy Herod mid-afternoon to review Austin testing. Seven psychologists tested 80 patients at Austin. Twenty patients were located for a possible Sunday group, and decided to call Joe Rickard and two U. of T. students, Laird and Klein to come Sunday afternoon. Sixty eight patients were scheduled for afternoon examination. Discovered one patient in the sample at Austin State School, and suggested Ralph ask Phil Roos to be responsible for that patient. Scheduled Kuekes and Johns to work Monday, and if indicated that Joy Herod remain in Austin. Joy later presented a summary of the Austin weekend assessment: 191 patients were tested.

All psychologists scheduled for the San Antonio phase of the Administrative Survey met in the San Antonio State Hospital Nursing Education Building at 7:30 am, Monday morning, July 25, 1966. The new personnel oriented were: Virginia Chancey, SMU; Lowell Grabau and Marvin Fogel, Temple VAH trainees; Bob Hetrick and Eric Theiner Baylor Medical School, Psychology Interns. I reviewed uniqueness of the San Antonio sample, and the possible necessary adaptations.

Examiners and assigned graduate student proctors by teams were: (1) Ralph Robinowitz, Walter Hooks and Eric Theiner; (2) Wayne Gill, Alan Brown, Bob Hetrick, Professor Chancey (Wayne's patient group was Spanish speaking); (3) Clarence Miller, Dick Lyles and Lowell Grabau; (4) Reese Kinser, Stan Sacks and Marvin Fogel; (5) Joe Rickard, Pat Yale and Joe Jackson.

The Hospital Superintendent ordered that all patients be collected and brought by bus to the test rooms and remain in the room until the bus returned. This requirement produced an hour delay in starting the examination; all five groups were off schedule. Buses returned for patients at noon long before examinations completed. I was able to arrange lunch for ten of the seventeen psychologists in the Nursing Education dining room, but buses began to arrive with the afternoon groups before all could complete lunch.

Afternoon groups were essentially full (twenty patients each), and began examinations by 1:30 pm. As the hospital administration expressed much anxiety about their maximum security patients, arranged for Joe Rickard to test sixteen patients under locked security plus an additional three non-security. Kinser's group was quite regressed; Gill's group was essentially un-testable; Miller had a smooth moving group; Robinowitz, a moderately good group.

We tested 184 patients on day one, and there were possibly 79 patients remaining for group assessment on Tuesday. San Antonio host, Wayne Gill arranged for a San Antonio River boat dinner that evening.

Family Arrived

There were perks within the demanding July schedule. Jean, Beth, Jackie, and Richard flew Braniff to San Antonio to visit during the final hours of the Administrative Survey. They missed Wayne Gill's River Boat Dinner when Braniff canceled the early flight from Dallas. But this was of no concern to the children for they loved roaming in the historic Menger Hotel next door to the Alamo. Jean recalled Richard coming in the hotel room saying, "I believe I'll run over to the Alamo for a little while."

Jean sent her mother-in-law a postcard: "Jackie and Richard have been riding the boats . . . went to the Alamo, shopping at Joskes, and swimming. Beth is with Jack. Had a nice ride down, but had to wait 2 hours for the plane."

Final Assessment Hours San Antonio

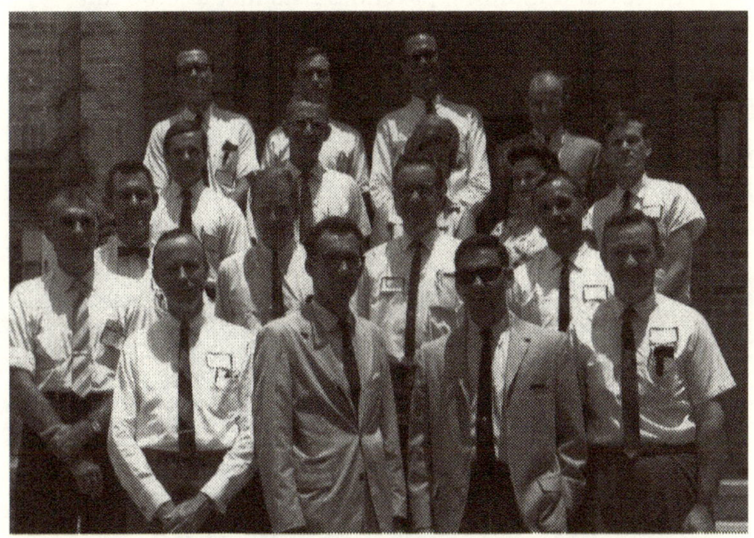

Front: Kinser, Lowell Grabau, Marvin Fogel, Jernigan
Second: Kuekes, Rickard, Alan Brown, Bob Hetrick, Eric Theiner
Third: Stan Sacks, Robinowitz, Pat Yale, Virginia Chancey, Miller
Back: Walter Hooks, Dick Lyles, Joe Jackson, Gill

I met briefly with the psychologists on Tuesday morning, July 26, 1966 to discuss strategies for examining the remaining chronic population. People were urged to use clinical judgment and improvise. Pat Kuekes appeared for individual testing, having completed assessment of all remaining Austin patients on Monday. Rickard and Miller attempted to examine two groups, but the morning became a one-on-one assessment and all psychologists used their skills in obtaining psychological data from 89 patients. Beth spent the morning assisting Mike Woods of C. O. examine the completeness of data from Monday's testing. I took the San Antonio psychology group picture before breaking for lunch.

All psychologists served as individual examiners in the afternoon. Team assignments composed of Ph.D. & Interns swept through seven wards. Seventeen psychologists assessed 63 patients making a total of 152 for the day. At the end of the day all but the Ph.D.s and Professor Chancey were dismissed.

The seven remaining psychologists met at 8:00 am Wednesday morning, July 27, 1966, examined 36 patients in the morning and 20 in the afternoon. The final test data turned in at 4:00 pm completed a total of 392 assessed at San Antonio State Hospital.

Examples of Group Psychological Assessment

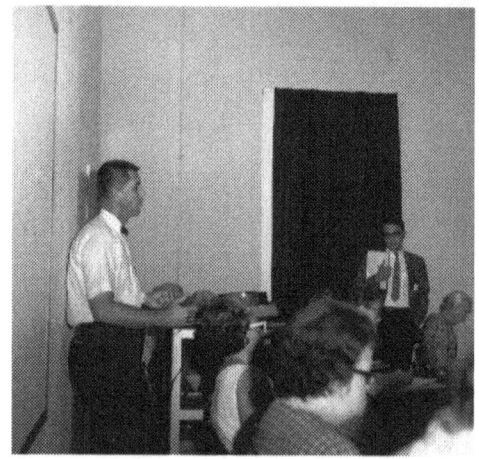

Joe Rickard and Jerry Sullivan

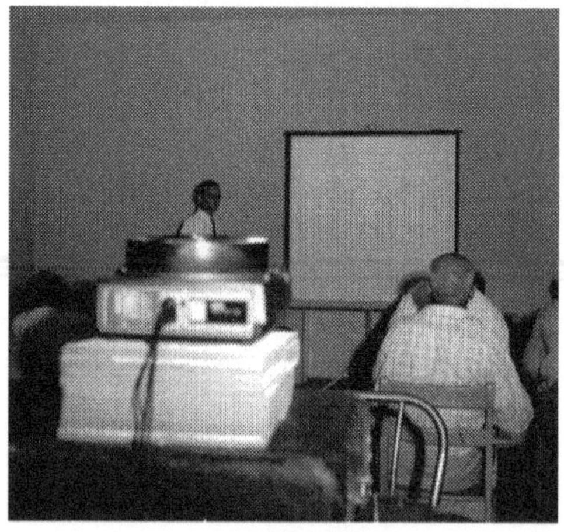

Ralph Robinowitz

Post Survey

The only personal references to family in the Administrative Diary were those related to entries when Beth and Jean assisted. Although I had little time to interact with the family, it was a gift to have them with me in San Antonio. On return from the State Hospital to the Menger Hotel, Jean reported a frightening experience of having been rescued when she felt she was drowning in the hotel swimming pool. We were thankful someone was there to rescue her. Our children, especially the boys, were comfortable swimmers, but neither Jean nor I felt confident in a deep pool of water. I had begun swimming lessons in May 1966 when called to coordinate the Psychological Survey, and never resumed training.

There was a call waiting from Hubert Reese when I arrived back at VAH on Thursday requesting a roster of people to be paid. (The Ph.D.s were paid $100 each consulting day and Interns, $35). A summary of days worked by 17 Ph.D.s, 21 psychology trainees, and Mrs. Ingram was mailed to Hubert. He announced the Commissioner of Mental Health wanted the first report of survey by August 27.

I had a work free weekend for the first time in over a month. However, I continued to respond to a number of Survey related activities including reports from those around the state who participated in the Survey. The VA Central Office requested a letter summarizing the role of the Veterans Administration in the State Survey. Excerpts from the August 18, 1966 two page letter to Cecil Peck:

"On July 7, I forwarded a copy of the first draft of the psychological test Manual . . . attached . . . the addenda to the Manual. . . . a copy of a test booklet with test forms used by the patients.

"The psychological survey of a 10% sample of the psychiatric patients in the Texas State Mental Hospitals. . .

completed in nine weeks. . . began with a group of psychologists meeting in Houston [in May]. . . .Approximately twenty psychologists participated in a variety of ways in developing the test battery . . . three pilot studies brought the project to its target date of July 10, 1966. . . sixteen psychologists met for a day of orientation at the Austin State Hospital.

". . . . In eleven days, the teams of psychologists tested, or attempted to test 1475 patients. This amounted to approximately 95% of the total sample. Fourteen Ph.D.s. (nine VA psychologists) and twenty-one psychology trainees (nine VA trainees) served as examiners or proctor-observers. Thus, eighteen VA psychologists and trainees participated in the actual testing. And it must be remembered, that a number of VA psychologists served in the background as counselors and advisors to the project.

"All who participated in this Administrative Survey feel a sense of pride in our accomplishments. . . Psychology had only one small segment. . . Dr. Alex Pokorny coordinated the total project and did an outstanding job in accomplishing a monumental task."

Chapter 9 - 1966

Quite a Year (Continued)

Two-day Vacation

The 100 day focus on psychological examination of 1475 Texas State Hospital patients came to a successful conclusion July 27, 1966. There was much "catching up" waiting at the office as well as many residual Survey details that required attention. The daily diary entry routine continued: August 17, 1966, "Reviewed J. Herod's work, prepared for 2-day vacation." However, before leaving town a call came from Dr. Pokorny asking me to be in Terrell the coming weekend (August 21, 1966) to work on the Commissioner's report.

The family took a mini-vacation in Oklahoma. We spent Friday night, August 19, 1966 at Ardmore Motor Lodge. Our Foster Hunt cousins were out of town, and not available to share dinner that evening. We made a brief tour of Turner Falls (where I lost my high school class ring in 1938).

A part of the next day was spent at Lake Murray. We had a pre-birthday celebration for Jackie's twelfth at Lake Murray as I was scheduled to be in Terrell on August 21st. I told the children that first-cousin E. S. Williams observed the construction of the dam that formed Lake Murray as he drove an Ardmore bread delivery truck in the 1930's. One of the communities where E. S. ("Redhot") Williams delivered bread was inundated by the water.

After retuning to Dallas, Jackie wrote his grandmother:

"Dear Grandma,

"Thank you for the three dollars. We are enjoying our new car very much.

"Last week when we went to Oklahoma we went to Turner Falls. While there we saw a bat in a tree.

"At Lake Murray there was a nice sandy beach. We rented a boat, driver, ski's and the jackets, and I went skiing for 30 minutes.

"Thank you again.

Love,
Jack [Jr.]"

The day Jean and the children flew to San Antonio, the hinge on the refrigerator door broke (again), and a new refrigerator was the first item purchased ($309) with the extra State Survey income. We were also in need of a better second car, and on driving to the VA Hospital one day along Illinois Avenue I spotted a "For Sale" sign on a tan, four-door 1964 Corvair. The second State Survey income purchase ($1097) was August 24 for a low-mileage, repossessed automobile from Republic National Sales.

In an August 25 letter to Mother, I told of attending a PTA Board Meeting as Treasurer, and added, "We bought another car this week - a 1964 Corvair. Not exactly what I would have bought, but there was considerable encouragement from the children. I am in the process of selling the old '54." The 1954 Plymouth sold four days later for $110.

A Second Call to Duty

At the August 21st Terrell State Hospital conference with Alex Pokorny, Hubert Reese, and Bob Humble, I was asked to assume responsibility for processing the psychological assessment data. Dr. Pokorny wanted psychological ratings by October 1, and suggested the evaluation project begin Labor Day weekend.

Only a tentative acceptance was given until I conferred with family and staff. The Survey was an invigorating experience, but for Jean, it was a trying time as she picked up the slack because of my absences from the home. We needed to discuss this additional request. Also, full approval of the Hospital Administration and Psychology Staff was necessary before assuming a task almost as formidable as the assessment project.

An eager acceptance of the challenge came from the Psychology Staff at the Monday staff meeting. Chief of Staff, Dr. Hinshaw gave his support as did the Hospital Director. Dr. Hinshaw indicated space for the scoring and processing project could be made available. Jean agreed I was the logical person to coordinate the project and should accept.

Ten Diary pages were required to document the steps taken between August 22 and September 28, 1966 when Hubert Reese came from Austin to retrieve 1475 test protocols, scores, and ratings.

Key decisions were necessary to determine a score for those tests typically evaluated by "Clinical judgment", e.g. Human Figure Drawings, Bender Gestalt, Description of Condition, etc. We discovered even the "Published Tests" required more detailed scoring guidelines.

The data processing phase of the Survey required no travel, but weekends and nights were again absorbed with project details. The coordination was time consuming. Again, Medical School psychologists and staff from other VA Hospitals assisted in the recruitment of necessary personnel.

Mrs. Ingram and I outlined the agenda to catalogue test booklets: (1) Identify each booklet by (a) name, (b) date, (c) am or pm, (d) code for examiner (1-5); (2) Dichotomize booklets into group or individually tested; (3) All tests except Otis Arithmetic to be scored by a Ph.D.

Mary Ingram, Beth Jernigan, and I received the mass of data from Hubert Reese at the VA Hospital Saturday, September 3, 1966. We three worked until 6:30 pm that day sorting each test booklet, assigning code numbers by group examiners, hospitals, etc. We returned Sunday afternoon to continue the work. Beth recruited her classmate, Claire Richards to assist Labor Day. The four of us worked from 8:00 to 4:00 with Jean joining us from 7:00 to 9:00 pm.

A brief note to Mother described our activity.

"I am spending a busy Labor Day weekend - they brought the data Saturday. Beth worked Saturday and Sunday afternoons and all day today. She will be paid $1.25 per hour, and is an excellent worker . . . I hate to have to get into this, but see I was the one to do it - no one else could figure out our notes and procedures. . . I expect I'll be tied up with this for most of the month. The children start school Wednesday."

By Wednesday, September 7, all patient records were coded and the rosters verifaxed. The Psychology Staff continued to work on scoring guide lines. Dr. Pokorny called and reported the Commissioner's interest in a new survey of all patients convicted of crime, as a result of the University of Texas Tower massacre. 1

Every member of the Psychology Staff found a unique area of creative contribution: Bill Hales developed a method for processing the Cornell Medical Index; John Geers and Bill Hales drafted pay scale proposals; Ralph Robinowitz wrote a Kent scoring guide manual; Walter Penk and AJJ developed Logical Memory scoring guidelines; Walter Penk and John Geers Human Figure Drawings guidelines; etc, etc. Jean Jernigan helped by running errands such as locating Goodenough-Harris Quality Scale Cards for evaluating Human Figure Drawings.

Wayne Holtzman suggested the development of a "bench-mark" technique for scoring Bender Gestalt (BG). Geers, Hales,

Penk and I selected 24 single page BG protocols from the June Pilot studies. From the psychology files, we pulled a random sample of BG protocols, selecting every fifth file until we located 24 single page records. Geers, Hales and Jernigan independently rank ordered from "best" to "poorest" the two sets of 24 protocols, using 2 of 3 agreements to select two extreme and one mid-point Bender protocol. Rankings continued until we reached agreement on three "Bench Mark Benders." These were photographed by Medical Illustration and duplicated for the test scorers. This effective scoring method was later adopted for Dallas VA Group Testing.

Data scoring began Saturday morning, September 10, 1966 at 8:00 am. Those on duty that first day: Ralph Robinowitz, Joe Garms (appointed as Level III Trainee from Texas Tech August 26, 1966), Mr. and Mrs. Frey (SMU students), Walter Penk, Millie Penk, Mrs. Ingram, Beth and Jack Jernigan. We began scoring the Kent Intelligence, Logical Memory and Otis Arithmetic in an assembly line flow.

Mrs. Genette Burris, Chief Psychologist, Dallas Child Guidance Clinic joined us the next day as consultant on the Benton Visual Retention Test scoring and the use of the Harris-Goodenough HF codes to score the Human Figure Drawings.

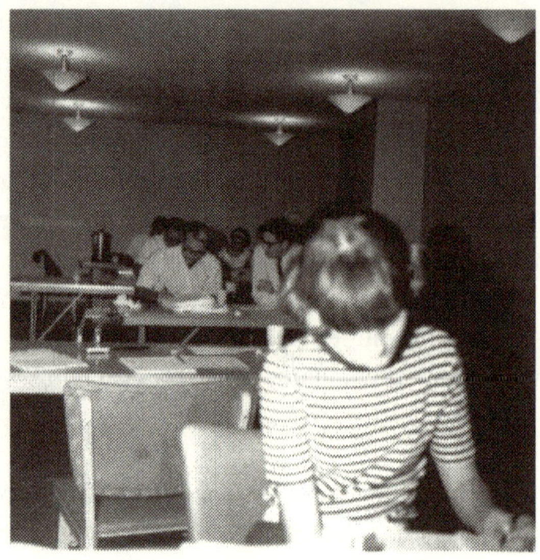

Beth Jernigan – Walter Penk to her right

Walter Penk began writing scoring guidelines for each test. Test scoring continued each night of that week. Jerry Sullivan, Medical School psychologist arrived Tuesday night to score Bentons, and Irv Gadol came later in the week.

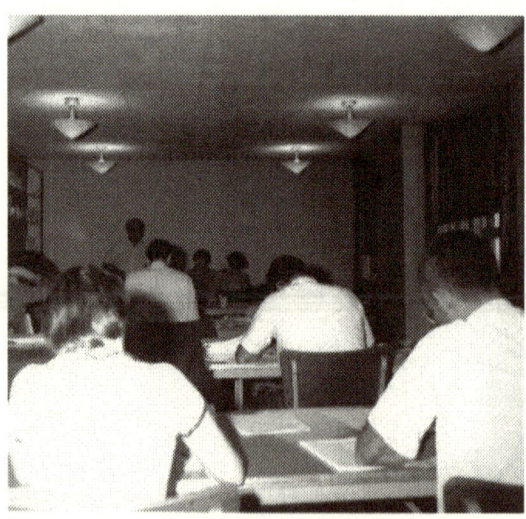

John Geers and Walter Penk devoted all day Friday scoring HFD protocols, returned Saturday, joined by Robinowitz, Gadol, Dale Dobbs and Alan Brown to score the Bender Gestalt tests.

Wayne Holtzman and Lou Moran were consulted throughout the week on scoring issues with the Holtzman Ink Blots and the Word Association Tests. I drafted an agenda for Saturday, September 19, 1966 to develop guidelines for rating each of the 1475 test protocols.

Dr. Pokorny, Hubert Reese, and Bob Humble flew to Love Field Saturday morning. I met their plane and drove them to the Medical School where we were joined at 9:00 am by Wayne Holtzman, Sid Cleveland, Maurice Korman and Bill Hales. This planning committee roughed out a rating scale, broke for lunch at the Mariott, guests of S. W. Medical, and completed the scale after lunch. The committee proposed 15 psychologists be recruited to rate the 1475 records the weekend of September 24 and 25, 1966. All the committee except Holtzman, Hales and Korman drove to the VA Hospital to review data scoring.

Robinowitz, Penk, Dobbs, and Jernigan worked all day Sunday, September 18, 1966, joined in the afternoon by Geers, Ingram, Gadol, and Sullivan. We completed the BG scoring and turned to Description of Condition (DOC). After running a number of reliability studies, made decisions that: "nerves" = physical; "nervousness" = psychological; "insomnia" = physical. John Geers served as reliability check.

Penk, Gadol, Dobbs and Jernigan completed DOC scoring Monday September 19, 1966. Some clinical observations: Austin patients were more expressive of feelings; Terrell patients relied more on denial. Passivity and poverty of ideation predominated with San Antonio patients. The Scale would have been improved by including a measure of "affect," and should have included a tally of patients who wrote: "The hospital can best help by discharging me."

Bob Brown, Maurice Korman, Sid Cleveland and others assisted in the recruitment-confirmation of fifteen psychologists from across the state. By Wednesday we located five VA and 10 non-VA psychologists, five of the latter were former VA staff. Mrs. Ingram mailed a letter to each with "Instructions to Raters."

A number of small details remained, e. g. Alan Brown and his father-in-law recorded BG scores one night until 9:45 pm. Mrs. Ingram and I checked each test booklet for code number accuracy (found a few errors). Gave test booklets four classifications ranging from "Completed all Tests" to "Impotent." Made random sorting of the 1475 booklets, equally divided into 33 piles, and stacked on shelves.

Walter Penk and I designed an index of scores to be found in each booklet and a map of room assignments for the rating psychologists. Alan Brown verifaxed the maps and the "Qualitative Rating Guide Lines."

Weekend Rating of 1475 Test Protocols

Hubert Reese and fifteen psychologists arrived at the Dallas VA Hospital's ninth floor at 9:00 am, Saturday, September 24, 1966. The fifteen psychologists were: Mac Sterling, Waco; Roy Long, Dallas; George Fabish, Houston; Marion Bishop, Houston; Clarence Miller, Houston; Charles Bounds, Austin; Don Wallace, Houston; Charles J. Black, Dallas; Robert Bates, Houston; Wayne Gill, San Antonio; Dale Johnson, Houston; Robert A. Brown, Dallas; James Baxter, Houston; Dale Turner, Dallas; Daniel Logan, Dallas. (Five of the psychologists participated in the July data collection.)

The recruited staff was given a general review of the Administrative Survey, a summary of scoring decisions, the scoring codes, and a copy of the score guide. The types of possible clinical content available in each protocol were summarized. The "Psychological Rating Sheet" was explained, and an operational definition given for each rating category: "Educational Level - Conceptual Disorganization - Personality Disorganization

- Rehabilitation Potential (Vocational)." A typical case was presented, and an agreement reached by group for rating each category.

Each psychologist was asked to rate 10 cases and return the rated sheets and protocols to the check-in desk. He would then pick up the next 10. It was believed this routine would reduce fatigue and give a physical and psychological break after a reasonable period of concentrated rating.

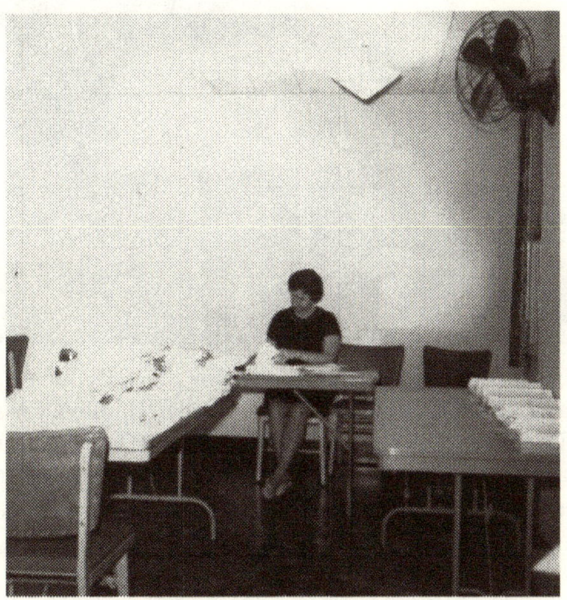

Mrs. Mary Ingram at Check-in Desk

All psychologists had completed a unit of ten cases by 11:45 am. The group assembled and shared experiences. Minimum questions were raised, and all seemed comfortable with the task. Rating speed increased in the afternoon and the staff completed 590 by 4:00 pm to end the first day.

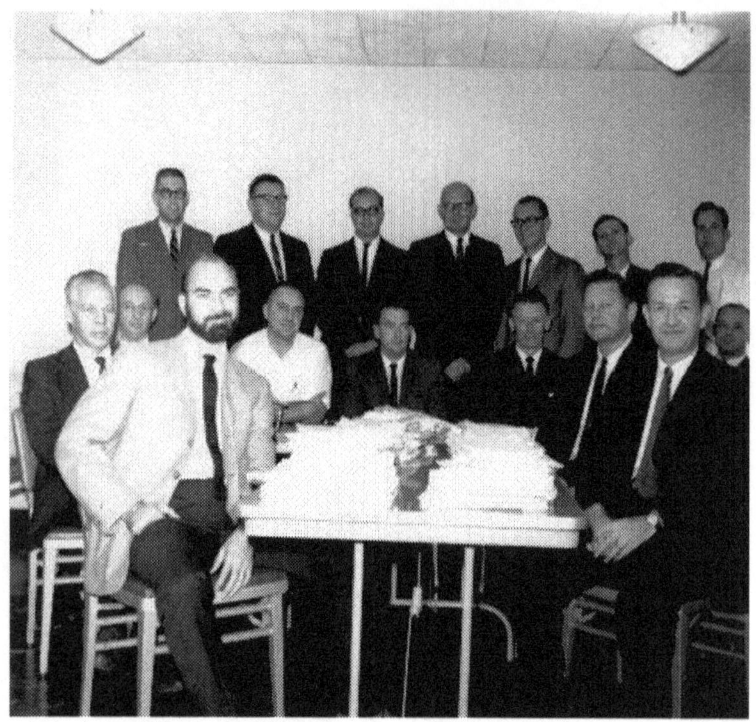

Sixteen psychologists: Mac Sterling, Waco; Roy Long, Dallas; George Fabish, Houston; Marion Bishop, Houston; Clarence Miller, Houston; Charles Bounds, Austin; Don Wallace, Houston; Charles J. Black, Dallas; Robert Bates, Houston; Wayne Gill, San Antonio; Dale Johnson, Houston; Robert A. Brown, Dallas; James Baxter, Houston; Dale Turner, Dallas; Daniel Logan, Dallas; Jack Jernigan

All raters were on duty at 8:00 am Sunday, September 25, 1966. We took a group picture of the raters at noon, and after lunch completed the entire process by 2:30 pm. Twelve of fifteen psychologists stayed to write a brief critique.

Early the next week we mailed Hubert Reese a detailed account of hours worked by each individual in scoring and rating protocols. The data were packed, and with a sigh of relief gave Hubert all the material on Wednesday, September 28, 1966 when he arrived to carry the boxes back to Austin.

I wrote Wayne Holtzman, Lou Moran and Don Gorham Friday, September 30, 1966, and released their data for further processing. A memorandum was forwarded to the Hospital Director to thank the Veterans Administration for its generous cooperation, and released Room A901.

Post-Survey

The post-survey diary indicated at least an hour each day was consumed for forty or more additional days on such items as clarifying pay vouchers, answering questions from Hubert Reese, Don Gorham, and others. In mid-December Hubert called and stated January 15, 1967 was deadline for final report.

I described the project in an article published in the October 1967 issue of the Journal of Clinical Psychology. The article's summary, quoted here: 2

"Between May and September 1966, psychologists in the State of Texas planned and standardized a psychological test procedure, completed a testing program, and rated the psychological assessment of 1475 psychiatric patients. Some 45 psychologists and 25 students contributed to a massive interdisciplinary project for the purpose of achieving a better understanding of the mental health needs of the state. Psychology was given an opportunity to make a contribution to this undertaking and at the same time test out certain assessment procedures and techniques. The special utility of the group test approach in assessing large numbers of psychiatric patients was demonstrated.

"Inasmuch as only a fraction of the psychological information was given in the report presented to the State Legislature on January 15, 1967, the psychological data will be analyzed and the findings published within the coming months."

A variety of presentations describing the State Survey and its findings were subsequently made at state, regional and national psychological meetings in 1966, 1967 and 1972. It was a great experience and brought much attention to the psychology staff and its programs at the Dallas VAH.

Back to the Family

Mother became 80 on December 6, 1966. Jack, Jack, Jr., and Richard each signed a birthday card to wish her a happy birthday with the following note: "Jean bought this card - she and Beth are practicing for the Lottie Moon play. We boys will sign and send."

Our "Christmas Greetings" to Mother postmarked December 20, 1966 included, ". . . The Christmas program at the church last night was excellent. Having all 3 of the children participate made the event especially enjoyable to us."

Jean wrote her Mother-in-law two days after Christmas:

"Dearest Mother J.,

"We all thought this was one of the nicest Christmases we've ever had. Richard is enjoying his guitar and will bring it up as soon as he learns a tune. Beth's hair dryer (the kind with a hood) matches her pajamas so she looks pretty sitting under it. We will go shopping for her sweater tomorrow!"

". . . We are lazy today. Naturally Richard is up going strong but Beth and Jackie are still asleep and it is 10 a.m.!"

Chapter 10 - 1967

Visiting Science Presentations

I spoke on the subject, "The 1966 Administrative Survey" on at least four occasions in 1967. Two presentations were made through the Visiting Science Program - the Texas Academy of Science.

The first Visiting Science presentation was January 18, 1967 to the Lewisville High School Biology II Class. The Science Department Instructor, J. G. Dieb and all his students signed a thank you letter a few days later.

"The Biology II class of Lewisville High School would like to extend our gratitude to you for taking time to come and speak to us. The topic of psychology was very interesting and the addition of slides made it even more so. The test was very new and thoroughly enjoyable to all of us."

The reference to "slides" suggests the Benton Visual Retention Tests was shown as State Survey example. The February 1, 1967 reply gave feedback to the class.

"You may recall, I explained a test procedure we employed in the 1966 Administrative Survey of the Texas State Mental Hospitals. Your students were kind enough to give me their completed protocols and, naturally, I was interested in their performance. Your students scored well above average. The performance of the seniors was slightly better than the freshmen, and girls scored some better than the boys. However, the differences in the scores of the girls and boys would not be considered statistically significant."

An invitation came from Jacksonville H. S. to speak a second time to their biology classes. (Do not recall date of first visit.) A February 17, 1967 copy of the school paper, "Drumbeat," included a photograph of me standing before the class and this notation: "Dr. Jernigan, chief psychologist at the V. A. Hospital in Dallas tests the 'Retention Factor' in Jacksonville High School Biology II classes." The headline read:

"Psychologist Tests Student Memory Fact

"Chief psychologist Dr. Austin J. Jernigan, of the Veterans Administration Hospital in Dallas lectured to the Biology II class of Mr. Billy Guinn on February 7. Mr. Jernigan is affiliated with the visiting Science Program of the Texas Academy of Science which is supported by the National Science Foundation.

"The Visiting Science Program is designed to improve science and mathematics understand (sic) by allowing professional scientists to come and discuss with various classes the current knowledge of his particular scientific field.

"Dr. Jernigan gave biology II students tests to determine their retention factor. He flashed drawings on the board for students to see and for them to recreate the drawing on paper from what they could retain."

Later in the month (January 26-27) I flew Braniff to Austin and stayed at the Crest Manor Motor Inn. The purpose for the trip was Psychology Training, TPA Committee, or State Survey follow-up or a combination of each.

Family Happenings

Jamie had his gall bladder removed January 30, 1967. We sent flowers and Frances reported he was doing well.

During the icy weather Jean slid into a car on West Kiest Blvd. We had our car repaired at a Lancaster Road body shop across from the VA Hospital. It was released in time for me to drive to Jacksonville.

A postcard to Mother later in February told of Beth returning from a "nice trip to Waco" and that Jean and I had an invitation to attend a breakfast meeting in Denton that coming Saturday.

A "Greedy" Saturday Afternoon

Cousin Sanders Coffey and his wife, Mae were administrators of Great Aunt Sis Coffey's "estate." Blanche Coffey Jernigan, Jean, and I visited Aunt Sis' old, vacant Anna house Saturday afternoon, February 25, 1967. We took some items thought discarded by Sanders and Mae. We discovered otherwise.

Two items were known to be for sale, Grandpa Jesse Coffey's dining room table and a musty day sofa. We bought the table from the Real Estate Agent, left the sofa, but took an "old press," a trunk with some clothes, a box filled with pictures and recipes. We "assumed" those were items not wanted by Mae and Sanders. It was late in the day so Blanche asked Russell Pressley to pick up the items and store them in the harness room at our Sedalia barn.

Soon thereafter, Mae and Sanders Coffey communicated they intended to sell the "old press" for $50. Mother discovered that a Mrs. Parker of Anna owned the trunk, neglected to take it with her when she moved from the house. Mrs. Parker wanted the trunk and content delivered to her current address in Anna.

Excerpts from my letter of confession and of contrition to Mae and Sanders that began with:

"One of the finest things I inherited from the Coffeys was to be honest. . . Jean fell in love with the sofa and table. She especially wanted the table after Mother told this story: 'I believe my Daddy bought this table for his mother and picked her up from her sick bed, laid her on it and said, 'Old Woman, you have always wanted a new dining table and here it is.' So we left a check for $10 with Miss Powell [Real Estate Agent] for the table. . . In addition, Aunt Sis's Bible and an old greeting card box filled with miscellaneous pictures and recipes were in the house. Mother has the Bible and I brought the box of pictures and recipes home to look at them."

Copy of the letter was attached to a note to Mother, March 2, 1967:

"Dear Mother:

"Didn't we get in a mess? Jean said that's what greed will do for you (us). I'm sorry you have to deal with all this. I hope you can satisfy the old lady and the trunk. I have a meeting Saturday and just don't see how I can come up. But I guess if she cared no more for it than to go off and leave such a valuable object there, she will just have to wait.

"I hope the letter to Mae and Sanders is satisfactory. I feel sure we don't want the old press (not for $50), but I may have to take it now that I have 'stolen it.' I'm sure glad we left that $10 check with Miss Powell.

"I sent the Pressley fellow a Zippo lighter today as a reward for his part in the crime.

"Jean said she didn't know when she had enjoyed herself more. We did have a good time with you and will have a lot to laugh about when we get everything straightened out.

Love, Jack"

Mae Coffey gave us the old "press" the day Jean and I took her to Jim Coffey's funeral. Family folklore is that Great grandfather Jesse Coffey made the pegged walnut press that now graces our dining room. The dining table resides in the Rectory, St. Mary's Episcopal Church, Houston, home of the Rev. Beth+.

I returned to the "scene of the crime," retrieved the clothes discarded from the trunk, restored them to their resting place, and delivered the trunk to Mrs. Parker's Anna residence. She was not at home. The trunk was left on her back porch. End of story.

Excerpts from a postcard to Mother on March 20, 1967:

". . . We were busy this weekend with church activities. . . I saw Uncle Sidney [Natalie Murray's Dad] at church again yesterday . . . I go to Houston Thurs. and return Friday. I may try to call Sanders Coffey. Love, Jack."

Come to Houston

The projected trip to Houston was in response to a request from Alex Pokorny. His March 7, 1967 letter is quoted in part:

"I am enclosing a letter to Earl Pollack [Chief, Demography and Epidemiology Section, National Institute of Mental Health, Chevy Chase, Maryland] concerning setting up a meeting in Houston for March 23rd and 24th to discuss subsequent steps in analysis and publication of the administrative survey. . . This isn't quite the type of meeting you had suggested earlier. . . I am not sure we can pay your way down. We might be able to swing something out of Austin, but in view of the new administration and the recently expressed sentiment that they would just as soon be done with the Administrative Survey, I cannot be sure of this."

The plane fare was reimbursed, but not the hotel.

In his letter to Earl S. Pollack, Sc. D., Dr. Pokorny outlined a seven point agenda. Item # 6 stated, "Findings on psychological testing of the sample and plans for further use of these findings, for publication, etc. All of this has barely been touched upon in the

January 15th Report. . .The persons involved will be Dr. Frazier at least part of the time, myself, Dr. Jernigan from Dallas, Hubert Reese, Bob Humble and your party."

Documents are no longer extant that give conclusions reached at the meeting. However, I had written letters in February to Pokorny, Holtzman, Reese, and Walter Hooks encouraging each to participate in a symposium on the Survey at the April 1967 annual meeting of Southwestern Psychological Association in Houston. The Pokorny meeting in March helped set the stage for the symposium.

Houston VA Psychology Intern, Walter Hooks responded to the letter with: "The material you sent has helped bring back into focus those three very hot weekends we spent trying to make order out of semi-chaos. . . My contributions to the SWPA symposium can, and probably will deal with all of the topics you suggested. Also, I have collected comments from the psychologist participants who are still in Houston. 1

While in Houston on March 24, 1967 I sent a picture postcard to Mother from the Tidelands Motor Inn, 6500 South Main, Houston, and told of a pleasant telephone visit with Mae and Sanders Coffey.

I flew Braniff to Austin April 17, 1967. There are no extant documents that tell the purpose for the trip.

Sad Notes

Telephone conversation notes written April 18, 1967 told of the death of a child of one of our "42 Club" families. The mother, Glenna Cason sought answers to the question, "Why did my child die." I listened as Glenna gave a series of symptoms that preceded the sudden death of their daughter, "aura of colored lights, seizures, convulsion," and the many tentative diagnoses made by physicians.

I listened, asked some questions, but was unable to help Glenna understand why her daughter died so suddenly. Jackie and the little Cason girl were classmates. All were saddened by the death of the beautiful child.

State Survey Symposium

Alex Pokorny, Walter Hooks, Hubert Reese, Wayne Holtzman and I discussed the 1966 Survey of Texas State Mental Hospitals findings, observations, and research opportunities at the April 1967 annual meeting of the Southwestern Psychological Association in Houston. The symposium title listed in the program: "Survey of Texas State Mental Hospitals: Psychological Assessment: Pokorny, Overview of Survey; Jernigan, Development of Psychology Test Program; Hooks, Psychology Trainee Views the Survey; Reese, Assembling Mass Data; Holtzman, Integrating Mass Data - Research Potential. "

I mailed a Hotel America postcard to the family on Friday, April 28, 1967.

Dear Family:

"I had breakfast this morning with Cassius Clay and his lawyers seated next to my table. My picture could be in the papers because they took a number. Is really a questionable distinction. Will see you tomorrow afternoon.

Love, Daddy - Jack"

Later in the day at the Hotel America I briefly met, shook hands, and obtained the autograph of Cassius Clay "Ali." My comment, "questionable distinction" reflected the then current sentiment about the Vietnam War. Cassius Clay had recently voiced his strong opposition to the war at the risk of losing his World Heavyweight Boxing title. He was very much in the national news.

We treasure his autograph.

Letters of appreciation were mailed to each symposium participant. The opening paragraph of the letter to Wayne Holtzman on May 1, 1967 stated: "Your presentation was superb and made the symposium. I appreciated the way in which you pushed to get the information you presented. The recording of the symposium is quite clear and our Research Department has agreed to make a transcript."

Many people requested a copy of the transcript.

Air Force mentor, Colonel Arthur W. Melton, spoke at the April SWPA convention. Excerpts from a May 1, 1967 letter to "Dr. Arthur W. Melton, Department of Psychology - University of Michigan: "It was worth the trip to Houston to see you again. I did not have an opportunity to visit with you after your Friday afternoon presentation. Do you plan to publish your address, 'Interference in Short-Term Memory?'. . . I hope you return to Texas again soon."

Dr. Melton replied from his University of Michigan office on May 31, 1967:

"Dear Jack:

"A thousand thanks for your rewarding letter. It was indeed good to see you again, and I hope we can have another shot of that soon.

"I do intend to put that paper into some form for publication, but it may be a while before I can get it done, because there are many more urgent things to take care of in the next two months. However, I will send you the first decent and reasonably complete copy I have, even though a draft.

"With best regards,

Sincerely yours,
(Art)
Arthur W. Melton
Director Human Performance Center"

May 1967 Happenings - Happy and Sad

Dr. Mac Sterling, Chairman, Department of Psychology Baylor University extended an invitation to participate in an "Honors Program" at the University. My notes indicated he needed "somebody from the outside" to judge the presentations of psychology students.

Excerpts from a May 12, 1967 letter to Mother gave other details.

"Jean and I had a very nice trip to Waco. Jean visited with Judy Sterling while I did my job at Baylor, then the four of us went to lunch. After lunch Mac took us through the new Science Building where the psychology department will be relocated this summer. It is a beautiful building - Baylor has really made great strides these last few years in their building program. . . I have been doing some house painting this week - will take some time to go all around the house. . . wish it was so we could come up this weekend, but can't because of the children's church schedules."

The house painting project was completed except for the high gables of our two-story home at 4012 Fountainhead. I contracted with one of the VA Hospital painters, Gilbert Rosson, a McKinney commuter, to come on a Saturday morning and complete the project. The following was written from memory thirty years later: "I waited until mid-morning Saturday, May 27, 1967 for Gilbert and finally called his home in McKinney. A relative answered the phone, and sadly reported that Gilbert (a young man) died suddenly that morning of a heart attack."

However, a Sunday, May 28, 1967 letter saved by Mother gave a different (and accurate) version.

". . . A sad thing happened: the painter, Gilbert Rosson, couldn't come yesterday because his brother-in-law was being buried yesterday afternoon. When I talked with him yesterday morning, Gilbert asked if I minded him coming on and doing the job today [Sunday]. I agreed under the circumstances. When he didn't show up, I called - his mother-in-law. She told me he died of a sudden heart attack last night at 9:00 PM. I don't know when I've had anything happen to sadden me so. I wrote his wife a letter and enclosed a check. He lived in McKinney."

A check was mailed to Mrs. Gilbert Rosson for the amount of Gilbert's contract. The discrepancy in recall of "the sad story" is an example of our dependence on ". . . . filtered, distant memory." There were two deaths, not one; Gilbert did not die on Saturday morning, but on Saturday night. 2

20th Anniversary

We five spent the 4th of July at Lake Texoma with Grady and Barbara Niblo, and their three children. The next day we bought a living room couch and two chairs to celebrate our 20th wedding anniversary. Later we ate out and went to a movie.

We visited Jamie, Frances, Jim and Laura in Kingsville July 21-23, 1967.

Psychology Trainees

Alan Brown, a significant contributor to the Administrative Survey, completed his internship at Dallas VA, and was awarded the Ph.D. degree from the University of Texas on January 28, 1967.

Dr. Wm. M. Hales supervised Alan's internship year, and concluded his evaluation with these sentences: "Throughout his [Alan's] stay at this station, the undersigned was impressed with Mr. Brown's maturity and high professional standards, his eagerness to learn and good work habits, and his ability to get along well with everyone with whom he came in contact. It is my opinion that Mr. Brown has good potential and will make a significant contribution to psychology."

Alan spent a half day a week at the Dallas Child Guidance Clinic for a brief period during his internship. Dr. Brown accepted a child psychologist position with the Division of Child Psychiatry, County General Hospital, Department of Health and Hospitals, Denver, Colorado February 6, 1967

Joe DeWayne Garms, our first VA Counseling Trainee from Texas Tech University came on duty August 26, 1966 in time to participate in scoring the Administrative Survey psychological data. Evaluation of his 1966, early 1967 training assignment is no longer extant. Termination summary indicated he was promoted to Level IV May 2, 1967 and became a "key participant in the development of the new Day Treatment Program, under the supervision of the Chief, Psychology Service." He also assisted in the supervision of a Third Year level psychology trainee.

The Psychology Staff gave Joe a 9th Floor Conference Room party on August 18. Dr. Garms resigned from the training program August 25, 1967 and was awarded the Ph.D. from Texas Tech the following day. He accepted a position with the Muskogee Guidance Center, Muskogee, Oklahoma.

Counseling Psychology Trainee Marvin E. Fogel, also from Texas Tech University, began a tour of duty June 5, 1967. He was assigned to Dr. Walter Penk, psychologist in charge of the Psychology Unit (Psychiatry). Marvin made satisfactory progress, and was promoted to Level III December 3, 1967.

In June 1967 I attended a Veterans Administration sponsored meeting at the Minneapolis VA Hospital, Minneapolis,

Minnesota. The purpose for the meeting may have been related to training or possibly a Cooperative Research project.

Death of an Uncle

We took a mini-vacation at Spanish Trace Inn trip in Athens, Texas August 21-23, 1967. While there, we had a call that Uncle George Coffey died August 22. We returned home to attend his funeral. 3

A note to Mother on August 28, "I know this has been a sad time for you. We hate to lose some one as loveable as Uncle George, but I'm glad that he didn't have to suffer and be confined to bed, helpless. I thought I would try to call on Aunt Gladys next week when I get back from Washington."

Aunt Bernice, Uncle George's first wife was pregnant when mother was pregnant with me. The parents' anticipated joy terminated in the eighth month with the still-birth of a baby boy. I was not a surrogate son, but received some attention as "the son they might have had."

A few months before Uncle George died he asked me to visit him so he could "pass on a few possessions" of his Dad, James Perry Coffey. These were: a large leather wallet filled with some of my grandfather's scribblings and other artifacts, and an inscribed gold-headed cane "From Bernice and George - TO DAD - Dec. 8, 1875 To Dec. 8, 1925" on the occasion of Mr. and Mrs. J. P. Coffey's fiftieth wedding anniversary. Jamie and I "carried the cane" during the photo-ops at our fiftieth wedding anniversaries, June 28, 1990 and July 5, 1997.

Uncle George made and lost two or three small fortunes. I first remember him in the 1930's when he was President of the Fox-Coffey-Edge Millinery business in Dallas. When WWII began he moved into heavy equipment sales for Galion Road Graders and from there into construction. He took part in the construction of Camp Howze at Gainesville, Texas.

Driver's License

State law in 1967 granted driver's licenses to children at age fifteen. The August 28, 1967 letter to Mother brought to memory Beth learning to drive and Jackie selling Tyler roses along Illinois Avenue.

"We are all well. Jackie sold roses again Saturday and will also sell this week. Jean plans to go to Waco Thursday to the WMU conference. Jackie will be selling and Beth and Richard will stay at the house. Richard goes to choir practice Thursday morning. Beth will probably take him. All of the choirs are "working out" four days this week - Beth and Jackie go in the evenings. This is something new and the children aren't too happy about it."

To Washington

Washington, D. C. was the site of the 1967 annual convention of the American Psychological Association. The 17th Conference of Psychologist Directors and Consultants in State, Federal and Territorial Mental Health Programs met August 30, 1967 at the Sheraton Park Hotel, a day before the convention began. I stayed at the Dupont Plaza Hotel and presented a paper to the Conference titled: "Assessment of Hospitalized Patients." The 1966 Administrative Survey of Texas State Mental Hospitals was of interest to many at that conference.

Dallas VA Medical Illustration Service developed slides from photographs of testing scenes at the three state hospitals; of the test forms; the Bender Gestalt bench-mark scoring examples; and six slides that defined the final rating categories.

Topics covered: “Introduction - Development of Test Battery - Psychological Assessment - Processing, Scoring and Rating.”

“Some interesting findings of the survey:

“(1) 25% of the patients are age 65 or more. Approximately 110 patients are 90 years old or more. Of this aged population, 43% have been hospitalized for five or more years.

“(2) 16% of all patients have been hospitalized for a period of 11 to 20 years. Nearly 14% have been in the hospitals for 21 or more years. An estimated 80 patients have been continuously hospitalized for 50 or more years.

“(3) A high percentage of patients (61.8%) had abnormalities in dental care.

“(4) 10% of the patients cannot care for their body needs.

“(5) 9% of the patients showed alcoholism; 0.4% showed narcotic addiction.

“(6) Approximately 3% (2.9) of all patients are under 19 years of age.

“Conclusions: (If local support facilities were available)

“(1) 25% of the patients could be released (3821 persons).

“(2) 32% of the patients could be transferred to facilities such as nursing homes, day-care hospital, half-way houses, etc. (4890 patients).

“(3) 43% should be retained in state hospitals (6573 patients).

A three page handout included these subjects: Goals - The Sample - Types of Examinations (10% sample) - Group Test Battery (suggested) - Individual Test Battery (suggested) - Development of Test Battery - Test Battery Selected - Psychological Assessment - Processing and Scoring of Data. The handout also included five references to recent papers and publications.

The presentation generated considerable interest by the number of requests for copies of the paper as well as the related article published in the Journal of Clinical Psychology. Texas was in the forefront of a nationwide effort of how to best treat and manage psychiatric patients.

In later years guilt feelings sometimes occurred when scenes of the homeless began to appear on national TV news channels. I felt our 1966 efforts may have encouraged a rapid treatment change before back up facilities and programs were developed. That is not to say all homeless are mentally ill, but the population does include many who need mental health care and protective facilities.

A picture postcard of the Sheraton-Park Hotel, 2660 Connecticut Avenue, Washington, D. C. mailed the family on August 30, 1967 carried the message:

"Dear Family - I completed the talk - believe it went fairly well. Bill Rigby Harl Young, Walter and Millie [Penk] were there. I'm a guest tonight (free) of the organization sponsoring the talk. Cecil wants me to have dinner Sunday with them. He is picking Jo Ann up at airport, they're just returning from vacation. Went to the Smithsonian this am. Wish you were here. Love - Daddy - Jack"

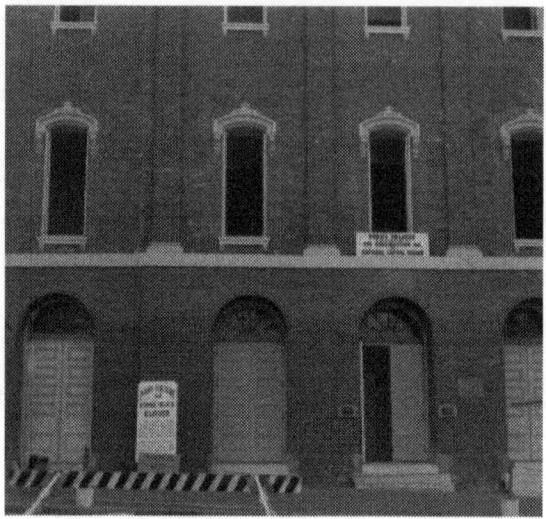

Ford Theater (under renovation)

"A picture postcard to Richard:

"I hope you receive this card Saturday. I went to the house this morning where President Lincoln died. I look forward to seeing you Sunday.

Love, Daddy"

And that same day to Jean:

"Dearest Jean:

"We had an informative V. A. meeting today. I have a refrigerator in my room, so bought some makings for supper and breakfast (found a Safeway nearby). I hope your day went well. I wish you and the children were with me. I love you.

Jack"

And to Jackie:
"Dear Jack

"This is the hotel where some of our meetings will be held [The Sheraton-Park]. Hope you sold a lot of roses today.

Love, Daddy."

Martin Luther King addressed the American Psychological Association's 1967 convention. In 1999, the APA publication, MONITOR printed Dr. King's 1967 address. I responded February 2, 1999 with the following letter, published in the Monitor's Letters to the Editor.

"MONITOR American Psychological Association
First Street, N.E.
Washington, DC 20002-4242

"Dear Editor:

"Thank you for reprinting Martin Luther King's address to the 1967 American Psychological Association's annual convention. I sat in the great ballroom near the aisle where this surprisingly small dignitary was escorted to the podium by the then current APA leaders.

"Today as I listened to MLK and read for the first time his speech to the APA Convention some of the tensions of 32 years ago returned. It was a vigorous message that made me an uncomfortable 'sinner' as I had not before considered myself prejudiced. Some of Dr. King's 1967 comments about America's role in Vietnam were perceived unpatriotic by an ex-GI of WWII, and I sat on my hands when the audience cheered his prophetic remarks. His speech was moving and I feel fortunate to have experienced that bit of Martin Luther King's legacy.

Sincerely,

A. Jack Jernigan"

Fall of 1967

After the convention, Wayne Holtzman wrote asking that we establish a meeting in October to further study the survey psychological data. He stated his office, Dean of College of Education, at University of Texas ". . . can furnish a certain amount of data analyses . . . it is important that you, Maurice Korman, Bill Hales or any others who have special interest in certain segments of the project get together and spell out their own interests so that whatever data analyses we undertake will have maximum benefit."

I gave a favorable response to an October meeting and indicated Walter Penk had an interest in making the meeting, but that Bill Hales was recovering from an operation and would be out of service for some time. Others would be contacted about the meeting, and added: ". . . have limited time and I must continually prod myself to keep at the task. There has been no lessening in motivation."

After several exchanges of letters, the October meeting was moved to November 11, 1967, the date of the Baylor-University of Texas game. Wayne offered to get tickets for all who came. I wrote October 27th that the family would not come, and added, "I will be the only person from Dallas."

Those who met November 11, 1967 in Wayne's office were: Alex Pokorny, Jack Jernigan, Lou Moran, Hubert Reese, Wayne Holtzman and his staff of Hugh Poynor, Don Witzke, and Jon Swartz.

Dr. Holtzman summarized the meeting in a two-page letter November 17, 1967. Since the meeting he learned that Jim Bieri and others in the Psychology Department were ". . . quite enthusiastic about using some of this valuable material for research projects by students and others." Wayne outlined the next steps:

"1. We will take responsibility for getting the basic data into final form for any additional statistical analyses and then for carrying out such analyses once they have been formulated.

"2. You will serve as liaison between Austin and any interests that develop in Dallas once they have been formulated.

"3. Alex will do the same for Houston and will also serve as our liaison to Washington in fulfilling the terms of the contract.

"4. Hubert will assist us with any financial and business matters, particularly with respect to paying any specialists who may work under our direction.

Wayne guessed that ". . . by early January, we will be ready to roll on whatever is requested."

A Note and a Certificate

The following note, dated September 19, 1967 from Grady Niblo:

"Thanks very much for this material which I have found most useful. Please give my thanks to Dr. Hales for lending it to me.

"It was good to talk to you today. Your encouraging words help a lot.

Grady"

Dr. Niblo referred to one of two Bill Hales' documents:

Paper presented at Southwestern Medical School Grand Rounds, 1967: "Hales, W. H., Jernigan, A. J., & Fuller, D. S., Demographic Study of Referrals for Psychiatric Consultation over a 5-year Period."

Or, to Dr. Hales' program outline that described a technique to help individuals quit the "smoking habit." He and Alan Brown introduced the procedure to patients on the TB Ward with some success.

A Service Award received: "Given at VA Hospital, Dallas, Texas - This 30th day of September 1967. This certificate is awarded to Austin J. Jernigan, Ph.D. by the Veterans Administration in appreciation of 25 years of faithful service to the United States Government." The certificate was signed by,

J. B. Chandler, M.D.

Hospital Director

Retirement - Resignation

Three men, significant to Psychology Service, were recognized with gifts, dinners and luncheons in the fall of 1967. The retirement events were: a dinner for Dr. Bill Hales October 11 and a lunch October 17, 1967; a dinner for Dr. Hinshaw, Chief of Staff, November 20, 1967; and a gift for Dr. Jim Uloth, Chief of Psychiatry December 11, 1967.

T. M. McDowell, M. D. was promoted from a Medical Service position to Chief of Staff upon the retirement of Dr. Hinshaw. There are no other extant documents to confirm, but it is my belief that Dr. Jim Uloth resigned about the time Dr. Isham Kimball transferred from Houston VA Hospital to Dallas as Chief of Psychiatry. Dr. Kimball was a member of Dr. Pokorny's staff in 1966 and active in the State Survey evaluations that continued into 1967. 4

Family

A note of thanks to Mother for her gift on my 46th birthday:

"Thank you for the lovely shirt. I received a tie from the JCJ's which goes quite well with your shirt. Received a modern language Bible from Mrs. Gibson, some tools from Jackie, a tie from Beth and Richard, and album and calendar from Jean. So, I had quite a good day. I appreciated your card and letter. Richard said he would write when he buys something with his dollar."

Mother came to Dallas in mid-November to attend a number of services at Cliff Temple Baptist Church conducted by Dr. Chester Swor. I took Mother home and visited Mr. and Mrs. Gibson; Mrs. Gibson was baking a fruit cake.

Excerpts from a letter Stewart sent to: "Cherished relatives in Dallas, Kingsville, Sedalia, Mobile, and Heidelberg."

"Uncle Jamie's Birthday, 1967

[December 20, 1967]

"Dear Family:

"I intended to write you all a long letter describing my visit to Honolulu and the Island of Oahu. Will you settle for a short one? That trip and the subsequent NDEA institute directors conference in Washington last week have put me almost permanently behind with the semester's work.

"The trip to Hawaii came as a result of a telegram from Albert Marckwardt, last year's president of the National Council of Teachers of English, which had its annual convention in Hawaii last year. Prof. M. said that he was calling a special meeting of 'recent directors' of NDEA English Institutes to discuss implications of recent trends in federal legislation for education. Although he meant only a meeting of those who would be there anyway, I showed the telegram to my department head, Lee Martin, and to Tom Cherry (our Vice President for Business Affairs--friend of Jamie's also), who thought I should go and found the money for the trip. NDEA institutes were discussed in several meetings, in fact, and we were asked to send concrete evidence of the value of institutes to NCTE headquarters, a project I'm still working on (came back, sent out a two-page letter to all 126 former participants, and am now sorting my mail).

"I saw quite a bit by stealing some time from meetings on a couple of occasions. I made the trip by boat to Pearl Harbor before meetings began on Thursday (Nov. 23), and I also made the bus tour of the island, covering about two-thirds of it. Everything I saw was interesting, and a lot of it tasted good, papayas for instance.

"And during my fourth and probably last trip to Washington on institute business, I also did some programmed sightseeing for the first time. One afternoon I went by tour-bus to Mount Vernon via Georgetown and Alexandria, Virginia. Then Saturday night, after the conference ended sooner than I had expected, I spent the night with Louis and Mary Lou Herndon, formerly of Bryan. Louis is in the USDA Soil Conservation Service was moved to Washington last year from the Fort Worth office. Sunday morning we hit high spots by automobile--went into Lincoln and Jefferson Memorial Buildings, the Capitol building, and one building of the Smithsonian, the natural sciences--and saw an awful lot before plane time.

". . . . We're going to miss seeing you all this Christmas. In a way, it's your fault, Mamma, we're doing what we were taught by example to do--putting our children first. We hope to be able to talk to David during the Christmas Season, but we have no schedule yet. MERRY CHRISTMAS AND HAPPY NEW YEAR, ALL! We love you.

Stewart (and Mary)"

Jean wrote her mother-in-law December 30, 1967.

"Dearest Mother J.,

"I have just gotten back from the doctor with Beth. She has another bad throat - hope she gets over it fairly quickly.

"Thank you so much for the nice pajamas. They are the prettiest I've owned in a long time. Beth has been wearing hers, too, and likes them so much. The boys have been sleeping in their pajamas and Jack wore his shirt yesterday. Each is a perfect fit and much needed and enjoyed!

"Dareen Heady and a friend of Richard spent last night. I didn't know Beth was as sick as she was. Jackie went <u>ice skating</u> with Mike, so we have had a busy time.

"Hope your cold is better. We had such good time being together.

Love,
Jean"

In the News Christmas Week 1967

Following are excerpts from Larry Powell's, December 25, 2000 <u>Dallas Morning News</u> summary of December 25, 1967 happenings.

"President Lyndon Johnson returned from round-the-world trip - asked Pope Paul to intercede with the North Vietnamese to gain humane living conditions for American POW's; Dallas Cowboy quarterback Don Meredith won NFL Eastern, beating Cleveland Browns 52-14 in the Cotton Bowl; Red Chinese set off a low-yield atomic bomb test; Ginger Rogers to star in "Hello Dolly" at Fair Park; Dallas Transit System bus drivers could make $6500 a year; female sewing machine operators, $2.00 an hour; 1968 Chevrolet Impala sport coupe, $2,398; a five-bedroom home in Highland Park, $54,500; one-acre home sites at Northwest Highway and Inwood Road, $20,000. On TV: "I Spy," "The Man from U.N.C.L.E.," and "The Monkeys." Opening at Northpark I: "The Graduate," and in its ninth week at Northpark II, "Gone With the Wind." Yuki, LBJ's dog, became excited at White House family

Christmas party, began to howl, so LBJ howled right along with her. 5

Chapter 11 - 1968

New Year – New Space Probe - New Car

Beth had a sore throat, but the doctor said she could attend her scheduled New Years Eve party. However, her throat was "worse" the next morning and we did not let her go to the Cotton Bowl game New Years Day with a recent admirer, Sunset High School Senior Jay Fain.

Surveyor VII Space Probe made a soft moon landing January 9, 1968. Man reached new heights with his instruments. A year later man rode into space.

Our 1965 Plymouth had a chronic electrical fault: The brake light unpredictably remained on and drained the battery. No one could correct the chronic problem. We usually kept an automobile for four or more years, but on Saturday January 13, 1968, with the '65 speedometer reading only 46,660, traded the 1965 for a 1968 four-door Plymouth, Fury III. 1

After completing the trade with Gene Hays in McKinney, I drove the twenty mile trip to Sedalia for a short visit with Mother. She wrote Wednesday, January 17, 1968:

"My dear ones,

"Hope all five of you are well and are enjoying your new car. I hope you children are half as proud of it as I was (and I suppose your uncles and Dad were) when we were able to own a brand new Model T! [The first new automobile I recall was a 1926 Chevrolet.] And when we got a second-hand car that had glass on the sides and back instead of curtains I felt positively rich. [In 1936 Dad purchased a 1933 two-tone tan, Pontiac, four-door, with spare wheel on each front fender.] But I feel sure that my three grandchildren appreciate all the many nice things their Mother and Daddy do for them. I heard or read somewhere that there were two essential things that every child needs - love and discipline and you have both. It's so good to have such wonderful grandchildren.

"I never think of any of my 7 grandchildren failing in their school work. Now all of you are Christians. That, after all is the most - by far- important step any human ever takes. You are all <u>smart, good looking, honest and dependable</u>. What a joy this brings to my heart!

"Monday it was so cold I never thought of washing until Mrs. Standridge said she was - so I knew she had to heat water in a kettle in the yard and decided I could certainly wash too. I had a fire in the bath room and also used some hot water in rinsing and by a little after 9 o'clock I had my two lines full - they froze but the sun was shining and every thing dried nicely. Of course I had a big washing but I've been washing out small pieces and my essentials so I made it fine.

"Surely did enjoy your visit Jack. Of course all of your visits when you come alone or with the family are much too short but I appreciate them all."

Professional Activities

The annual report of the Texas Board of Psychological Examiners dated December 15, 1967 announced Wayne Gill and I were elected to serve a three year term as members of the Board - Wayne as private practice representative, and I, the institutional representative.

The first 1968 Board meeting was scheduled for March 10 in Austin. There were two meetings scheduled that week in the Austin area. The second Annual Clinical Psychology Training Conference sponsored by the University of Texas Psychology Department was to meet in Kerrville on Thursday and Friday, March 7 and 8, 1968. I wrote Wayne Holtzman to ask if we might schedule our delayed State Survey data evaluation follow-up that same weekend.

Three hundred miles were added to the new '68 Plymouth speedometer. Home movie film documented the Kerrville Conference. The Thursday evening session included group techniques in developing trust among group members. Janet Spence, a recent addition to the UT Faculty, was a "guinea pig" in the demonstration. Dr. Janet Spence was elected President of the American Psychological Association in 1985.

Minutes for the March 10, 1968 meeting of the Board of Psychological Examiners noted the ". . . following persons present: Iscoe, Wheeler, Andreychuck, Gill, Jernigan, and Smith, and Secretary Betty Cleland."

The Board approved five applicants for certification, three by examination and two by reciprocity. Three applicants were not approved. One certification was delayed because of insufficient experience. The Board discussed changes in the By-Laws; cut-off for acceptable scores on the written examination; and complaints brought against three psychologists.

The background for the following paragraph may have been an Ad Hoc Committee report.

"Dr. Jernigan reported on the meeting of TPA to discuss the relationship of psychology to the Texas Education Agency. The members of the Board expressed strong feeling that this is a matter in which the Board should be involved. Dr. Jernigan was asked to relate the Board's position to Dr. Korman, current president of the Texas Psychological Association, and to inform him that the Board would be happy to serve as a committee to work with TEA in establishing the standards in question. The Board feels strongly that the Texas Education Agency should place on their staff two certified psychologists to assist in the establishment of the program contemplated in the school service centers; and that all psychological examiners utilized in the program should be supervised by a certified psychologist."

Board President, Ira Iscoe, made a significant recommendation at the March 10 meeting, ". . . that one of the years of experience required for certification by the Board should be post-doctoral." This qualification carried forward into the 1970 State Law.

Staff and Trainee Changes

Dr. Bill Hales retired in October 1967, and he and Mrs. Hales moved to La Jolla, California. That same month, Anthony M. Gallagher was appointed as a Level II Clinical Trainee from U. T. Austin. His evaluation stated: "Mr. Gallagher was supervised during most of this second year by Dr. Donald K. Smith."

Dr. Don Smith, a Ph.D. in Clinical Psychology from Rutgers University was hired in late 1967 or early 1968. Dr. Smith occupied the office vacated by Bill Hales on the A-wing, 9th floor, Building 2. This quiet, gentle young man would bring unwelcome publicity to Psychology in a law suit that went to the 10th Circuit Court of Appeals in New Orleans.

Level III Counseling Psychology Trainee Marvin Fogel returned to campus (Texas Tech University) 1st of February 1968. Final evaluation dated February 6, 1968 stated in part: "During the past two months, Mr. Fogel has continued to function in a training capacity on the Psychiatric Service, under the supervision of Dr. Walter E. Penk. Psychotherapy training has been confined to the group approach . . . has continued to participate in the assessment of all new admissions." The staff had a small "going-away" party for Marvin February 2, 1968.

I mailed former classmate-mentor, Dr. Richard M. Griffith, Lexington, Ky. a copy of the 1967 State Survey Symposium transcription April 1, 1968, and included the following note:

"Received the Form 57 on Dr. Tucker and am impressed with his experience and background. Our Position Management people will review funding this week and, hopefully, will know more within the next day or so."

The Position Management review was favorable. Jean and I and Walter and Millie Penk entertained Robert "Buzz" Tucker with a dinner at the home of Walter and Millie Penk and a visit to the Dallas Theater Center May 2, 1968. Buzz sought a transfer from the Lexington VA Hospital because of Dallas' cultural attractions, especially opera. Buzz brought with him long time friend, Bill Minor, an optical technician.

Dr. Tucker was assigned the Psychological Unit (Psychiatry) position vacated by Dr. Penk when Walter began training as a Psychology Research Associate.

Anticipated Data Analyses

Those of us interested in State Survey data analyses continued to seek support for computer service. Dr. Bill Hales was contacted in La Jolla, California, to inquire if he wished to continue the analyses of the Cornell data.

Retired Psychologist, Bill Hales sent a detailed analyses of the 195 Item Cornell Medical Index Health Questionnaire. I dictated a letter of appreciation and current news to Bill, April 10, 1968.

". . . recognize the amount of time you spent, because Walter and I devoted almost a day making what we thought was a cursory set of recommendations relative to the other psychological test data.

"This next week I will be in New Orleans and possibly see Wayne and some of the other people interested in the Survey data. The VA is having a one-day meeting prior to SWPA of the chiefs [of Psychology Service] in states surrounding New Orleans. This last month John Overall [Research Psychologist, Galveston Medical School] paid a visit and expressed great interest in the State Data. I sent a copy of your letter to Wayne, so that your ideas are a matter of record.

"No new developments since I last wrote you. Dr. Isham Kimball is now on duty as Chief of Psychiatry. I believe we may be near filling the position Walter vacated as Dr. Buzz Tucker, Staff Psychologist, at Lexington, Kentucky, is interested in a lateral transfer. Have two or three good leads for students this summer that will be graduating and will consider the Day Treatment Center and the projected Day Hospital position.

"Best wishes to you and Mrs. Hales, and do keep in touch with us."

Attended the VACO sponsored Veterans Administration meeting April 18, 1968 at Jung Hotel, New Orleans. When in New Orleans I always visited Preservation Hall where elderly black and some white musicians played jazz into the night. There were no seats, but the charge was only $1.

A History Lesson Repeated

Jackie brought home a well pulley from his grandmother's shed without permission from either his grandmother or parents. Grandma Blanche's April 3, 1968 letter suggests one of Jackie's parents encouraged him to write a letter of apology or explanation. The event was reminiscent of the time I brought home a wooden spool retrieved from Mrs. Lane's yard, and was required to return the object with an apology.

"Dear Jackie and Richard:

"I appreciated your nice letters. Richard, I am glad you have a saving account. Think that is so nice. I always wish I could make all of your birthday checks much larger.

"Jackie, I am glad that you know it is always right to ask anyone about anything, however trivial, that does not belong to you before taking it. If you had asked me for the pulley I would have asked your Daddy about it for I do not consider any of these <u>old</u> things around belonging to me. I mean the things that he and your uncles might want. But any time you find anything about this place that you think you might use just tell me and you will certainly get it unless your Dad or uncles want it. I am so very proud of you two boys and <u>also</u> of my other two grandsons. I believe all of you are dependable, honest and Christian gentlemen and I know all of you are <u>extra</u> smart and good looking. Of course my three granddaughters are just as fine.

"I wish I could keep a horse or something up here that you could enjoy when you come. What about <u>digging</u> a <u>pool</u>. There is plenty of water to fill it at present.

"I am sure no grandparent ever had finer grandchildren than I and no one ever loved them more than do I.

Grandma Jernigan"

Kimball High School Annual

Beth was a staff member of Kimball High School's 1968 annual yearbook. I accompanied Beth and other members of the staff to T.C.U. in Ft. Worth for an all day High School Pictorial Annual workshop. Tax return mileage indicates there were additional workshops that spring. 2

Beth attended a yearbook training course in San Antonio at Trinity University in June. She mailed three undated picture postcards to her family.

"Dear Rich - Went to HemisFair today and got you and Jack a little something. This Campus (Trinity U.) would be perfect for your skate board – it's so full of hills. HemisFair is a big disappointment, so don't get real excited, 6 Flags is better. We never could get to the top of the Tower - lines too long. Love, Beth."

"Jack,

Hi, we went to HemisFair today. I've now got blisters on top of my blisters from doing so much walking on campus. Our dorm is so far from everything and it's all so hilly. The food is really pretty good. We've had steak twice but Linda and I've decided to buy donuts at the coffee shop for breakfast from now on - eggs were raw - but ate toast and jelly and bacon and juice and choc. milk and was good. Love, Beth"

"Dear Mother and Daddy,

I hope you don't mind if I don't right (sic) too much cos it's 12:00 and I've got an 8:00 class. I've been really busy - mainly walking. I've been having some kind of trouble in the chest or something but it seems to be going away. I wish it were Fri- I'm having fun but I miss clean sheets and dry towels and a bath tub without years of grime. (We keep a towel in the bottom of it just in case.) Lines are so long I got donuts for breakfast. Tooth brush bought for dentures couldn't get in mouth some bristles off - [ ] O.K. Love, Beth."

The 1968 San Antonio HemisFair extended from April 6 to October 6.

Extra Professional

Dallas Mayor Erik Jonsson was the guiding light for the Goals for Dallas program of the 1960's. The Mayor's team made its introductory presentation May 14, 1968 at a downtown hotel ballroom filled with Dallas citizens. Each of us was given a zipper brief case embossed with, "Goals for Dallas" as we entered the ballroom. I served as a Team Leader, Goals for Dallas in 1969.

Dallas Psychologist, Dr. Cliff Jones, and Lawyer Jerry Gilmore, Deacon at Cliff Temple Baptist invited me to join them in establishing a Suicide Prevention Center in Dallas. I became a member of the board and participated in the development of a training program and the training of the first lay volunteers to answer telephone calls from suicidal individuals. Two documented Suicide Prevention meetings occurred October 27 and December 17, 1968.

Dr. Cliff Harris of Dallas Baptist College extended an invitation to teach an early morning undergraduate Psychology course in the summer of 1968. Income Tax statement: "Dallas Baptist College, 25 trips @ 10 cents per mile plus $4.00 parking fees, $34.20."

Family Happenings

Beth began dating Jay Fain regularly in the spring of 1968. His mother, Jeanne Fain, Dallas elementary school teacher was responsible for four sons, Jay, Bubba, Pete, Joey, and two daughters, Jill and Julia. Jay's Dad was no longer in the home.

Jay was a handsome, courteous, friendly teenager, with an outgoing personality. He and his younger brothers had part time jobs. Jay owned a moderately dependable, older model automobile.

One night Beth and Jay wanted to attend an event in north Dallas, and Beth asked if they might use the '68 Plymouth as Jay's car was not running well. Jay was reliable, and we felt secure in turning over the keys to our new automobile. As expected, the car and young couple came home safe and sound. We liked Jay. Beth ordered her 1969 Senior Class ring.

Jean was busy as a volunteer in 1968. She was President of WMU at Cliff Temple Baptist Church, and worked in the children's nursery. Jean also served as a volunteer at "Block Nursery" (United Fund), near Cliff Temple. The nursery playground was devoid of trees, and she suggested we use left over vacation Travelers Checks to purchase two trees. The entire family participated in planting the trees at the entrance to Block Nursery.

Mother wrote July 3, 1968, "Do you know until this very minute I'd forgotten it was your anniversary . . . Too late to call but I shall before the day is done. Jean - I am so <u>very very</u> glad Jack persuaded you to become his wife. He could not have found a sweeter, finer girl in all the world." True.

We bought tickets for "Girl of the Golden West" playing at Fair Park for our 21st wedding anniversary.

HemisFair

The family stayed at the Park Motel in San Antonio when we attended the HemisFair in August 1968. An IBM Pavilion postcard told of, "The lively spirit of the Latin American market brightens the two IBM Pavilions at HemisFair '68 - the Durango Pavilion and the Lakeside Pavilion - where visitors can experience for themselves the exciting world of computers." I wrote on the postcard to Mother, mailed August 22, 1968:

"Wednesday
Dear Mother
We are enjoying the HemisFair.

"IBM furnishes the equipment but not
the mistakes. Am tired but it is
worth the trip."

Back home, a postcard to Mother August 30, 1968:

"I'm glad the [Democratic] convention is over. Now I may be able to do something else. I am pleased with our selection [Hubert Humphrey and Edmund Muskie]. . . Beth spent last night with some friends. Jackie is continuing to work out for football. Richard has accepted returning to choir practice this week, with grace . . . am back on a heavy work schedule. Jean has been sewing. I hope to see you sometime soon.

Love, Jack"

Psychology Trainees

Helen Kay Ludeman, Level I Psychology Trainee from the University of Texas entered Dallas VAH training program July 15, 1968. Kay served as an observer in group testing and administered the Holtzman Inkblot Techique to fourteen patients. She began to have reservations about a professional career as a psychologist, and left to return to the University September 13, 1968 to take a terminal masters degree rather than a Ph.D.

Tony Gallagher was recommended for promotion to Third Year level training and assigned to Temple VA Hospital. Dr. Donald K. Smith's final paragraph of his two page evaluation stated:

"From my experience with Mr. Gallagher this summer, I am inclined to predict that he will have a productive career in psychology. His promise is reflected in his intelligence, imagination, and interest which should all serve as assets in his professional pursuits. Another quality which should engender a successful future is his open-mind ness to new ideas which is accompanied by a sharp critical faculty. He has an evaluative and judgmental set which is highly objective. Although he shows a tendency to procrastinate in the fulfillment of certain duties less attractive to him than others, it is suspected that he will become more conscientious with increased maturity."

Level I Counseling Psychology Trainee David T. Lane from Texas Tech was appointed to Dallas VAH on May 22, 1968. John Geers assigned a variety of psychological tests for Tony Lane to learn (WAIS, Strong Vocational Inventory, Rotter Sentence Completion, Guilford-Zimmerman, and Kuder). Mr. Lane developed a questionnaire to gain information about a patient's vocational history and attitudes toward vocational choices past and future. The questionnaire was administered as a final task in group testing. To enhance the trainee's interviewing skills, each patient was followed up with an interview designed to evaluate the adequacy of the data.

Mr. Lane was assisted in the design of a rating scale completed by members of the nursing staff and a corrective therapist that provided some measure of the ward adjustment of patients previously evaluated by questionnaire.

Mr. Lane returned to the University in September, but terminated from the Psychology Training Program in November. We documented, "It is the understanding of the [VA Training] Committee, that he terminated from the program for academic reasons. . . Should this trainee, in the future, make application for V. A. Psychology Training program, it is recommended he be considered for reinstatement."

A Surprise Announcement

We knew Jay and Beth had become quite fond of each other. Jay, a University of Texas Freshman, called Beth from Austin. They talked and let their families know they wished to marry. After extended counsel we accepted their decision. Jay came home and resumed his work at Coca Cola.

Announcements were made to our families that these two teens had fallen in love, declared their wish to marry, and we gave our consent.

The new Texas A&I Library was named the James C. Jernigan Library. Blanche, Stewart and I attended the September 1968 dedication.

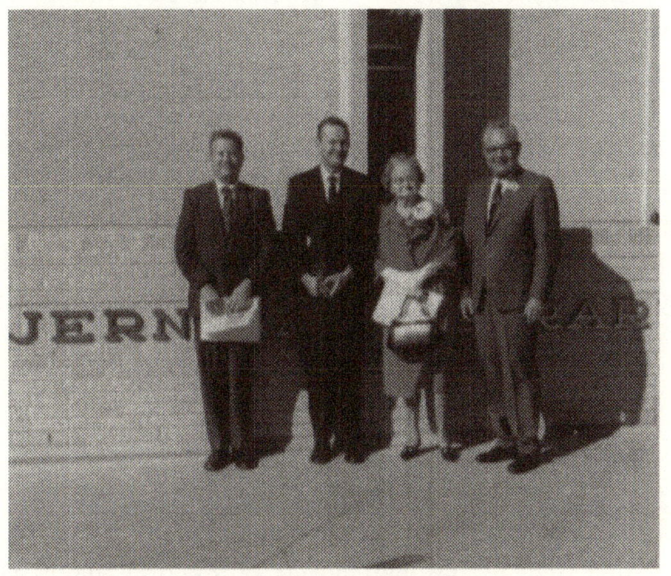

Stewart, Jack, Blanche, Jamie

Mother sat next to me at the dedication program and we talked about Beth's marriage. I referred to the wedding plans in a letter to Mother, Monday, Oct. 7, 1968,

"We thought about you yesterday [her 62nd wedding anniversary] with many fond memories. . . This weekend we went with Jay and Beth to look at an apartment. We are beginning to get accustomed to the idea of Beth being married."

Jamie came for a visit in October. I wrote Mother:

". . . We discussed the wedding plans with him and told him we hadn't intended to go much beyond the brothers and sisters of Jay and Beth . . . our thinking has begun to change. Today I wrote Clyde and Stewart - told them of the impending marriage - and extended an invitation. I believe the date will be next Friday night (Oct. 18). We have not yet been able to directly confirm Dr. Morgan (he is holding a meeting in Missouri).

"This weekend we all will be working on painting the apartment.

"I feel you and she would feel better if you could visit before hand. Of course as you and she have "seen each other a thousand times" maybe it isn't necessary. 3

". . . We are all feeling well and in good spirits. Jean has just about completed Beth's dress. I hope you are feeling well.

Love, Jack"

Jay Fain and Beth Jernigan were wed October 18, 1968. Beth's pastor, Dr. Darold Morgan, Cliff Temple Baptist Church performed the ceremony in our home at 4012 Fountainhead. Grandmother Blanche Jernigan played the wedding march as the bride came down the stairs. She was given in marriage by her father. Those present: Jay's five siblings, mother, father, grandparents, and Aunt Thelma as well as Beth's parents, aunts and uncles, brothers Austin and Richard, and some friends,

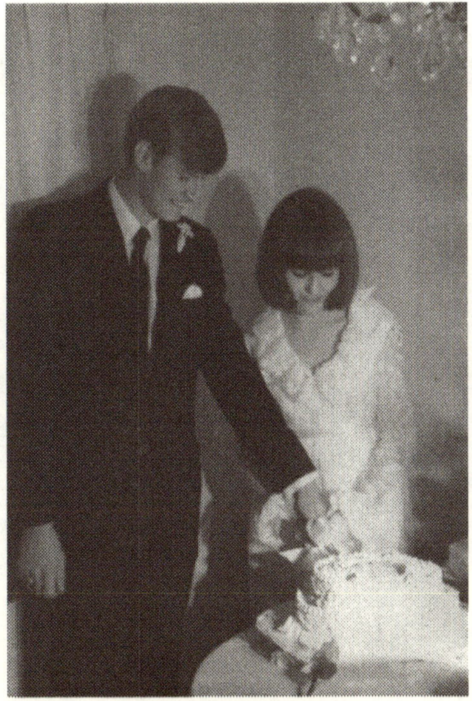

Jay and Beth cutting cake

Clyde Tilton volunteered to take photographs of the wedding. He incorrectly installed his flash so that only one of the 72 exposures was printable, and that by coincidence, a perfect picture of Jay and Beth cutting the wedding cake. It so happened that my movie camera floodlights were on them the precise moment Clyde took his still photograph of the event. It was a perfect photo of a lovely wedding.

They rented an upstairs apartment owned by Jay's grandfather. Beth continued her part time job at a variety store and her senior year at Kimball High School. We loaned them the '64 Corvair.

Following is a "Thank You for Your Wedding Gift" note from Beth to Grandma Blanche. Blanche wrote on the envelope: "This corsage was worn at Jay's and Beth's wedding October 18, 1968. What a beautiful wedding!"

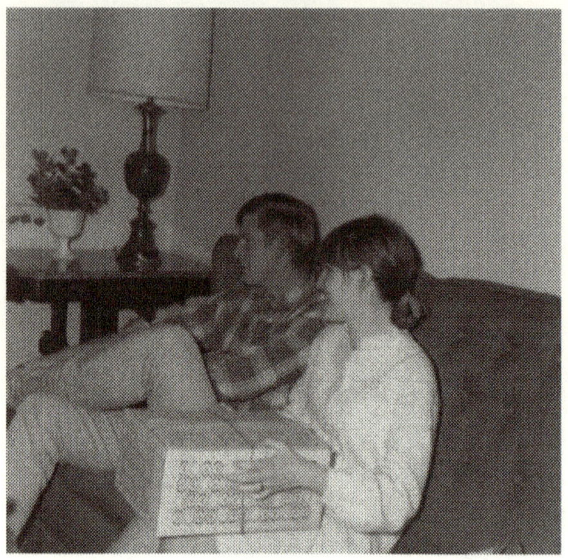

Jay and Beth receiving a wedding gift

"Dear Grandma,

"Jay and I just got in from church and I thought I ought to right [write] you and finally thank you for the $30. It's going into our savings account - which means it'll be an education fund.

"We want you to come down and spend the night now that the apartment is shaping up. With the curtains and rugs Jay's Aunt gave us (Aunt Thelma - you probably met her at the wedding) its really looking pretty. We'll be up the next free week-end. O. K.?

Love,
Beth & Jay"

"P.S. Thanks for the beautiful wedding music. Don't worry - I'm doing fine in school. I made all A's, 1 B in English History. I'm going to pull that B up next time. Love, Beth"

A postcard to Mother, 11-15-68:

"Have you considered Thanksgiving? What do you think of inviting the Gibsons and let us bring the food and do the work? We all went to Frances' [Waller] last year - think it would be fun, if you would promise not to overdo yourself. We are all doing pretty well. We had some real fine reports on Jackie at school this week. Glad your car works, most of the time."

A letter from Beth postmarked 22 Nov 1968 from 221 South Oak Cliff Blvd.

"Dear Grandma,

"Today I got inducted into the National Honor Society. I was proud and pleased. It's the [?] percentage of seniors - so it's a real honor.

"Jay and I certainly enjoyed your letter. We usually just get bills or announcements of the latest sales, so we really appreciated it. We're coming for Thanksgiving, if you don't mind. I miss all the family and I want Jay to see the farm. He's never been there, you know. Would you like me to bring anything? I have a can of pumpkin and one of apple, so I'd be glad to make a pie, or anything you wanted me to.

"Jay got a raise last week and so did I. Two very nice surprises. It all adds up doesn't it?

"Tonight we had dinner with Mother and Daddy. I feel bad going over there but they want us to come so badly and I do miss them. They and so many others (including you) have done so many nice things for us. We've gotten so many beautiful gifts. I'll never get all my thank you notes written!

"By the way, I was saving you grease for your cats but . . . we have bugs and one morning I woke up to find, I think, a whole nest (or whatever) of them. The cats might not have minded, but I did, so I threw it out.

"Last week Barbara's [Bowers] friend Malcolm, from England came to America. She met him on the trip over there several summers ago. He had been in Mexico for the Olympics for his company, and stopped in Dallas on his way home. Lat Fri. nite the 4 of us spent an enjoyable evening together. He was very interesting.

Must go,
Love, Beth"

"P.S. Jay sends his regards."

Friends and relatives were most generous in their love to Beth and Jay. Jean and I were members of an informal "42" Group composed of parents of children attending Webster Elementary, Browne Junior High School, and Kimball High School.

Don and Barbara Jarvis gave Beth and Jay a lovely wedding shower. This ecumenical group of friends surrounded us with Christian love.

Professional

Psychology Service Secretary, Mary Ingram resigned in November 1968 when her husband, Pearly Ingram retired as a Dallas Transit Bus driver. They moved to Jacksonville, Texas. Mrs. Susan Gallo, mother of three lovely children was selected to replace Mrs. Ingram. Her husband, Joe Gallo was a career Federal employee with the Post Exchange System, headquartered in Dallas. Mrs. Gallo reigned as secretary until my retirement

I flew to Austin November 9, 1968 to attend a Psychological Board meeting. The five page summary of the Board Meeting minutes indicated it was a comprehensive agenda. Some of the highlights: ". . . approving certification renewals, reviewing new applicants, reciprocity grants, certification on basis of examinations, informing two individuals not to use the title 'Doctor,' etc. The Board decided to discuss the decision to certify only graduates of departments of psychology or educational psychology at the upcoming annual business meeting of TPA."

"Report of the committee to count ballots for persons nominated by membership to serve on the Board beginning in 1969 was read: Carl Hereford, institutional; George Kramer, private practice. The Board nominated two individuals to oppose these two in the final election: Joe Rickard, institutional, and J. Ralston Kennett, private practice."

The next meeting date of the Board was set to take place on the same December day that TPA held its annual business meeting.

Houston, Texas was the site of the Texas Psychological Association annual meeting, December 5-7, 1968. (Tax record: "520 mile round trip, with '68 Plymouth speedometer reading 14,898 miles on return.") The Texas Board of Psychological Examiners met as scheduled, and gave its yearly summary to the TPA membership. Excerpts from the minutes:

"Present at the closed Board Meeting: Ira Iscoe, John I. Wheeler, A. J. Jernigan, Wayne Gill, Laurence Smith, George Kramer, and Secretary, Betty Cleland. It was announced that Carl P. Hereford and George Kramer were the new Board members. Election of officers resulted in: John I. Wheeler, Chairman; A. J. Jernigan, Vice-Chairman; and Theodore Andreychuk, Treasurer."

Thanksgiving and Christmas - 1968

All the Melissa members of the Gibson family were present for Mother's Sedalia Thanksgiving dinner. She wrote a ten page letter January 5, 1969 to her life-long friend Mary Lance documenting experiences for the previous three months. Excerpts from the letter are identified: Mary Lance:

Mother wrote us before Thanksgiving, ". . .I want Jay and Beth to come and will feel honored but knowing how their time is budgeted I want them to do exactly as they wish and I will understand if they have other plans but I hold them to a visit before long."

Then, a few days before Thanksgiving (November 19, 1968), Mother caught her hand in the washing machine wringer. Friends assisted in helping her get to the Wysong Clinic where she received three stitches in her mashed left (preferred) hand. She told all the details in her letter to Mary Lance.

"Mary Lance The past two Thanksgivings Mr. and Mrs. Gibson have had me eat with their families. (That's Jack's in-laws.) So Jack and I decided it would be nice to have them all up here this year. Just that morning I had written one of the sisters and family who live in Shreveport that they were invited. At first I thought I couldn't go through with it and of course could not if Jack and Jean had not taken charge. They came up on Saturday and did some house cleaning one of Jack's boys ran the vacuum - Jean cooked the turkey and brought salad and all that came brought a dish. It had been raining but that day it was nice and clear so we all had a good time and I was glad I went ahead. I managed to make a cake and two apple pies."

Mother wrote after Thanksgiving, "I'm so glad we had our day together Thursday. I believe all enjoyed it and I would not take anything for having had Mr. and Mrs. Gibson and Beth and Jay especially."

We invited Mother to spend Christmas with us. She wrote her friend:

"Mary Lance Jack and his two boys, Jackie and Richard, came for me and I stayed with them through Christmas. Jamie's family came Christmas evening. We all spent the night at Jack's. Jamie's family brought me home Thursday and stayed until

Saturday. Jack's family came up Friday and we had our Christmas meal Friday night. Every body had a good time. Mary and Stewart called us Christmas Eve. They were leaving for Alabama to spend Christmas with Susan, husband and 2 year old Lisa. Susan is expecting another baby in April. David is still in the service in Germany. He sent me a very pretty Candle holder.

"Mary Lance I think one reason Jack and Jean were so glad to have me with them for Christmas, Beth Ann their 17 year old daughter got married in October. I believe I told you about it. We had a pretty home wedding and I played for it. She married a very nice young fellow. Beth is finishing high school - is an A student. He has a good job and they have an apartment about 4 miles from Jack's. She got worlds of lovely gifts but they surely did hate for her to marry so young but they like the boy very much. So they are reconciled to what can't be helped. Beth and Jay came up for Thanksgiving. They came over Christmas Eve night for exchanging of presents but Beth was not there Christmas morning and I made a very good substitute I think. At least - it helped. They've always had their tree on Christmas morning."

Jean wrote her mother-in-law December 30, 1968.

"Dearest Mother J.,

"It was so good to have you with us during Christmas and we especially enjoyed being at Sedalia Friday. We took Jim [Jernigan] to Forney and it was almost like going to Williamsburg to see Florence Reagin's lovely home.

"I've never enjoyed anything more than the lovely robe. Jack is working on getting comfortable in the trousers; Jay and Beth have been making waffles and like the other gifts, too.

"Richard has enjoyed the pretty blue sweater and we went to town today and got Jackie a green sweater. Both he and Jim enjoyed the records - so it's been a nice Christmas.

"Beth quit her job today and is feeling better. I'm glad she will have a little more time to spend on the house and her school work.

"Hope you are well. The cake was delicious. I found the recipe in Kimball Cookbook and it said to leave in pan overnight. I am sure the recipe is the same and I want to make one - the two Jacks liked it so well.

Love, Jean"

Chapter 12 - 1969

A Granddaughter – A Man on the Moon

Richard received a rocket kit at Christmas. The first Saturday in January Beth and Jay came for lunch and Jay helped Richard launch his rocket. Jay promised to come back the next Saturday, and I wrote Mother ". . . we may have to get Jay a rocket too."

We sold the Corvair to Jay and Beth. We became a one car family, but not for long. 1

Dr. Donald Smith announced he was selling his 1963 Pontiac Tempest for $300. I drove the two-door, blue, slant-4 cylinder, four on the floor "Tempest", and bought it January 15, 1969. Jean and I were again able to go our independent daily routes without bothering the other's schedule. The boys loved the "new" car and later took it over as theirs when they reached driving age.

Jackie and I had colds and stayed home the weekend of January 19. Jean and Richard attended church; Beth and Jay came home with them for lunch. Read a book purchased for the children, America's First Civilization - Discovery of the Olmec, by a Dr. Coe. I was amazed to learn there was a civilization equal to the Greeks and Romans in Mexico, centuries before Christ.

It was a Dallas Independent School District policy in 1969 that a pregnant student could not remain in school. Beth began "to show" pregnancy in January. There was an option: Dallas ISD designated the night program at old Crozier Tech High School for exceptional students. Beth was an "exceptional" student in many ways.

Crozier Tech was across town from Kimball High School. I drove Beth to her night classes, and Jay picked her up after class.

Jay worked each day as a Coca Cola truck driver. It was an active schedule.

A note to Mother, "We had a busy weekend. I was in church related meetings all Saturday afternoon. Saturday night Jean and I went to her S. S. Class dinner."

Jean had a curettement in late February at Baylor Hospital.

Richard thanked his grandmother for a March 4, 1969 birthday check. He added: "I'll probably save some then spend the rest on model rockets."

Work Rewarded

Jackie, Richard and I went to Sedalia the weekend of daylight savings time change in April, and as usual, did considerable work "around the place" that Mother believed should be rewarded financially. A Monday letter to her:

"Surely did enjoy the day with you. Jean was put out with us for accepting the check but she agreed we can't do 'anything with you.' It is always a pleasure to do something there, especially when it looks so pretty afterwards. I gave the boys a portion of the money, and then will put $5.00 in each of their education accounts. Later when they are in college they can say their grandmother helped them earn some of their tuition money.

"We all got off to church an hour earlier. I had to give a talk and also help in the 11th grade department. Hope Jack and I didn't foul you up - we set your kitchen clock wrong - it is now 2 hours off - we thought about what we had done on the way back."

Professional

The University of Texas Psychology Department held its 1969 Clinical conference at the Million Dollar Hotel on Padre

Island March 6-8, 1969. The family went with me, and after the meeting we drove from Padre to Kingsville for a short visit with Jamie and family in the President's House.

The following week I flew to Austin for a Texas Board of Psychological Examiners meeting at the Capitol Room of the Commodore Perry Hotel, March 16, 1969. We renewed certification for six psychologists, granted inactive status to three, and noted that 225 psychologists had renewed as of March 16. Certification by examination was granted to six and ". . . tentatively to Robert Lovett when his degree is a year old in May." Bob Lovett participated in the 1966 State Survey.

Noteworthy Texas Psychology history: "The Board discussed the current Legislation attempt by the Texas Psychological Association and expressed its support for the endeavor." That attempt would be successful.

Fourteenth Annual Conference

Cecil P. Peck, Ph.D., Chief, Psychology Division, VACO mailed an invitation February 16, 1969, to attend a meeting of VA Psychologists to begin at 7:30 P. M., Tuesday, April 1, 1969, ". . .in the Massanet Room on the 3rd floor of the Sheraton-Lincoln Hotel, [Houston]. Jack Davis and Hal Dickman of VA Central Office Psychology Division will be present."

Eugene M. Caffey, Jr., M. D., Chief, Psychiatry Division, VACO also wrote members of the nationwide research project, "The Principal Investigators of Project 19: The Validity of a Typology for Psychotics. . .will meet at the Fourteenth Annual Conference, VA Cooperative Studies in Psychiatry which will be held at the Sheraton-Lincoln Hotel, Houston, Texas, March 31 - April 2, 1969. . .Three hours have been scheduled the first day of the meeting for discussion of the project."

Dr. Alex D. Pokorny of VAH, Houston, and Dr. Maurice Lorr of Catholic University in Washington were Co-Principal Investigators of Project Nineteen. Dallas was one of ten participating VA Hospitals. Former classmate, Bob Ferguson of Murfreesboro, Tennessee was also a Project Nineteen investigator. "The purpose of the whole series of studies is to establish subtypes among the functional psychoses and determine the important correlates with antecedent conditions and treatment outcome."

I was assigned fifteen minutes from 8:45 to 9:00 A. M. Wednesday, April 2, 1969 to present a paper by Jernigan, A. J., Penk, W. E., & Tucker, R. B., "An Empirically Derived Group Assessment Approach." The following summary statement appeared in the program:

"A standardized group assessment method is reviewed, comparing 1436 state psychiatric patients with 146 veteran psychiatric patients. Group assessment is a relatively untried technique which seems to reduce examiner difference, increases productivity of patient subjects and permits a level of standardization of data collection impossible in individual testing."

Charles A. Berry, M. D., Director of Medical Research and Operations, Manned Spacecraft, NASA, Houston, Texas, gave an Invited Address at 10:15 A. M.

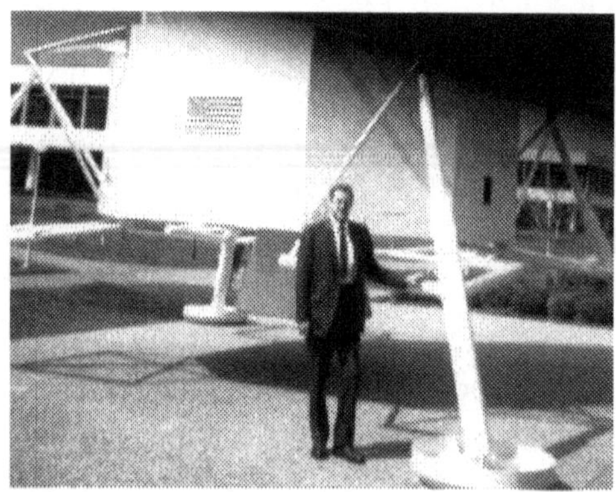

Cecil Peck at NASA

All attendees were given the opportunity for a NASA Tour of the Manned Spacecraft Center organized for Wednesday after the conference closed. My photographs taken on the NASA tour included Cecil Peck and other conference attendees. We also made two trips to the Astrodome during the conference.

Two weeks later I attended the Sixteenth Annual Convention of the Southwestern Psychological Association held April 17-19, 1969 at the Hotel Driskill, Austin, Texas, and served as Chairman of a group of papers entitled, "Studies of Adult Psychopathology."

I was promoted to a GS-14 on April 20, 1969.

Sail On - Sail On and On

Our neighbor, L. E. Manns placed a "For Sale - $350" sign on their wooden, twin hull catamaran sail boat, built by an airline pilot. Tommy Manns gave us our first sailing instructions on nearby Mountain Creek Lake.

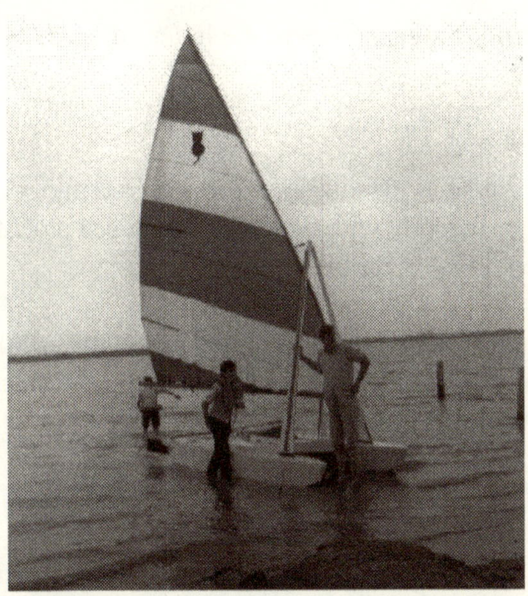

Richard, Jackie and Jay at Mt. Creek Lake

During the spring and summer we enjoyed sailboat outings on Lake Texoma with our '42 Club members, at Grandpa Gibson's Lake at Chambersville July 4th, and later at Lake Bardwell. We were sailing at Lake Bardwell on that great historical moon landing moment in July 1969 (more later). We stored the boat during the winter months at the Sedalia barn.

Letters from the Governor

I began a review of a book owned by Grandpa Andrew Jackson Jernigan, titled, The Civil War - Tennessee - Roll of Honor, and discovered Tennessee had a Brig. Gen. Preston Smith. A photocopy of the General's photograph and related data were mailed to Governor Preston Smith along with a reminder of our March 18, 1969 conversation during breakfast at the Driskill Hotel. Jack Wheeler, two other psychologists and I were having breakfast together, and the Governor stopped briefly at our table as he made his habitual early morning rounds to greet each table in the Driskill Coffee Shop. We encouraged the Governor to support the Psychology Certification Act then before the Legislature.

Governor Smith answered the letter, May 15, 1969:

"Dear Doctor Jernigan:

"Just a note to personally express to you my gratitude for your nice letter recently with which you enclosed a photo of the late Brig. Gen. Preston Smith.

"I enjoyed very much meeting you recently while you were in Austin and also the information as contained in your letter relative to General Preston Smith.

Sincerely,

Preston Smith
Governor of Texas"

Another letter came from the Governor's office May 29, 1969.

"Dear Doctor Jernigan:

"Dr. James L. McCary of Houston [President of Texas Psychological Association] has recommended to Governor Smith that you be considered for appointment to the new Texas State Board of Examiners of Psychologists.

"In the event you are interested in being considered for such an appointment, you will please be kind enough to fill out and return the enclosed biographical form.

"Upon receipt of same, your name, as well as all others who are recommended, will be presented to Governor Smith for his consideration.

Sincerely,

Bob Bullock
Administrative Assistant"

I responded June 3, 1969, ". . . honored to have been recommended . . . am especially pleased that the Legislature . . . passed the Bill concerning Certification of Psychologists . . . attached is the completed biographical form."

In addition to usual demographic data, e.g. family, education, etc. gave the following current information: "Member of Board, Suicide Prevention of Dallas; Representative in Region #1 (Kimball High School Area) 'Goals for Dallas'; Member of Advisory Committee, North Texas Planning for Hospitals & Related Health Facilities; member of the Democratic Party."

The requested five references: T. A. McDowell, M. D. (Chief of Staff, VAH); Mac Sterling, Ph.D. (Baylor University); Darold H. Morgan, Th. D. (Cliff Temple Baptist Church); Thomas S. Sligh, Jr., LL.B (Dallas lawyer); Maurice Korman, Ph.D. (Southwestern Medical School).

Happy Events

Mother wrote May 26, 1969:

"Tell Beth I was proud of her [H. S. graduation] invitation. (Also glad I'd sent her gift ha). Am so very happy that she stayed in school and was an <u>A</u> student.

". . . Of course the main thing on our minds at this time is Beth's trip to the hospital. I'll be so happy for all concerned when that is over. Of course - a lot of women much younger go through such but that is not our Beth."

Jean and I were also very proud of Jay and Beth for their discipline in making certain that Beth completed her senior year of high school. Although Beth completed the academic work at Crozier Tech, she graduated with her class at Kimball High School.

Jean wrote May 27, "Beth and Jay are getting anxious but are doing fine. Jackie is having exams. He and Richard will be out of school Friday."

The well remembered call from Jean came June 3, 1969: "Beth and I are on our way to Baylor Hospital. Go get Jay!"

A fast run ensued from Veterans Hospital to the Coca-Cola plant - then to Baylor Hospital with the expectant father urging increased speed. Beth "waited" until Jay arrived and very soon afterwards (5 pm) delivered a beautiful little girl named Lisa Jeanette Fain. From the day of her arrival onward, Lisa Fain became a joy and a blessing to all who have the privilege of being a part of her life.

We began a busy schedule: Jay enrolled as a freshman in the night school at University of Texas at Arlington; Jean stayed with Beth at their apartment the first few days after Beth and Lisa came home from the hospital. I taught a summer Psychology course at Dallas Baptist; the boys were out of school.

A Monday note to Mother: "We (the boys) went by after Sunday School and Jean came home for a couple of hours. Otherwise she has been with Beth. She and the baby are doing fine (I haven't heard today, but I don't call because the phone is right by Beth's bed).

"I guess the boys got off today. Richard was going to church [VBS] and Jackie was to visit with a neighbor. He is to cook supper tonight [chicken on the grill].

"Jay starts his course at Arlington tonight - so he will have a busy day. I was pretty dull at my 7:30 class this morning [at Dallas Baptist]. Was good to talk with you Saturday."

Psychology Training - Expectation

Gus Roberts, Level I, Counseling Trainee from Texas Technological was one of our assigned trainees for 1969. Excerpts from a two page letter to Gus:

"Early in the summer, you will be assigned a selected patient to follow in some depth on a daily basis. This is not a psychotherapeutic assignment, but one in which you will be given an opportunity to enrich your observations of human behavior. On alternate weeks, you will serve as an observer and participate in the test scoring of our group assessment battery for psychiatric patients. (Attached is a copy of paper recently presented at the 14th Annual Conference VA Cooperative Studies in Psychiatry,

Houston, Texas). The staff will meet with the trainees on a weekly basis to lead discussions on a variety of subjects, example of which are included in the following: (1) Conceptual Area Analysis of Object Sortings by Dr. Walter Penk. Book Review: Neiseer's <u>Cognitive Psychology</u>. (2) Clinical Inference by Dr. Donald Smith. Emphasis might be placed on the treatment of this topic by Sarbin, Taft, & Bailey in <u>Clinical Inference and Cognitive Theory</u>. (3) Techniques of Psychotherapy and Milieu Therapy - the Therapeutic Community by Dr. R. B. Tucker. (4) Role of Psychotherapy in a Total Treatment Program by Dr. Ralph Robinowitz.

"Dr. John Geers, away on vacation has not given a subject area, but most likely will select a topic in the general area of vocational rehabilitation. I will discuss with the trainees some of our current thinking on Assessment of Human Behavior by Group Methods.

"For several years, we have followed the policy of encouraging trainees to select a brief research project which can be completed within the 3 month period. . . The following [topics] have been proposed: (1) Survey of the records of patients maintained over a long period of time on minimal treatment (Mental Hygiene Clinic). (2) The relationship between visual perception and visual memory. This could be ascertained by giving each subject a test of visual perception and a test of visual memory. This might provide information about performance on the Benton Visual Retention Test. (3) 'Cognition of Palpable Objects.' Assist in data analysis for an on-going research project. Research design is completed and much data has been collected. Goals for the summer could include: (a) analyzing data; (b) refining research instruments; and (c) collect cross-validation sample. (4) Development of rating scales for relevant psychological dimensions, e.g., dependence-independence, active-passive, etc., based on patient's responses to Sentence Completion Blank. [The topic selected by Gus.] (5) Develop questionnaire and rating scale for patients leaving hospital in reference to rehabilitation gains (or deficits) resulting from patient's participation in I.T. programs.

". . . There will be conferences led by consultants in Psychology, Psychiatry, and Neurology during the summer. . . We look forward to having you with us, and expect to see you June 2."

The evaluation summary for Trainee Gus Roberts: "Mr. Roberts designed a project utilizing content from the Rotter Sentence Completion Test. Taking the responses of patients to the stem "I need" -- Gus developed a classification of content into categories "active," "passive," and "neutral." . . . 100 case records from Psychology files and submitted the stems for rating by five Ph.D. psychologists. He related the ratings to patients' length of stay . . . patients who project a sentence classified as "active" spend significantly fewer days in the hospital."

One Small Step for Man

Our family went with the Burrells to Bardwell Lake near Ennis Sunday afternoon, July 20, 1969. We carried the play pen so Lisa could observe all the happenings.

By radio we heard that Apollo 11 landed and a member of the crew would be descending later that evening. We raced back to Dallas under a bright, full moon, and remarked, "Just think, men are up there on the moon."

We watched Apollo 11 hour after hour on the television screen as the ship sat on the moon with the three astronauts inside. And then - those exciting moments as Neil Armstrong exited from Apollo 11 with his historic statement, "ONE SMALL STEP FOR MAN- - ONE GIANT LEAP FOR MANKIND!"

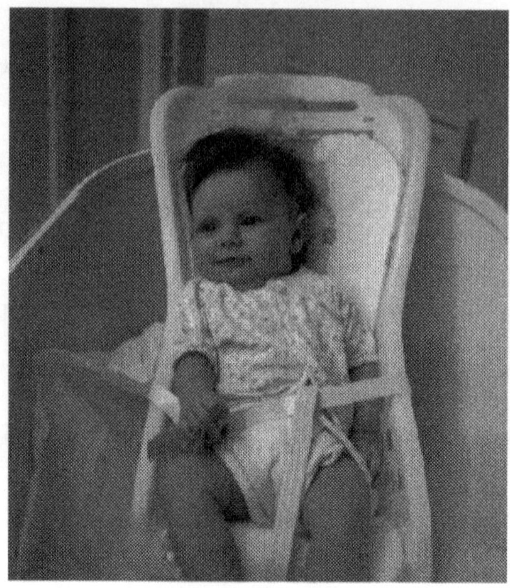

Lisa Fain – 2 months

It was Monday, July 21, 1969 when Jay, Beth and Lisa returned to their apartment. A new world era was born (thirty-seven days after Lisa's birth).

Jean recorded a check July 28 to "Jay L. Fain (SAT) - 16.25 for Beth to enter University of Texas at Arlington."

Jay thanked Grandma Blanche for his birthday check (July 16, 19th birthday).

"Dear Grandma Blanche,

"It was certainly nice receiving a birthday present from you. It was very thoughtful and it was certainly appreciated. I used it to take Beth to the movie. It is very seldom we get out these days. Both girls and myself are well and we are looking forward to seeing you soon.

Love, Jay"

Beth received six hours of college credit because of her excellent SAT score.

Two weeks later, another letter to Mother, "Last evening we came by after church, picked up Beth and Lisa so Jay could study for his final exam. We bought a 1/2 [gallon] of ice cream, took Jay a dish, and then the rest of us came on to the house. Jay picked them up around 10:00 PM. Beth was thrilled with her box of [baby] clothes from Susan."

In the fall Beth joined Jay in night school at University of Texas at Arlington. Lisa stayed with us during the nights they were in class.

Board of Examiners

The Texas Board of Psychological Examiners (TBPE) met August 3, 1969 at the Forty Acre Club in Austin.

The Board followed the usual pattern: Approval and denial of certification of applicants; review of correspondence. I was asked to serve as Board representative to the American Association of State Psychology Boards to meet in Washington, August 30, prior to APA. And the Board ". . . officially recognized the work done by Larry Smith and Betty Cleland in the legislative attempt."

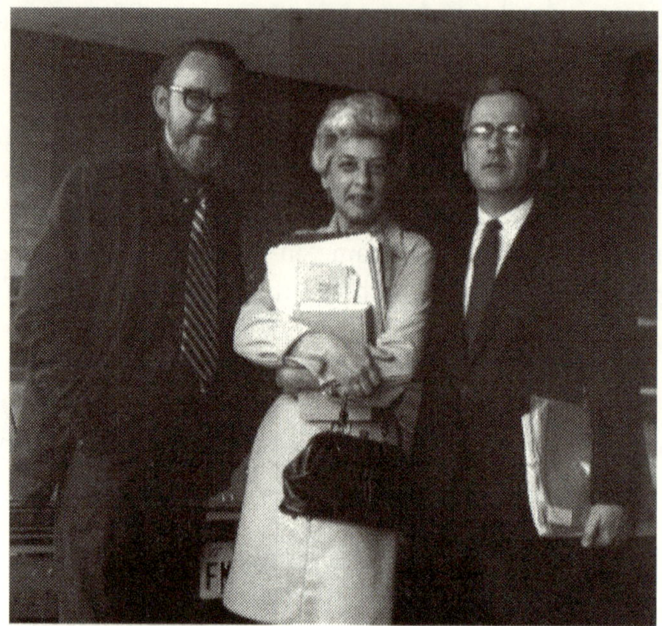

Carl Hereford – Betty Cleland – Jack Wheeler

The afternoon session was devoted to a discussion of the structure and regulations of the prospective new Board, and the process of changing from TBPE to the new State Board. In light of the pending transition, ". . . the Board decided to mail a substitute ballot asking certificands to extend the terms of the out-going Board member for one year to allow for the transition."

A Professional and Family Outing

Jean, Austin, and Richard accompanied me to the annual meeting of the American Psychological Association in Washington, D.C. in August 1969. We flew American Airlines, and stayed first at the Washington Hilton, and later at the Statler Hilton. The Veterans Administration funded my cost of the trip to attend a VACO Psychology's meeting and recruit staff. I represented the Texas Board of Psychological Examiners at the annual meeting of the American Association of State Psychology Boards.

Congressman James M. Collins' Texas 3rd Congressional District office scheduled a White House tour for our family for Thursday, August 28, 1969 at 8:15 am. Congressman Earle Cabell's, 5th Congressional District Texas office scheduled a tour of the FBI Building and a special Congressional Tour for August 29 at 9:30 am.

We documented the trip with 8mm movie and still film and in picture post cards saved by Blanche. The first card, "Manassas National Battlefield Park, Manassas, Virginia" mailed August 27, 1969:

"Dear Mother:

We rented a car and drove by the park on way to Washington from airport. We have a lovely room and look forward to our conducted tour of the White House in the morning. Richard and Jackie seem to be enjoying the trip. We have already viewed a number of historical places.

Love, Jack"

And a picture postcard of Washington's church and "Washington's Prayer is the closing paragraph of a circular letter addressed to the Governors of all States on disbanding the Army in 1783."

"Today we visited this church and Mt. Vernon. We are having a very fine time. Tonight we go to the Peck's home for supper. They are old friends from Ky. days. We called Beth and Jay this morning. We will be back Tues."

And on reverse side: WASHINGTON'S PRAYER

"Almighty God: We make our earnest prayer that thou wilt keep the United States in thy holy protection; that thou wilt incline the hearts of the citizens to cultivate a spirit of subordination and obedience to government; and entertain a brotherly affection and love for one another and for their fellow citizens of the United States at large. And finally that thou wilt most graciously be pleased to dispose us all to do justice, to love mercy and to demean ourselves with that charity, humility and pacific temper of mind which were the characteristics of the divine author of our blessed religion, and without a humble imitation of whose example in these things we can never hope to be a happy nation. Grant our supplication, we beseech thee, through Jesus Christ our Lord. Amen."

Jackie and Richard discovered the Annual Convention's hotel accommodations interesting places to explore. The convention offered exhibits and films attractive to youths. It was a fun trip and most educational.

A brief note in early September, "The boys are getting settled down to school. Richard is going out for football, but Jack isn't. I sometimes wish we were in a smaller school. . . Jean had her Sunday school class meeting last night - had 12. Beth and Jay are well."

A Tragic Accident

John and Bea Geers left in the early afternoon of September 19, 1969 for a weekend at Lake of the Pines in east Texas. They stopped within a mile or so of their destination to purchase a few items, but Bea did not attach her seat belt for the final fatal mile. John did. As they crested a hill, a drunk driver crossed the median and hit them head-on. Bea was thrown through the windshield with a broken neck. John suffered a broken leg and many body bruises.

Several trips were made to a hospital in Gilmer between September 20 and September 28, 1969 to visit John and assist in some of the funeral details, as well as John's rehabilitation needs. He asked me to take photographs of the wrecked automobiles for insurance liability.

John's Mother came from Iowa (?) to stay with him for several weeks after he returned to Dallas. It was a sad occasion. Everyone loved Bea Geers.

The tragic event had a positive effect for our family: It increased self discipline to always wear seat belts. One would say to the other on seeing a loose seat belt, "Remember what happened to Mrs. Geers."

Sedalia Homecoming

Jean, Richard and I attended a Sedalia School Homecoming Sunday, October 12, 1969. A postcard to Mother the next morning,

"We had pouring rain all the way back but got in safely. The Fains spent the afternoon with Jackie but left soon after we arrived as Lisa was getting sleepy. We had such a good time. I continue to be amazed with all the contributions you make year by year. I'm not sure I'm interested in an annual affair but I do enjoy on occasion seeing all my old friends. The food and everything was so nice. Sorry we didn't get to talk with you more. Hope you have plenty of butane this morning."

A Trip to Austin with Guests

Jay and Beth rode with me to Austin and visited the campus while I attended a Texas Board of Psychological Examiners Board meeting at the Forty Acres Club Sunday, November 9, 1969. Lisa stayed with Jean and the boys.

It was announced at the meeting that the membership voted to extend current board member composition for one year. The president of the Tarrant County Psychological Association wrote Governor Smith requesting appointment to the soon to be announced Texas State Board of Examiners of Psychologists. He wrote a similar letter to Dr. Beeman Phillips, President elect of the Texas Psychological Association.

"Jack Jernigan brought a lengthy statement from the APA in response to HEW's Medicare study . . . for review and discussion at the next [Board] meeting."

Some forty psychologists received certification renewal. The Board agreed to meet at TPA on Saturday, December 6, 1969, ". . . at about 9:00 A. M. in Jack Wheeler's room. If Board business cannot be completed on Saturday, the Board will continue in session on Sunday. By that time the Texas State Board of Examiners of Psychologists should, by law, be appointed."

Goals for Dallas

A letter from Mayor Erik Jonsson's office alerted recipients of the Neighborhood Committee meetings for the fall. Mr. Jonsson made reference to ". . . 600 Neighborhood Committee volunteers [and]. . . 50,000 citizens from every section of the Dallas area [who] attended the Goals meetings." Goals for Dallas Neighborhood Meetings were scheduled for October 28 through November 25, 1969.

Neighborhood meetings were held at Justin F. Kimball High School Tuesday evenings October 28, November 4 and November 18. Jean and I attended at least one of the three meetings. I served as a Discussion Leader for both the Goals for Dallas Information Meetings and Neighborhood Meetings according to a December 22, 1969 letter of thanks from Mr. Jonsson.

I also served as Discussion Leader for the "Welfare Panel" at Pinkston High School, and sat on the platform with Mayor Jonsson, and three others. Mr. Al Lipscomb, then in the early stage of his activist role in the City of Dallas, filled the night with questions that Mayor Jonsson tactfully answered. In a friendly conversation with Mr. Lipscomb during the break, discovered he was a Veteran. He remarked he could use my services. His eyes appeared dilated.

A transcript of the Pinkston proceedings indicates I was the first Discussion Leader to speak following the small group meetings. The other panels were: Recreation and Entertainment, Rev. B. L. McCormick; Transportation and Communication, Mr. Charles Purnell; and Health, Mr. Ed Tiffin. I served a similar role at Roosevelt High School later that fall.

The Discussion Leader was asked to complete a Report Form. I submitted a report of "Neighborhood 11 (Pinkston)," dated November 4, 1969. A personal critique of the Pinkston and Roosevelt meetings was submitted later to Bryghte Godbold, Staff Director for Goals for Dallas.

Bryghte D. Godbold responded on December 8, 1969:

"Dear Dr. Jernigan:

"Thank you very much for your letter containing the valuable suggestions about the Welfare Goals. We will certainly use them as we revise the proposals for achieving the Goals, as well as the Goals themselves.

Many thanks for serving as a Discussion Leader."

Planned Parenthood of North East Texas

I do not recall from whom, how or when the invitation came to become a Board Member of Planned Parenthood. Beth's pregnancy precipitated an increased sensitivity of need to become better informed about family planning and available educational tools. That interest came to the attention of active members of Planned Parenthood, and fulfilled a desire to have a psychologist as a member of the board.

Four Planned Parenthood Board meetings were attended in 1969. Sixteen meetings were attended in 1970.

Jay and Beth moved to a new apartment in November. Their address: Apt. 201, 426 Walton Walker, Dallas, Texas.

Open house visits to Jackie and Richard's school brought good reports from teachers. During that same season, Jackie made $42 building a backyard fence for disabled veteran, Ben Roseman.

The Canceled Debate at SMU and Walter Penk

The Friday, November 7, 1969 issue of The Daily Campus, Southern Methodist University, reported a speaking invitation to controversial psychologist, Timothy Leary. SMU President Willis Tate responded:

"To some of us, Mr. Leary is a discredited man who is not a fit subject for testing academic freedom. . . I am denying the permission to have Mr. Leary speak on our campus until the ambiguities of our rules on outside speakers can be considered. . . I am making a strong personal appeal to the University and its friends to support me in this decision."

Walter Penk insisted we communicate our displeasure and jointly write to Bill Bell the Program Chairman. The November 10, 1969 letter was written by Walter, and signed by both of us. Some excerpts from Walter's two and one-half page letter, with a copy to Dr. Willis Tate:

"We grieve for our recreant peer Timothy Leary. . . Several years ago, his self-described new religion, his new discoveries, and his unique view on certain drugs were given judicious forum and judged inadequate by the same colleagues at Harvard who once championed his early ideas. His peers in the American Psychological Association counseled with him and finally rejected him because his actions and his exorbitant claims did not meet criteria of professional responsibility.

"... .The deterioration of Timothy Leary is indeed a sorrowful history to follow . . . [he] is a disturbed man who does not need to be put on public display . . . prevent further deterioration of Timothy Leary as a person.

"We have cited Dr. Leary's book <u>The Interpersonal Diagnosis of Personality</u> it may be read and discussed as a memorial to the talent he once possessed. For the area of creative thinking, J. S. Bruner of Harvard and E. Torrance of the University of Georgia are more in vogue, are available for speeches. . . In the area of psychopharmacology, Gardner Lindzey, a resident of Texas and a Vice-President of the University of Texas ranks as an internationally recognized scholar."

President of SMU, Dr. Willis M. Tate responded November 28, 1969, enclosed an official policy statement issued on November 4, !969, and added: "As you probably know, Leary cancelled his appearance on November 18, so his debate with Dr. Jerome Lettvin of MIT did not take place. They had already appeared in public, and their debate was shown on Channel 13 in Dallas a few weeks ago. . . Again, thank you for your interest in SMU."

GOV. SMITH RECALLS THREE APPOINTMENTS

Never before were Texas Psychologists so well organized as when Gov. Smith appointed three "quacks" to the newly legislated State Board of Examiners of Psychologists. Psychologists from across the state wrote, called, and did whatever necessary to call attention to the fact that three men who identified themselves as psychologists, "Hugh Howell Buice of Dallas, Charles Elden Stovall of Arlington and Raymond Lee Ruhlem of Houston" were not qualified to serve on the Board.

Smith said he was withdrawing the names of the men in response to a telegram from the Texas Board of Psychologists (sic) Examiners, a private organization, which questioned whether the appointees held degrees from accredited colleges.

The Governor claimed there was no legal question about recalling the nominations, since Secretary of State Martin Dies, Jr. had not issued their commissions. . . .Bob Bullock, the governor's aide in charge of screening appointments, reportedly was out of town and not available for comment. 3

With this fiasco settled the self-certifying Texas Board of Psychological Examiners set the agenda for its December meeting. The Governor's Board appointments were not on the official agenda.

First Research Grant in Psychology

An unrelated "News Release" (1969) by the Dallas VA Hospital concerned the award given to Dr. Walter E. Penk, Research Psychologist - a grant ". . . in the amount of $104, 500 to support an individual research program." The Veterans Administration Department of Medicine and Surgery, Washington, D.C. further stated: "This is the first research grant in psychology awarded to the Dallas V. A. Hospital under the direction of its Research and Education Committee. During the next three years, Dr. Penk will be working to devise measures of cognitive change in psychological disorders."

Thanksgiving

The Thanksgiving Prayer, published in the Dallas News the morning of November 27, 1969, was read as grace prior to our Thanksgiving Dinner. It was Lisa's first Thanksgiving.

Mayor Erik Jonsson sent a copy of his Thanksgiving proclamation and this note: "I appreciate very much your thoughtful letter of December 2 and your kind words to me. I am pleased to send you a copy of the Thanksgiving proclamation. 4

THANKS-GIVING PROCLAMATION
Dallas, 1969

HOW BLESSED WE ARE AS A PEOPLE TO HAVE A SPECIAL SEASON FOR A WHOLE NATION TO THINK ABOUT HOW GOOD GOD IS TO US! HOPE IS VERY REAL FOR THE CITIZENS OF A COUNTRY THAT HAS GRATITUDE AS ITS OLDEST TRADITION.

AND NOW, THIS YEAR WE HAVE BEEN GIVEN THE REVELATION OF A WHOLE NEW VIEW OF HUMANITY FROM THE MOON, SEEING IN ONE BEAUTIFUL WORLD A VISION OF MAN'S PLACE IN THE HAND OF A LOVING CREATOR.

BUT WE ARE ESPECIALLY GRATEFUL FOR THE SIMPLE ACT OF ONE ASTRONAUT WITHIN THE FIRST HOURS ON THE MOON IN OFFERING HIS PERSONAL THANKSGIVING FOR ONE MANKIND UNDER GOD. BY THIS HUMBLE ACT OF GRACE WAS THE FIRST THANKS GIVING ON ANOTHER SPHERE CELEBRATED.

SO IN THIS YEAR OF DAILY THANKSGIVING, IT IS APPROPRIATE THAT AS MAYOR OF DALLAS, I, ERIK JONSSON, DO APPOINT THURSDAY, NOVEMBER 27, 1969, AS A SPECIAL DAY OF PRAISE AND JOY FOR THE DIVINE POWER THAT SUSTAINS US.

An "ESPECIALLY FOR YOU" birthday wish and a note on the eve of the Texas Psychological Meeting:

"Dear Mother:

"I begin three days of meetings today and want to get this card to you before I become engrossed in something else. I hate it that I have to work Saturday and can't come to see you on your birthday. (Texas Psychological meets here in Dallas.)

"We surely did enjoy your visit last week. Then Tuesday afternoon Jamie came out from his meeting and visited until about 7:30. I took him by Beth and Jay's apartment.

"Wish you could have been at the program last night. We were so proud of Jackie - he did an exceptional job and received a number of compliments.

"Have a wonderful birthday.

We love you, Jack"

Texas Psychological Annual Meeting - Dallas - 1969

The Texas Board of Psychological Examiners met December 6, 1969 at the Statler Hilton Hotel, Dallas during the annual TPA meeting. All six Board members were present and, "Guests (appointees to the Texas State Board of Examiners of Psychologists) Drs. Murray Kovnar and Alvin J. North. Also present were Dr. Laurence Smith, Legislative Chairman for TPA, and Betty Cleland, Secretary to the Board."

In addition to renewing certificands for 1970, I moved and Carl Herford seconded that the present officers of TBPE be retained for the coming year. TBPE normally followed the pattern that the Vice-President moved to President, but as 1970 would be the last year for TBPE, the recommendation passed that Jack Wheeler continue as President, Jack Jernigan, as Vice-President, and Ted Andreychuk as Treasurer.

The Board "formally commended Laurence Smith for his work as Legislative Chairman for Texas Psychological Association and the Texas Psychological Association for its cooperation in the attempt to gain acceptable appointees to the Texas State Board of Examiners of Psychologists."

Good News - The Good News Accepted

Blanche's Guest Book recorded that the three families were at Sedalia December 24, 1969 with all grandchildren present but David and Susan. There are also many home movie scenes of each member, receiving and giving gifts.

One memorable event for Christmas 1969 was the planting of the balled cedar indoor Christmas tree. After Christmas we planted the tree in the front yard, and a photograph tradition began with me holding Lisa in front of the tree. Relatives looked forward each Christmas to their annual card that always included a photograph of the previous year's Lisa-Grandpa living Christmas tree scene.

A second memorable event was told in a letter to Mother on Monday, December 29, 1969.

Dear Mother:

"You will be pleased to know that Jay joined the church and was baptized last night. Beth told us last week he had reached this decision, and would make his profession on Sunday. It was such a bad day, raining, that we thought he might postpone, but here both of them came at the end of the service. Dr. Morgan announced the baptismal service. Jay was the only one baptized. It was an impressive and moving event.

". . . We have not heard directly from Jackie but another boy called to say they arrived on Friday @ 4:00 P.M. [Colorado ski trip with Young Life]. It's lonesome around our house - just glad we have Richard.

"Jay and Beth are buying a new Ford Maverick this week. We are so pleased for them.

"Hope you have a Happy New Year.

Love, Jack"

Chapter 13 - 1970

Family Happenings - Trips

Jay and Beth enrolled as freshmen at University of Texas at Arlington. Beth attended full time, Jay, part-time at night after a day on his Coca-Cola route. Jean cared for Lisa during the day, and wrote her Mother–in-law: "Lisa and I are getting along fine. She is a sweet baby and is very easy to care for."

Jackie attended Browne Junior High School. Richard attended the 7th grade at Daniel Webster Elementary.

We drove to Waco Sunday, January 25, 1970 to a wedding shower for Mike Sterling and his bride. Mike was a small boy when we were in graduate school at Kentucky with Mac and Judy Sterling. A postcard to Mother the next day:

"I hope your butane tank is full. The weather has caused us no great inconvenience. The boys showed their movies this past weekend; had a small crowd and those who came said they'd come again. We enjoyed our trip to Waco; saw a number of old friends. This Friday I go to Austin for two days."

Jackie and Richard adapted the upstairs den to show rented "old movies." In time the room became their "Bijou Motion Picture Palace." And it wasn't long before they started making movies.

Jackie began driver training. He drove to church one night, and I prophesied he would become "a good driver." Prophesy fulfilled.

The trip to Austin may have been to attend the University of Texas Psychological Department's annual Clinical conference.

Richard celebrated his 13th birthday and wrote Grandma Blanche March 10, 1970 on his letterhead stationery:

Richard Jernigan
4012 Fountainhead
Dallas, Texas 75233

"Dear Grana,

"Thank you for the three dollars. I haven't spent it but I will soon. That time I launched the camera rocket, the picture did not turn out but I launched another. I am expecting good results.

"I'm now developing my pictures with a developing outfit I got for birthday.

Love, Richard"

Presentation to UT Seminar in Psychology

Dr. Norman (Jim) Prentice, Director of Clinical Training at University of Texas extended an invitation to speak at a "Meeting of the Seminar in Clinical Psychology on Friday, March 13th, at 3:00 P.M. in Meses 301." He announced, "Dr. Jernigan's topic will be: 'Certification of Psychologists: The Case Example of Texas.' All interested clinical students and faculty are cordially invited."

Jim Prentice suggested: "I think we can just talk fairly informally about stuff like why psychologists seek certification, who started the ball rolling in Texas and why and what objections were raised to it, in and out of psychology, how well the voluntary program worked and why that was tried first, what problems encountered in passage of statutory legislation, and why and so forth. I'll be on hand and perhaps can throw in some comments about other states. Also we can take a look at the bill itself. O. K.?"

The eight page (double spaced) paper, "Certification of Psychologists: The Case Example of Texas," responded to most all of Jim's suggestions. It historically traced the period from 1948 when APA drafted its first Code of Ethics to December 1969 when the Governor of Texas appointed the first psychologists to the Texas State Board of Examiners of Psychologists. The referenced documents are no longer extant. See Appendix.

It was a pleasant afternoon discussion with students and faculty. Dr. Jim Prentice and I maintained a cordial relationship through the years.

The Texas State Board of Examiners of Psychologists met the following day. Betty Cleland arranged for a "single at Forty Acres Club for March 13th and 14th.

Texas State Board of Examiners of Psychologists
Texas Board of Psychological Examiners

"The Texas Board of Psychological Examiners met on Saturday, March 14, 1970. Board members present were: John I. Wheeler, A. J. Jernigan, Carl F. Hereford, and George Kramer. We reviewed eight applications for certification and all scored above the "cutoff" on the Professional Practice in Psychology Examination, and thus approved." The minutes continued:

"A financial report was presented, and the Board agreed that while the by-laws of the Board require that all property of the Board must revert to the Texas Psychological Association, the Board will request TPA to give this material to the Texas State Board of Examiners of Psychologists.

"A report will be mailed to all certificands in April, 1970 and the Board will continue to exist until the end of 1970. It is anticipated that a meeting at Texas Psychological Association Annual Meeting in December will constitute the remaining business of the Board. Balance in treasury, $31.50.

Respectfully submitted,

Mrs. Charles Cleland, Executive Secretary"

Texas Psychologists anticipated that members of the Texas Board of Psychological Examiners would become the nucleus of the new board for Texas State Board of Examiners of Psychologists. The Governor's office rejected my name, stating that State law prohibited Federal employees from serving on any state board. Later, this ruling was modified, but I declined to let my name be resubmitted.

Betty Cleland suggested I pass on to TSBE Board Member, Dr. Alvin J. North, SMU Professor, the copy of the Handbook for Members of State Psychology Boards, published by the American Association of State Psychology Boards. The transition between the two Boards was nearly complete.

An undated announcement card from the Texas State Board of Examiners of Psychologists indicated it was ready to provide "applications for certification of psychologists as required in Senate Bill 667, passed by the regular session of the 1969 Texas Legislature. . . .The Board meets again in March, 1970."

Mr. Gibson's Leg and Other Happenings

Jean's father, Jake Gibson was in the hospital with a broken leg. He walked across Highway 5 from the grocery store late one afternoon on his way back home. A young man in a VW struck Mr. Gibson and knocked him to the pavement. The devastated young man went often to visit him in the hospital, and after Mr. Gibson returned home.

Because of his age and nursing needs, Mr. Gibson was subsequently transferred to the Wysong Nursing Center on University Drive in McKinney, Texas. By the end of March he was becoming very restless, and urged the doctor to dismiss him. Mrs. Gibson told Mother that "Jake wants so much to be home in time for his birthday, March 29th." He had been at the Center for 12 weeks.

Mr. Gibson left the Nursing Home AMA (against medical advice). After the Doctor made his rounds one morning, Mr. Gibson called a cab and went home.

Uncle Sidney Matthews visited Cliff Temple Baptist Church with his sister Alice Moore in April 1970. As we helped them down the steps after church services, Uncle Sidney told me he had been with Natalie at Lamplighter the day before and complimented the growth of the Jernigan tree.

Soon after the dedication of Lamplighter I asked Natalie if she would like to have a tree from her Grandfather's land. Of course, she said yes. Jackie and I dug an elm from the Jernigan woods and transplanted it in the school's front circular drive. Elms are slow growing, and the groundskeeper eventually replaced the elm.

Beth wrote Grandma Blanche a postcard "between classes" at the University.

"Dear Grandma,

"Jay starts his vacation this weekend so we're coming up this weekend. We'll probably be up around noon Saturday. We're really looking forward to this much overdue visit. We can't wait to show you how much Lisa has grown.

"Well I'm writing this during a break between classes and now must go to class.

Love,

"See you Saturday!! Beth"

The Peace Pin

The most public documentation of my role as a Service Chief at Dallas VA Hospital came for: "Sustaining a direct order to a Staff Psychologist not to wear a Peace Pin while on duty."

The nation was in great conflict in 1970 over the purpose of the Vietnam War. Many of us of the WWII era were disturbed when citizens behaved in a way that could cause distress among our men and women in the uniform of our country. The Veterans Administration began to recognize that hospitalized Vietnam veterans required different treatment modalities from those used in treating veterans of WW I, WW II, and the Korean War.

I was a member of a special study committee to review the distinct needs of the young Vietnam veteran patients. An example of one decision was to change "lights-out" to a later hour on wards with large numbers of Vietnam Vets. The effect was a reduction in need for certain restful medications. Later the Veterans Administration established off-site offices to respond to the special needs of the Vietnam Vet. In some ways the nation (and to some extent the young veterans themselves) perceived these brave ex-service people as second-class veterans. That mood carried over into the treatment center.

Into this environment walked Dr. Smith wearing a peace pin in his lapel, a symbol opposed in essence to what many veterans had made great sacrifices in time, body, and spirit. Dr. Smith was counseled the pin reduced his objectivity as Ward Psychologist, and directed not to wear the pin while on duty. 1

The pin was a dove with a simulated U. S. flag on the side of its body with one wing extended above. The Peace Pin became a Vietnam resistance symbol.

My counsel to Dr. Smith as his supervisor proved fruitless and the Chief of Staff and Personnel advised documentation of each directive and Dr. Smith's response. Eventually Don was given written notice to either remove the pin while on duty or be removed from his position because the symbol of resistance to the Vietnam War was potentially distressing to some hospitalized Vietnam, Korean, and WW II veterans. He held fast to his position. The media picked up the conflict.

A late night telephone call came Saturday evening, March 28, 1970 from a <u>Dallas Times Herald</u> reporter asking questions about "the breaking story." The reporter inquired if Dr. Smith was told he could never wear the Peace Pin, and I replied to the effect, "When Dr. Smith is on duty as a Psychologist at the Dallas VA Hospital he is not to wear the Peace Pin. I don't give a damn where he wears the pin when he is not on duty."

The response was quoted in the Sunday morning <u>Hearld</u> and <u>Dallas Morning News</u>. I was a bit uncomfortable at church that day for the "damn."

A personal file, "Public Responses" has some eighteen references to telephone calls, personal letters, newspaper articles, Letters-to-the Editor, a <u>Times Hearld</u> Editorial favorable to Smith, etc. The April 6, 1970 <u>Dallas Times Herald</u> article was written after Don's removal from his Consultation Service position and reassignment to a research activity devoid of patient contact:

"I wish to express my disappointment over the reassignment of Dr. Donald K. Smith. His personal beliefs should not be grounds for removal as long as they do not interfere with the performance of his job at Veterans Hospital.

"If we may believe the report in your paper, Dr. Smith displayed a mature outlook toward his actions, indicating a willingness to concede his constitutional freedom of expression, should it hinder his work as a psychologist. Under the circumstances, neither the attitude nor action of Dr. A. J. Jernigan is reasonable.

"As Dr. Smith stated, 'Peace and patriotism are not incompatible.' Such a stance should not be considered disrespectful of the country; rather, it is an expression of faith in the potential of our nation. Yet this attitude - because of the affiliation between the peace movement and the New Left - is effectively repressed and condemned by the Establishment (or, if you prefer, the Silent Majority). Stephen L. Samusson - Dallas."

Some of the callers misperceived the articles to mean that Dr. Smith was prohibited from wearing a U. S. flag pin. When explained that it was a distortion of the U. S. flag, they quickly agreed with the Veterans Administration's position.

Times Herald Staff Writer, Dick Shaffer wrote under his byline, "Face in the Crowd" a sub-heading on March 31, 1970: "Dr. Donald K. Smith - 'I wore it to express that peace and patriotism are not incompatible.'" Excerpts from the reporter's interview:

"It surprises you to see Don Smith making waves, but then he has changed a lot lately. . . He is still a mild, nearsighted single man who wears a calendar watchband and always rests his drink on a coaster. . . He mixes his V.O. and water with a jigger and as carefully as a pharmacist compounding a prescription. He is president and membership chairman of the single adults group at the First Unitarian Church - although he was raised a Southern Baptist - and his favorite sports are an occasional game of tennis or Frisbee.

"He drives a 1969 Tempest with automatic transmission and carries a gold-plated pen and pencil set (a Ph.D. graduation gift) in the pocket of his button-down shirts. . . Don Smith is a 30-year-old psychologist who voted for Barry Goldwater in 1964 and likes to read Ayn Rand and C. S. Lewis.

". . . Maybe it all started when Smith opened a Saturday Review of Literature one day in New York and saw an ad for the pin which is sold by Save-the-Flag, Inc. He ordered two. . . Or maybe . . . last summer when Dr. Smith abandoned the crew cut he had worn since 1957 and began to let his hair grow. Or did it start in November with wire frames? Or two weeks ago when he started growing a moustache?

"'I wouldn't call myself a liberal - but I seem to have been adopting their life-styles lately.'. . . Perhaps the walls of the Turtle Creek apartment reflect the transition or balance he is trying to achieve. Mail-order peace and love posters decorate the rooms. On one wall a barefoot couple embrace on a vacant beach beneath the word 'love.' On the opposite wall is a decoupage copy of the Declaration of Independence.

". . . .'I consider the request to take the pin off unreasonable.' He smiled. 'You know, the funny thing is that I've never done anything like this before.'"

The April 24, 1970 issue of The San Diego Union printed an earlier Dallas Times-Herald editorial and a copy by an unsigned California reader was mailed to my VAH office.

A Matter of Opinion
Lapel Pin Has Point

"From the Dallas Times-Herald

"The lapel controversy at the Veterans' Administration Hospital in Dallas apparently boiled down to a difference of opinion about the pin's effect on patients.

"Dr. Donald K. Smith, who wears a pin consisting of an American flag surrounded by a dove, said in an interview he said he would take it off if he thought it interfered with his work as a psychologist. Dr. Smith's supervisor, Dr. A. J. Jernigan, says the pin does disturb the war veterans in the wards and has transferred the official to research duties.

"Dr. Smith says he believes he should be free to wear his dove-flag pin anywhere 'as long as it doesn't hurt anyone else.' As a psychologist, he should be able to determine quickly whether any of the Veterans Hospital patients are affronted by the political pin."

The person who sent the articles wrote, "And he knows it does. Good for you. Glad to know of an Administrator with common sense and the courage to enforce it. Our Veterans need people like you, and the country does too."

Dr. Smith, a non-veteran, began a tedious appeal process as outlined by Personnel's Rules and Procedures. A note to Mother on Friday, May 8, 1970,

"Have tried all week to drop you a note but this has been an unusually busy week. We held a grievance hearing on the staff psychologist and I was testifying from 10:00 to 3:00 PM. Am glad that is over."

Fifth Circuit Court of Appeals

Dr. Smith hired a lawyer and brought suit against me and the Veterans Administration. VA lawyers took charge at that point. I was never required to testify. Don lost the appeal to the 5th Circuit Court of Appeals, New Orleans.

The Dallas Morning News for October 10, 1974 reported: "Appeals Court Upholds Psychologist's Firing." Quotes from the decision: "Smith was fired from his job at the Dallas Veterans Administration hospital May 27, 1970, 11 weeks after he began wearing a small pin showing a white dove superimposed over an American flag. Hospital administrators had warned Smith on several occasions against wearing the pin in front of emotionally disturbed veterans."

Said the 5th Circuit, "The controversy involved did not arise on the hustings, in a classroom, at a political gathering, on a public street or in a public park. It arose in a veterans administration hospital. . . We feel that the action of the veterans administration in insulating its patients from what the hospital administration considered to be potentially harmful stimulus was well directed and free from constitutional imperfections."

In June 1975 Kentucky classmate, Bob Ferguson, Chief, Psychology Service, Murfreesboro, Tenn. wrote: "Thought you might find [this article] amusing, particularly the, 'aged supervisor,' bit." The Article:

St. Petersburg Times, [no city identified] Wednesday, May 21, 1975:

"BALANCE OF JUSTICE
What Happened?

"Doctor Smith a young clinical psychologist treated emotionally disturbed war veterans in the VA Hospital. While on duty, he wore a 'peace pin' in his lapel - an American flag with a white dove on it.

"His aged supervisor was infuriated, 'You can't wear a peace pin in a VA Hospital while treating Vietnam veterans,' he yelled. It's against regulations.'

"The psychologist refused to remove it. 'My right of free speech would be violated if the hospital forced me to take it off.'

"'Wear it as long as you want,' said the supervisor. 'You're fired.'

"The psychologist filed suit in federal court demanding his job back.

"Who won?

"Donald does not get his job back, ruled the judge. 'Freedom of speech is not absolute,' he said. 'Wearing a peace pin could be harmful to the care and rehabilitation of boys who have been severely injured in Vietnam.'

"(Based on a recent federal appeals court decision in Texas as retold by Law Prof. John Ritter and Atty. Paul Levine. Smith v. U.S. 73-2435, 5th Cir. 1974.)"

Sadly, I lost track of Don Smith, and never again had contact with him professionally or personally. I regret we were unable to reach an acceptable resolution of the conflict with this likeable young man.

Black or White

Group test findings from the State Survey, VA group test data, and high school student responses stimulated an interest in racial differences. Of special interest were racial differences by students in verbal and non-verbal recall, and the human figure drawings made by black and white subjects.

Dr. Don Smith expressed interest in developing a research project to determine if there was a similar recall difference among our black and white patient population. His exploratory research lay dormant, and the project became Dr. Smith's duty assignment during the Peace Pin issue. My interest in the incomplete research subject continued after his firing.

The Goodenough-Harris Drawing Test elicits projective qualities from an individual's drawing of human figures. The question: "Do individuals express racial characteristics in the Draw-a-Person (DAP) so that the race of the Ss can be identified?" The answer was a qualified yes. The results were accepted for publication by the Journal of Projective Techniques & Personality Assessment. 3

Students from Dallas Baptist College (white) and Bishop College (black) served as judges as did the psychology staff of Southwestern Medical. Reprints of the article, "Judging Whether a Patient Is White or Black By His Draw-A-Person Test" were sent to Dr. Cliff S. Harris, Jr., Dallas Baptist College, Dr. Barbara Wilcox, Assistant Professor, Bishop College, and Dr. Maurice Korman, SWMS with the notation:

"I thought perhaps you would like a copy of the attached reprint as you and your students participated in the research. Again, thank you for your help in making this paper possible."

May Events

Brother-in-law, Jim Wysong extended an invitation to play golf with him at Hurricane Creek Country Club, a new rural course near the Grayson-Collin County line. Jim was a member. It was a fun afternoon.

More than 35 individuals came to a shower for Sandy Seaman, hosted by Jean at our home in May. Sandy and Mark Gutzler received many beautiful gifts.

A card mailed in July to Blanche from Jack and Jean.

"We're enjoying this pretty weather, but will need rain soon. We have our annual church picnic tomorrow night - wish you were here to go with us. We took the sail boat out after supper by the lake at Dallas Baptist College - the boys really did enjoy it. We surely had some good services at our church Sunday - a youth choir from Alabama and a drama group from State B.S.U. Jean is feeling well - hope you are too."

Jean wrote on opposite side of card: "We're fine - enjoyed Stewart's visit. We had a quiet weekend . . . want to get rid of the sinus drainage before we go to Colorado. The Fains came over last night and had supper . . . They are busy studying; Beth takes her finals this week." (July 6)

At the VAH

Dr. Jack Davis, a member of the VACO Staff, Washington, D. C., called to ask if I would consider accepting the transfer of Staff Psychologist George Haven from the Waco VA Hospital. Do not recall if the telephone call was pre or post "Peace Pin" dilemma. The request had an "out of the frying pan into the fire" aura, but agreed to consider after discussing the request with the staff.

Dr. Haven was a disabled Korean War veteran, who suffered a head wound in battle resulting in loss of one eye. (He wore an eye-patch). Dr. Davis described Dr. Haven as a well trained, friendly psychologist (and he was), but unhappy at Waco. Jack Davis believed Dr. Haven would be better adjusted with the Dallas VAH or words to that effect.

Our staff interviewed Dr. Haven and with some reservations, agreed to the transfer. He was assigned the office previously occupied by Drs. Bill Hales and Don Smith.

We received two University of Texas Psychology Trainees for the summer of 1970: Charles A. Pierce, Level II Counseling Psychology Trainee, and Joanne Sheahan, Level I Clinical Psychology Trainee. Charles came for two weeks during semester break in January 1970 and returned May 18, 1970 to accumulate 500 hours of training by August 1, 1970. His evaluation summary:

"Mr. Pierce was supervised by Dr. John Geers . . . and had frequent contact with other Unit Psychologists . . . participated in group testing, the Industrial Therapy program, individual evaluation of patients from the Medical, Surgical, and Psychiatric Services, individual counseling with patients presenting a variety of problems and a limited research project.

"In all of his work, Mr. Pierce demonstrated a mature, well-motivated and interested approach. He relates well to patients . . . and hospital personnel. He hopes to complete his academic work, and dissertation during current academic year, and devote two years to work in a hospital setting."

Joanne Sheahan began a 40-hour-a-week tour of duty on June 1, 1970 and completed 500 hours of experience on August 20, 1970. Following are excerpts from her evaluation:

"Miss Sheahan was assigned to the Consultation Program . . . was an observer-participant in the weekly group assessment program . . . was asked to individually follow a psychiatric patient she had observed in group testing. She averaged two new individual cases a week. . . was an alert, eager student. . . accumulated additional skills in such techniques as the WAIS, Human Figure Drawings, Bender Gestalt, TAT, and Rorschach. . . using the Beck System. She was introduced to the Cornell Medical Index, Ravens Progressive Matrices, Roos Time Reference Inventory, Description of Condition Test (DOC), etc.

". . . She was a participant-observer in a once-a-week Mental Hygiene Clinic group led by Dr. Ralph Robinowitz . . . led the group during Dr. Robinowitz's absence. She met weekly with Dr. R. B. Tucker's group psychotherapy seminar.

"Miss Sheahan. . . completed a brief research project. . . chose the Description of Condition technique. . . selected from the clinical files a group of 48 patients for detailed study. Following a careful review of Novinger and Kessler's two volume work, Measuring Ego Development. . . applied their scoring system to the DOC and correlated the results with the rating scale for the DOC currently in use. . . found they are significantly correlated. . . Miss Sheahan is an above average clinical psychology trainee."

Ronald V. Kidd came on duty November 1, 1970 at the Dallas VAH as a Level III Trainee on the Psychiatric Service, under the direct supervision of Dr. Tucker. His appointment began August 30, but through a training contract with the University of Texas, the first 180 hours of training at Level III were accomplished at the Counseling-Psychological Services Center, University of Texas at Austin, Texas.

National Wildlife Conference

The National Wildlife Federation was to inaugurate a full week of activities for families at a National Wildlife Summit in Estes Park, Colorado in July of 1970 featuring Roger Tory Peterson. Jackie and Richard were not especially excited about the idea at first, but agreed that it might be O. K.

We mailed a deposit of $160 March 9, 1970. The boys bought a two man tent so they could participate in an overnight event at Estes Park.

It was a great experience for the four of us. There were times Jean did not feel well, but didn't complain as she participated in all the outdoor activities. One of the high-lights was an early morning bird walk with Roger Tory Peterson.

The Summit gave each visitor an opportunity to study nature in Estes Park's outdoor classroom through the guidance of distinguished teachers in subjects such as geology, biology, botany, wild life preservation, photography, etc. All four of us thrived on the week of learning, fun, and relaxation.

A frightening high-light was our being awakened one night and informed Richard had been cut accidentally by his brother while erecting their tent during their overnight campout. Richard was taken to a local physician for stitches on his arm. He carries a prominent scar.

Jackie began his creative film making at the Summit. He asked and was given permission to take brief close-up 8 mm movie shots of a dozen or more out-of-state automobile license plates of Summit participants.

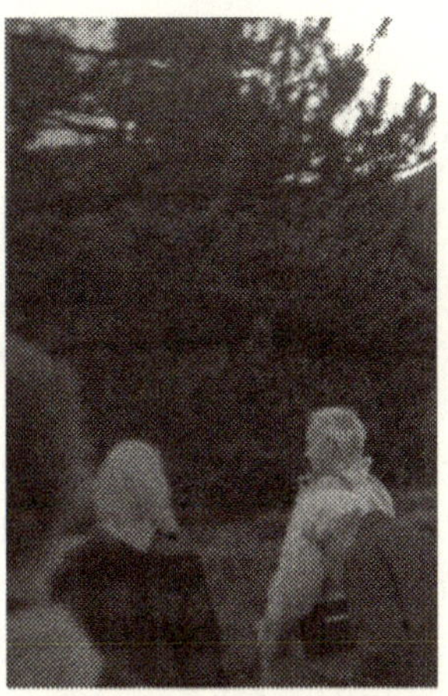

Roger Tory Peterson

Back Home – Hospital - Cards and Letters

Jean underwent hysterectomy surgery at Baylor Hospital in August 1970. Jean wrote her mother-in-law after her discharge from Baylor Hospital August 12, 1970.

". . . . We are grateful to be getting along so well. Jack, Sr. is getting the worst of the deal, I'm afraid.

Love, Jean -August 17, 1970"

The Fains began their fall studies at U. T., Arlington. A postcard to Mother:

"Your card to Jackie was so nice and he appreciated it and the gift. We hope to have a good birthday for him tomorrow. Beth is helping with it. Jean has been up and down but is making strong, steady progress. She gets bored just sitting still. We are trying to get ready for school next week. My, this has been a short summer."

Jack, Jr. sent his grandmother a thank you letter August 24, 1970, and told how he obtained his drivers license.

"Dear Grandma,

". . . On my birthday I got my driver's license so when I come up to your house I can drive you wherever you want to go. I had no difficulty when it came to taking the test but we encountered a few problems otherwise. Beth was on her way over to take me to the place where I was to take the test and she had a flat. With Mother in the front seat with me, I drove over and got Beth and Lisa at the gas station. We went on to get my license, but when we got there, I discovered I had forgotten a document saying I had passed driver's training. So we drove back home. We couldn't find it, so we went to my school, where they made me another one. Halfway back I discovered I didn't have my parent's signatures on another paper I had to fill out. We didn't want to go home then. Anyway, as you know, I got my license.

"I don't know where the summer has gone, but it's all but over now since school starts Tuesday (the 25th).

"Well, I've got to go now. Thanks again, and come see us sometime when you can.

Love,
Jack, [Jr.]"

In a brief letter to Mother, early September, wrote:

"Jean is continuing to get her strength back. She did too much over the weekend and felt it some on Monday, but was fine by Tuesday. We kept Lisa Monday and Wednesday nights and she was so good. She is a very remarkable baby."

"The boys are enjoying their school. For sports, Jack is taking tennis and Richard swimming. Richard doesn't want to go out for football and if he doesn't that is fine with us. Jackie is enjoying experimenting with movie taking. He will have to bring them sometime so you can see them. His car driving is coming in handy now."

Jackie was involved with movie making while Richard's interest for the moment was the repair of small motors. Richard overhauled a lawnmower motor in belief he would make a profit. Jackie presented one of his movies to class on September 24, 1970. The three Fains came for lunch on Sunday, the day after Beth's nineteenth birthday. She received many nice gifts.

Beth sent her grandmother a thank you letter September 30, 1970.

"Dear Grandma Blanche,

"Thank you so much for the $3.00. I need a belt to wear with a couple of skirts, so I imagine I'll use it for that. And today I received my first issue of "Contengo." I've only had a chance to thumb through it, but it really looks like a fine magazine.

"I had a very nice birthday. Jay took me out to dinner and to a show. Something we hadn't done in months.

"Jay and I are both studying hard. Tests always come in cycles - and this next week is the time. We really are enjoying our classes, but it seems we have more reading than we ever have.

"Lisa is really getting around - trying to do everything. After you left, I took her to the foot doctor, and he put a slight correction in her shoes - she was slightly pigeon-toed. Tonight Lisa tried to brush her teeth. Right now she's back in the bedroom telling Jay some tale.

"I got put on the telephone committee in Sunday School. Like grandmother, like granddaughter! Ha! Ha!

"Well must get ready for class. Jay and Lisa send their love, Thank you again for all your thoughtfulnesses.

Love,
Beth"

Jackie and Richard mowed for Inez Coffey Alexander (a third cousin) during 1970. Inez and Dr. Nelson Alexander divorced, and the house was for sale.

In early October I wrote: "Beth and Jay studied all weekend - they have tests this week. Jay came over Saturday, changed the oil and washed his car. The boys mowed for Inez Saturday. I went over to see how they were doing and visited with her. She is planning to sell her home she gets 1/2 of it. . . We have tickets to the play '1776' which starts this Friday at the State Fair."

Southern Research Support Center

The Veterans Administration opened a "Southern Research Support Center" at the Little Rock VA Hospital and offered research services to all VA Hospitals in the region. Four years after the Texas State Survey, we believed there was an opportunity to complete a statistical analysis of the mass of psychological information gathered in 1966. Walter Penk and I outlined twenty-six questions concerning survey data scores that required means, standard deviations, etc. A copy of the October narrative went to Dr. Alex Pokorny with an invitation for him to also submit questions for analysis of interest. Walter's eight page narrative, directed to Mr. Dennis Robinettee, Biostatistician, Southern Research Support Center, included a review of analyses prior to October 1970. 4

In the letter to Dr. Pokorny it was noted that Wayne Holtzman would be informed. There had not been any communication with Wayne about the State Survey since 1968, and remarked to Alex that ". . . the last time I talked with him, Wayne seemed rather discouraged about the data." It is my recollection that Wayne's staff discovered flaws in the State's recording of the raw data.

That was the last grand effort to complete analyses of the data.

Back to the Family

My forty-ninth birthday was celebrated at Sedalia. Each member of the Fain and Jernigan family (except Richard) signed Blanche's Guest Book, 10-24-70. Jay wrote: "Jay, Beth & Lisa Fain Dallas Wonderful lunch on Jack's Birthday." A. J. Jernigan, Sr. wrote: "Thank you for the 1st 49 years. You have sent me into the 50th with the same love and kindness as you did on the 1st."

Jay stayed home and visited with Lisa during his vacation. Jean wrote, "Jay and Jack played golf yesterday. I miss Lisa, but she is really enjoying Jay from what they say."

I wrote the first week of November that the release form for Civil War Headstone for Andrew J. Jernigan arrived and required the signature of an official of the cemetery. (Mr. Standridge signed as owner of the land surrounding the Jernigan graves.) The letter concluded, "Last night Jay locked his keys in his car and Beth, Lisa and I went over to Arlington with Beth's set. We enjoyed the trip."

On Their Way to Vietnam

We waxed floors at 4012 Fountainhead in preparation for the November 22, 1970 "Open House" for Captains David and Pat Jernigan. Mother told all the details in a letter to her friend Mary Lance.

"Stewart's son, David got married Nov. 7th to a young lady whose home is in Washington, D. C. David had been writing me that I <u>must</u> come to the wedding but I did not go but of course Mary and Stewart flew up and Susan and her husband and 2 children drove up. . . David and Patricia are in service - both are Captains. They went for a few days honeymoon. Then drove through to Alabama for a 2 or 3 day stay with Susan. Then came on to Bryan to see the parents. Then on Sunday afternoon Jack and Jean had an Open House for them and invited <u>all</u> the cousins and some of Mary's relatives and some friends from McKinney. It was all so nice and we all got to be together but Pansy was not able to come. She says it makes her nervous to get in a crowd. Natalie and <u>all</u> four of Claude's children were there. Also Mozelle (Pansy's daughter) - Kermit's family didn't come. He called and said he had to practice some music they were using at their church [First Baptist, Dallas] that night. Some of <u>my</u> kin came too.

"David and Patricia brought me home and spent the night. The next day they went to San Antonio to visit <u>her</u> sister's family. Her sister and husband were both in the wedding party. Then they came back to Bryan and spent Thanksgiving with Mary and Stewart. They flew to San Francisco and on to Vietnam. Patricia will be in Saigon but David had not been given his assignment. Of course they are hoping they would be together. I think Patricia is going to stay only the one year as they both want a family. O, how I wish this war could be terminated but in the right way if there is one."

Texas Psychological Association Annual Meeting

Betty Cleland sent a memo to: "Members of this lovely Board" on November 2, 1970: "We will meet in my room at the St. Anthony Hotel in San Antonio, Friday, December 4, 1970, at 12 noon. . . Jack [Wheeler] will make the final report to the TPA business meeting Friday afternoon."

Jack Wheeler mailed each member a draft of the report. Excerpts presented by Jack at TPA:

"As most of you know, this is the final report of the Texas Board of Psychological Examiners to the Texas Psychological Association. The passage of Senate Bill 667 (Psychologists' Certification and Licensing Act) in the 1969 Legislature created the long-sought statutory certification and licensing of psychologists in Texas and established the Texas State Board of Examiners of Psychologists. Thus the need for the voluntary certification Board has passed. When those persons certified to the end of December, 1970, are no longer certified, because their certificates are not being renewed by TBPE, the Board will, in all respects, cease to exist. (See Appendix for more information.)

". . . . The Board will continue to answer letters from other state boards seeking verification of certification, but will, effective December 31, 1970, dissolve as an entity. The tax-exempt status of the Board rested on its agreement to give all remaining assets, in the event of dissolution, to the Texas Psychological Association. The executive committee of TPA has voted to give those assets to the new Texas State Board of Examiners of Psychologists.

". . . . The profession of psychology in Texas owes a debt of thanks to those twenty-one psychologists who have been members of the Board during its lifetime. These men and women served without compensation and largely without recognition through the trying years while the profession attempted to establish a vehicle through which it could exercise its responsibility to the public. The profession also owes unceasing gratitude to the indispensable efforts of the Board's executive secretary, Betty, Mrs. Charles Cleland. [Betty added: 'A bit thick!']

"Past and present members of the Texas Board of Psychological Examiners:

Gordon Anderson	Earl Koile

Theodore Andreychuk
Richard B. Austin
Gladys Guy Brown
Wayne S. Gill
Harold Goolishian
Carl Hereford
Ruth Hubbard
Ira Iscoe
A. Jack Jernigan
Irwin Jay Knopf
Maurice Korman
George Kramer
John MacNaughton
Harry Martin
Glenn Ramsey
Laurence Smith
Joseph Thorpe
John Wheeler
Harold Weiner

"For twenty years--from 1949 to 1969--the profession of psychology attempted to obtain statutory regulation of psychological practice. Finally, Senate Bill 667 was passed by the 1969 Texas Legislature and this goal was achieved. No psychologist should forget the twenty year struggle, nor fail to recognize the vital role in that effort played by the Texas Board of Psychological Examiners during the 1960's. The present and final members of this Board wish to congratulate the profession of which we are members on so ably exercising its responsibility to the people of Texas.

Respectfully submitted,
John I. Wheeler, Ph.D., Chairman"

Christmas 1970

We had open house for VA Psychology Staff, Trainees and their families 12 days before Christmas.

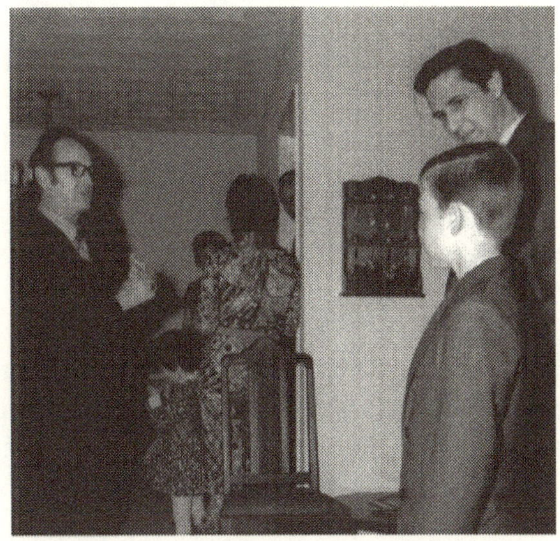

Buzz Tucker – Mark and Walter Penk

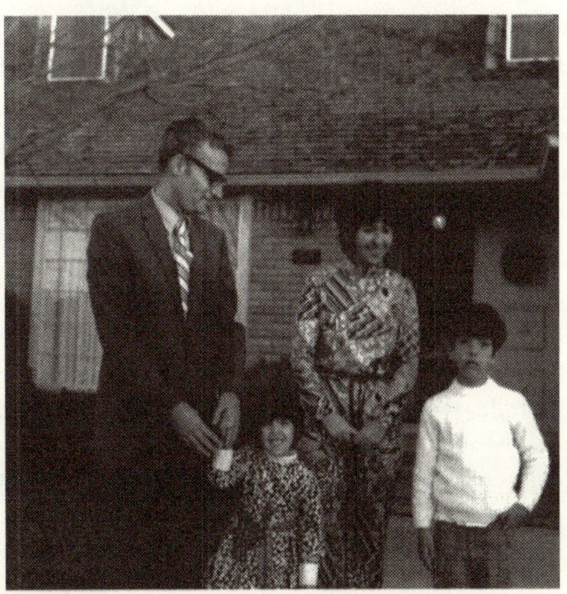

Ralph – Jill – Hanna – Howard – Robinowitz

The Robinowitz family was photographed in our front yard. Because of our schedules we had not "put-up" the Christmas tree. Hanna reported the children were disappointed for they were looking forward to seeing our Christmas tree.

Blanche wrote her friend Mary Lance December 15:

"I'm going to Kingsville to spend Christmas with Jamie and family. Guess I will go Sunday. Jack's coming for me Sunday morning. I am going to fly and Jamie will meet me at Corpus Christi. I've always gone by bus except one time I flew back. I can't do much flying. It is too expensive for me.

"But after this I'm staying at home for Christmas. I miss the getting ready for at least some of them to come. Jamie and Frances come every Christmas and they wanted all of us to come down there but I am the only one going, I believe.

". . . . I'll write again before too long. May God continue to watch over you. Isn't it wonderful to know our Heavenly Father loves us and never fails us as we so often fail Him. I love my Bible reading of mornings. Wish I had read it more when I was young. I have read it through every year since 1954 but O I know so little about it's great treasures compared to what there is to know."

Civil War Headstone

A Government Bill of Lading arrived announcing that the Office of the Chief of Support Services Department of the Army, Washington, D. C. was shipping "Non-Military, Crated Headstone Cut and Lettered, -----, Hand Rubbed - Andrew J. Jernigan."

The stone was shipped December 29, 1970 from Hillsboro, Texas. We stored it in our garage and set at the foot of Andrew Jackson Jernigan's grave in March 1971.

Chapter 14 - 1971

The family enjoyed some of Mother's canned black eyed peas New Years Day, 1971. An extant record indicated we exchanged the 1968 Plymouth for a 1971 Plymouth at Gene Hays Motors in McKinney for $3867 that same day.

Jamie was in town the first week of January for a professional meeting, and while waiting his return flight to Corpus took Jean and the boys to Kip's restaurant for hamburgers. I tested a private client, and did not join in the festivities.

It was tree pruning time and I spent one weekend moving plants and shaping trees. There was an accumulated seven years growth for those trees we transplanted on our barren 4012 Fountainhead lot in 1964.

The word was out about Jackie's movie making interests and skills. His Sunday School class invited him to assist in the creation of a movie film. The group met at our house for a Saturday session.

Jay, Beth and Lisa came for Sunday lunch the 17th, and we watched the afternoon Super Bowl. Beth transferred to Texas Woman's University mid-term, and made her first drive to Denton Monday morning, January 18, 1971.

Jackie (Austin) printed a letter to Grandma in bold letters on both sides of an 8 1/2 by 11 inch sheet of paper. The front side was in bold blue and the reverse side in bold red. Grandma was pleased with his name identification switch.

Jan. [20] 1971

"DEAR GRANDMA,

"I HOPE YOU ARE IN GOOD HEALTH AND HIGH SPIRITS. BUT I AM MAINLY WRITING YOU TO EXPRESS GREAT APPRECIATION FOR THE CHRISTMAS GIFT YOU SENT ME. IN CASE YOU ARE WONDERING, I SPENT IT ON MY TRIP TO COLORADO, WHERE I HAD A GREAT TIME. THE SKIING THERE WAS [changes color to red] GREAT, NOT TO MENTION EVERYTHING ELSE WE DID. AND I DON'T THINK I COULD HAVE MADE IT WITHOUT THAT CHECK FROM YOU.

"I HOPE TO SEE YOU SOON AND UNTIL THEN, GOODBYE,

LOVE,
AUSTIN"

Richard bought a new bike with his savings. His Sunday School youth group took a church sponsored trip to East Texas the first of February. Austin and Sunday School members worked on their film that weekend at our house. They finished the film February 26.

Beth wrote her grandmother 16 Feb 1971.

"Dear Grandma Blanche,

"How are you? Jay, Lisa, and I are all well. Jay is going to UTA 4 nights a week and studying hard. He says he doesn't mind the work because he's enjoying his subjects. I like TWU. The drive isn't bad because it's a much better road and only takes about 10 minutes longer to get to Denton than it does to Arlington. I am particularly enjoying a course, "Speech Handicaps in the Classroom." Not only is it very helpful in my field of study (Special

Education) but it's particularly interesting in the descriptions of language development in children. I enjoy using what I know in helping Lisa with her sounds.

"In March I will be working with a handicapped child either mentally or physically. It will be good experience.

"We so often think of you and wish we could be with you. You know that you are one of our favorite people and we love you so. Jay will be on vacation in two months. I know it's a long time but we plan to see you then at the very latest.

"We had some bad news. Jay is going to have to have his wisdom teeth cut out, whenever he can work it into his busy schedule.

"Well I must study while Lisa is asleep. I apologize for the shortness of the letter, but I did want to say hello.

We love you,
Beth, Jay and Lisa"

Dr. Darold Morgan, Pastor at Cliff Temple Baptist Church resigned February 14, 1971 to become Chairman of the Southern Baptist Annuity Board. Assistant Pastor, Les Morris served during the interim.

The Fains came for hamburgers on Friday night. Jean and I saw "Fiddler on the Roof" starring Robert Merrill at State Fair Music Hall, Sunday afternoon, February 19, 1971.

Jean spent two days with her Aunt Betty Muse at the McKinney hospital. We had very complimentary reports on Austin and Richard during Open House the first week in March. Austin's algebra teacher proclaimed him "her best student."

Richard thanked his Grandma Blanche on March 10, 1971 for her gift to him on his fourteenth birthday

"Dear Grandma,

"Thank you very much for the five dollars. As you know I got a new bike. Friday I had two blowouts [overfilled with air] on it so your money will come in handy.

"I haven't been down in a while so I'll be down soon. I might ride my bike down.

Love,
Richard"

I wrote March 19th: "Lisa got some braces this week to correct 'toe-in'. She wears them during the day and she is quickly adapting (they cost the kids $80). We are doing well. The Fains have invited us over for Saturday night supper, barbecued turkey. I plan to go to St Louis Sunday after S. S. (leave at 12:15)."

Professional Meetings

I stayed at the Chase Park Plaza Hotel in St. Louis March 21, 1971 while attending the Veterans Administration meeting.

I explored the grounds of the 1904 St. Louis World's Fair in Forest Park and collected information about the site. Photos taken by my Dad and his brother Jim were stimuli for the interest. Jean's Mother, Mary Chambers attended the 1904 Fair with Otho Harris and his two sisters.

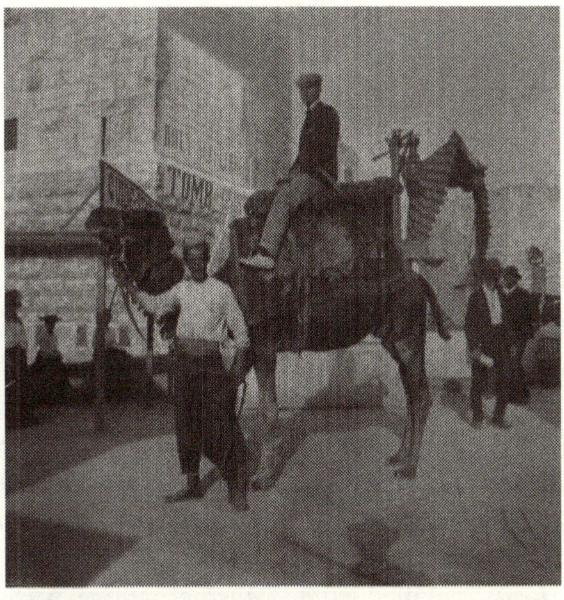

(Above) Austin Jernigan on Camel, "Church of Holy Sepulcher" St. Louis Worlds Fair, photograph by Jim (note shadow).

I mailed the family a Picture Postcard March 22, 1971 of the "Statue of Saint Louis - in Front of City Art Museum in Forest Park, St. Louis, Mo."

"Dear Family,

It is 29 degrees here. Yesterday I walked thru the Park and visited the Museum. I took a picture of 'The Rabbit,' but will probably not appear as I needed a flash. Took the patch off but need to keep it covered. Glad you sent the round band-aides.

Love - Jack – Daddy"

The "Rabbit" by Durer then on display at the City Art Museum in St. Louis was mentioned because during a professional trip to New Orleans I purchased a copy of Durer's famous painting.

Professional Territory

Psychological assessment and its interpretation are considered a sacrosanct function by Clinical Psychologists. Minnesota Multiphasic Personality Inventory (MMPI) profile sheets began to appear in Dallas VAH patient clinical files. We discovered that at least one physician was using the technique most inappropriately to treat patients, and soon learned other psychiatrists were following his pattern. Psychology Trainee Ron Kidd documented a conversation with one of the psychiatrists about her attempt to use the test findings. This behavior was reported in the annual "Psychology Service Narrative Report" to VA Central Office. Dr. Oliver J. Harris, Regional Medical Director, Region #3, VACO, Washington, D. C. requested more information.

Dr. Harris' detailed letter of further inquiry was discussed with Dr. Isham Kimball. Six areas were covered: The physicians may lack necessary formal training; test being used to determine drug dosage, to grant passes, etc.; "cook-book" interpretations made; test data should not be in clinical file; the tests were not purchased through hospital Supply - profile sheets were verifaxed; etc.

The final paragraph of Psychology's response to Dr. Oliver Harris:

"Psychology has had a centralized group assessment service for psychiatric patients for a number of years. For a period of two years every patient admitted to the Psychiatric Service was routinely assessed with a battery of tests within the first week of admission. Approximately 16 months ago, in agreement with the Psychiatric Service, the group assessment program was placed on a referral basis. Ph.D. psychologists assume responsibility for the program. These psychologist do not approve of making judgments regarding the functions mentioned in paragraph b [diagnose, grant passes, determine drugs to be prescribed, etc.] or on the basis of any single instrument. Psychology does frequently employ the

MMPI or a variant, the Mini-Mult, in the assessment of patients as part of the battery of tests. However, Psychology does not accept specific prescription for the administration of any psychological test."

The hospital's well meaning physicians were redirected by the Chief of Psychiatry. The conflict was an example of the type of necessary alertness and initiative required in a hospital setting to maintain balance among professional disciplines. It was and is a never ending battle.

A Florida Conference

Scheduled to leave for Bay Pines, Florida on April 19 and be in Houston April 30th, wrote, "I'm beginning to feel like a salesman."

I flew to Tampa, Florida Monday night, April 19, 1971 to attend a VA sponsored Conference on Automation at St. Petersburg VAH: "Psychological Assessment and Programming." The participants stayed at Tampa's Happy Dolphin Inn near the Gulf of Mexico's beautiful white sandy beach.

It was a timely meeting considering the recent Dallas VAH assessment conflict. The St. Petersburg Conference was one of the early discussions on practical computerized psychological assessment. I reviewed the current group assessment program at Dallas VAH and was a participant in another presentation according to a letter written before leaving for Florida. Our papers were later published in the VA Newsletter for Research in Psychology: Vol. XIII, No. 2, May 1971, 35-36.

Film Festival

A note to Mother Tuesday, April 27, 1971, "Jackie and I go to Austin early Friday. I hope this turns out well for him. Your place looks so pretty. I'm proud of the way you keep it up and are able to care for yourself, and continually amazed at your energy."

The second annual Texas Student Film Festival at St. Stephen's Episcopal School, Austin, Texas came the weekend of the annual meeting of the Southwestern Psychological Association in San Antonio, Texas, April 29, through May 1, 1971. I attended sections of the Film Festival and some of the San Antonio meeting.

Austin [Jackie] won an award in special effects for a film that featured Lisa, titled "Wabbit Chasing." The award read: "Congratulations for having won a prize for Best Optical Effects in the second annual Texas Student Film Festival. Your outstanding entry prompted the judges to create a new category for future entrants."

Austin's prize was a "50 x 50 beaded wall type screen" (pull-down movie screen) of such quality that we continue to use it into the twenty first century. He has been making creative films ever since. We both learned much and had a most enjoyable time at the Saturday night presentations May 1, 1971.

Preserving the Wounded

There are no extant records about the purpose for the Houston trip. Records document a room at the Tidelands Motor Inn, on May 6, 1971 with reimbursement and an airplane ticket from the Veterans Administration. 1

The May 6, 1971 Houston VAH meeting may have been the occasion of the nation-wide effort by the Veterans Administration and the Defense Department to educate VAH Professional Staff on the U. S. Army Medical Service heroic efforts to preserve the lives of men and women wounded in battle in Vietnam. We were briefed on medical and psychological triage of the wounded by an on the spot, uncensored film of dramatic battlefield rescue scenes "To

Save a Soldier." We returned to our VA Hospitals with renewed incentive to develop new treatment programs.

New Staff

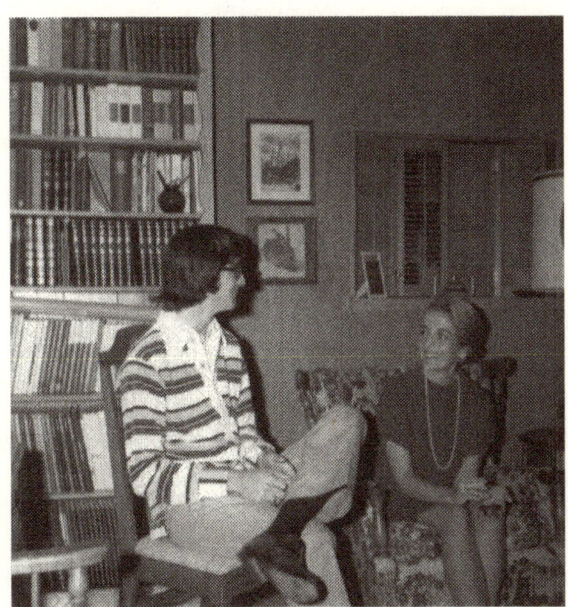

Mary Louise King Toland was appointed in 1970 to develop the Psychology Unit at the Day Hospital. This charming Tennessee Belle joined the Dallas VAH Staff directly from graduate school. The photo is Joe Gallo (son of Mrs. Gallo) and Mary Louise Toland at Open House, December 1970.

Mary Louise was subsequently placed in charge of the Psychology Unit in the Mental Hygiene Clinic.

Dr. Toland requested an appointment with the Chief of Psychology from time to time. She would quietly close the door, smile sweetly, and drawl, Dr. Jernigan, "I am pregnant." The purpose for the announcement was to request a special tour of duty at the Mental Hygiene Clinic. She made four such requests, and I soon caught on that Mary Louise and Tom were expecting a new addition when she closed the door, and with a grin, drawled, "Dr. Jernigan!" We were usually successful in establishing a special tour of duty for Mary Louise.

New Trainees

Don Minnick and Ron Kidd were two very active Psychology Trainees during the summer of 1971. Donald J. Minnick, Level I Trainee from University of Texas was in a training status from May 10 to August 13, 1971. Don had a split assignment under the supervision of Dr. Robinowitz in two Psychology Units: Inpatient Psychiatry and Outpatient (Mental Hygiene Clinic).

Following is Dr. Robinowitz's description of Mr. Minnick's MHC training.

"In the Outpatient Service he was assigned three patients for individual psychotherapy: a young veteran of Vietnam service struggling with choices involving schooling, career, home, etc.; a WWII veteran who previously had maintained a quite adequate adjustment but was now experiencing overwhelming feelings of doubts and fear; a married couple (who he saw together) where the veteran's difficulties emanated from and contributed to marital instability. He was able to see some change in all three of these cases. The Outpatient Service by its very nature gave him the responsibility for 'his' patient - such as writing a report for a State Employment Commission, setting up and arranging appointments, handling files and records, etc.

"Mr. Minnick is a bright, perceptive creative individual who gains much and contributes a great deal to the opportunities afforded him for learning. He sees every situation as a potential classroom or laboratory and stimulates those about him by his interest and enthusiasm. . . If there was <u>a</u> most important lesson for him to learn in psychotherapy it was that behavior tends to be consistent and major personality changes are unlikely to happen over a thirteen week period. It was felt that all three of his patients benefited considerably from his interest, his sincerity, and his warmth, as well as his knowledge. Overall, I would regard him as equal to the most capable trainee I have worked with."

I shared Texas Film Festival observations with Donald Minnick and Austin's experience in film making. Don became interested in giving patients an opportunity to produce an 8mm film as a "metaphor of their lives." This interest was described in an excerpt from Dr. Toland's evaluation of Donald Minnick:

"In addition, Mr. Minnick worked with a number of other psychologists, but showed special interest and creative thinking in assisting Dr. Mary Louise Toland in a pilot study designed to determine the merit of 8 mm film making as a therapeutic medium. He did considerable literature review, wrote a tentative prospectus and assisted in setting up the beginning guidelines for the introduction of the project to patients."

Ron Kidd began Level III training in November 1970, was promoted to Level IV in April 1971 and resigned September 10, 1971 to accept a faculty position as Instructor at the University of Texas at El Paso. He subsequently returned to Dallas to become a member of the Psychology Staff

Ron began a "rap group" for Vietnam Veterans from the Medical and Surgical wards. During the summer of 1971 he accomplished one of Psychology's goals: Survey every Vietnam Era Veteran admitted to Dallas VAH during a four month period. I shared some of the interview load with Ron, and as Chairman of the Station Vietnam Era Committee invited him to make a verbal report of findings to the Committee.

Ron completed a rough draft of the research during his last week at VAH and continued to evaluate the data at the University. He and I published the findings in 1972, titled, "Jernigan, A. J. & Kidd, R. Interview Survey of 220 Vietnam Era Patients. VA Newsletter for Research in Psychology: Vol. XVI, No. 1, February 1972, 40."

Dr. Tucker's evaluation of Trainee Ron Kidd concluded with: "He is a highly intelligent and personable young man . . . relates easily and with poise to professionals of other disciplines and to patients."

Family Matters Summer 1971

Richard's bicycle was stolen and Grandma Blanche gave him ten dollars. Richard responded in his thank you letter to her: "This summer, some friends and I want to ride our bikes to Lake Bonham. We'll stop at your house maybe overnight if you don't mind."

We made a weekend trip to Shreveport to visit Clyde and Margaret Tilton. Clyde had a new boat he wanted to show and share.

Jean froze 16 pints of beans picked from Mother's garden in June, and "gave Beth a mess."

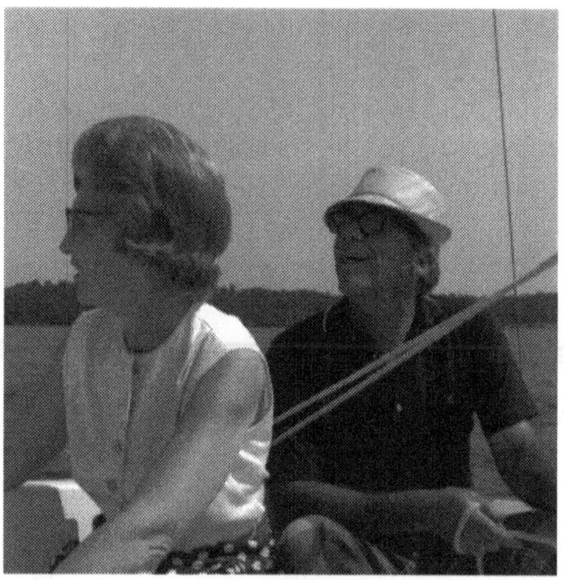

Margaret and Clyde Tilton

Beth and Jay began summer school: "The Fains are on a busy schedule. It is like the Pony Express, one gets in from school, and the other goes. Beth brings Lisa every morning. Jay is taking two night classes. Made all A's last semester. Jackie made a straight-A report card on his finals. Richard and Beth did almost as well but a B or so . . . The boys have been busy mowing yards and planting grass. Jackie is enjoying his film course at SMU."

Late June, to Mother: "Richard's new bicycle came Friday, a bright orange. He is so proud of it and thank you for your part in helping him get it. He brings it in the den each night as boys are losing bicycles in this neighborhood. . . Lisa had a mild ear problem but is now over it. The Fains are keeping up with their busy schedule. Jackie got back one of his films and it was another funny one."

Early July: "Beth started her 2nd 6 weeks today - must be in Denton by 7:30, so she and Jay had Lisa here by 6:15. They move to their new apartment this weekend. We will help them move. . . We've enjoyed the black-eyed peas; froze a good many of them."

Beth wrote Grandma Blanche, July 27, 1971.

"Dear Grandma Blanche,

"Jay told me to send this thank you note over a week ago and I kept forgetting. I'm so sorry.

"We're sending you a picture we had made for the church pictorial directory. We wanted you to have one.

"Things are really hectic around here, what with moving and going to school. We're really enjoying our new apartment. There's a room for a washer and dryer, so we got a washer and dryer. It certainly is a convenience. There is about twice as much storage space. We have closets we're not even using! There's a nice backyard. We put a little plastic pool back there for Lisa - she just loves to go swimming. Please come see us.

"In two more weeks will be through for the summer. Jay is really studying his brain off. He's taking Economics and Accounting and just loves his economics course. I'm taking a remedial reading course that's really a lot of work and a course in child growth and development.

"Lisa is getting cuter everyday. She copies everything we do.

We love you,
Beth, Jay & Lisa"

And the "week old thank-you note" from Jay:

"Dear Grandma Blanch[e],

"It was very nice to hear from you. It's always a pleasant surprise to have you remember my birthday. I haven't yet decided how I'm going to spend the money, but I will let you know.

"We are all moved into our new apartment now. We are looking forward to having you down to visit us. Beth and Lisa send their love,

Love, Jay".

New Hospital Director

Mr. Earl P. Whitaker, Director of VAH Shreveport (1965 - 1971) transferred to the same position at Dallas VA Hospital in July 1971. All previous Dallas VA Hospital Directors were physicians. Mr. Whitaker received his Bachelor of Arts degree from Doane College at Crete, Nebraska, and was a Naval Aviator during WWII. Mr. Whitaker replaced Dallas VAH Acting Director, Banks Paul.

Mr. Paul returned to his former position as Assistant Hospital Director.

A Southern Tour

The planned August trip to our second National Wildlife Conference at Ashville, North Carolina included a preliminary tour through Civil War sites with stops at Shreveport, Vicksburg, Tuscaloosa, and Lookout Mountain. Grandfather Andrew Jackson Jernigan, a member of the 30th Regiment, Tennessee Infantry fought at most of those locations. Men of the 30th from Sumner, Robertson, Smith and Davidson Counties in Tennessee trained at "Red Springs" in Tennessee in 1861. The return trip included a stop in Nashville, Tennessee.

On the possibility that "Red Springs" and "Red Boiling Springs" were one and the same, I wrote the "Postmaster, Red Boiling Springs, TN" July 25, 1971 to inquire if there had been a Civil War training camp site near his town. He replied August 3, 1971: "Dear Mr. Jernigan, We can find no one that knows anything about this at all. Sorry, Frank Sadler, Postmaster."

When away on vacation we attempted to enhance Mother's security by giving our itinerary, as in this August 4, 1971 note:

"Our address will be: c/o Conservation Summit Blue Ridge Assembly, Black Mountain, North Carolina, 28711. Telephone 704-669-8422. We leave Thursday spend the night with Clyde and Margaret. Friday, we stay at Holiday Inn, Tuscaloosa, Ala.; Saturday we will be at Holiday Inn (#1), Chattanooga, TN. We will be in Asheville, N. C. from Sunday Aug. 8 to Saturday noon Aug. 14. We spend the night of 14th in Nashville, Tenn. area and probably get home late Monday."

A Holiday Inn picture postcard message, Sunday August 8, 1971, 2100 Market Street, Chattanooga, TN:

"We have had a good trip, went thru Vicksburg Friday and Chattanooga Saturday. We saw friends [the Frank Horners] at Tuscaloosa, Ala. Friday night. We leave this morning for Ashville, should get there by noon. I took a picture of the same cannon Daddy photographed atop Lookout Mt. Hope you are feeling well.

Love, Jack"

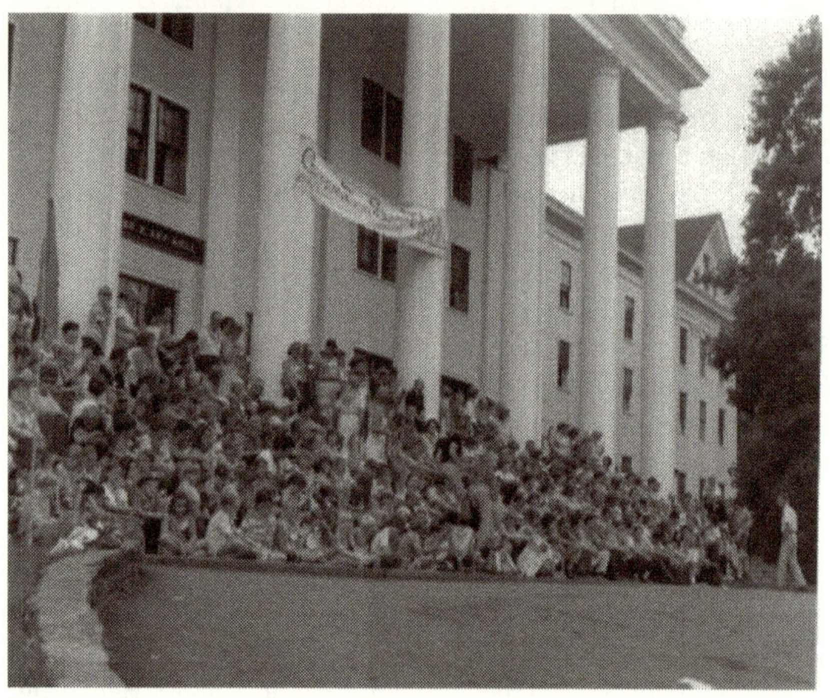

Group Photo at Summit 1971

Robert E. Lee Hall

Jean mailed a picture postcard August 9, 1971 of: "Robert E. Lee Hall - Blue Ridge Assembly, Black Mountain, North Carolina - Robert E. Lee Hall, and vacation center founded in 1912."

"Jack got to see Vicksburg, Chattanooga and Chickamauga. This is where we are staying. It is cool and damp.

Love, Jean"

Another picture postcard of Robert E. Lee Hall: "Main building at Blue Ridge Assembly, dated 8-12-71, was addressed to Mr. and Mrs. W. M. Gibson.

"Dear folks:

"We have had a very good week here. Our trip up with Clyde and Margaret was such a good way to begin a vacation. We leave Saturday for the return via Nashville. We probably will be home sometime Monday, and later in the week we will see you.

Love, Jack"

Following are some of the staff photographed at the National Wildlife Conference: Arthur Stupka, Retired Naturalist, Great Smoky National Park (Bird walk); Dr. J. W. Duffield, Professor of Silvi Culture, North Carolina University; Dr. A. Murray Evans, Department of Botany, University of Tennessee; Professor Stanley Mulaik, Emeritus Professor of Biology, University of Utah; George Harris, Managing Editor, National Wildlife Magazine; Nancy Ignatius, President of Concern, Inc. and wife of former Secretary of the Navy; Dr. Harley E. Jolley, Director of Environmental Education, Mars Hill College, N.C.; Edsel Martin, local wood carver and dulcimer maker. 2

And there were others. All were master teachers who filled minds with new ideas about the need to cherish and preserve our environmental heritage. We considered purchasing a dulcimer from Edsel Martin, but instead decided to buy one of his hand carved mockingbirds. The dulcimer came later.

At Home in Texas

Back home, we learned Beth and Jay made "straight A's" in summer school. Remarkable! Jean and I began the restoration of the "old press" from the Aunt Sis Coffey estate, and discovered that Great-grandfather Jesse Coffey assembled the walnut piece with wooden pegs.

Grandma Blanche sent Austin an extra dollar for his seventeenth birthday for being late, she thought. Austin responded:

"Dear Grandma,

"Thank you for the check you sent me. It got here right on my birthday, so if you want I'll return the extra dollar. If not, I'll put it in on the bicycle I'm trying to get. I hope you are doing alright. We are all in good health, and Daddy's back seems to be just about well.

"I don't know where the summer's gone to, and now for the first time I can remember I'm looking forward to starting to school, with the new photography course at Skyline [High School].

"Come down and visit us sometime.

Love, Austin, Jr."

The back pains were attributed to hundreds of miles of driving during the vacation. Austin attended Kimball High School in the mornings, and rode the school bus across Dallas to Skyline High School in the afternoon to attend the cinematography program for 1971-72. He was the only student to get an "A" both semesters. His instructor, Mr. Collier, took the Skyline class to the 1972 Texas Student Film Festival. Austin won two awards.

We "called" a new pastor at Cliff Temple Baptist Church, Dr. Douglas Watterson. Billy Graham held a Crusade in Dallas.

TPA Executive Committee

I attended a Texas Psychological Association Executive Committee meeting September 18-19, 1971 at the Menger Hotel, San Antonio. I recall listening to a piano player one evening at the famous Menger.

Executive Committee meetings in the 1970's were usually composed of the chairman or one representative from each standing committee, any ad hoc committee members, the President Elect, the current President, and the immediate Past President of the Association. Secretary Betty Cleland was always present.

Jack Wheeler was the 1971 President-elect. My name was mentioned as a possible candidate for President-elect for 1972.

Crusade - Church - Birthday

Billy Graham held his Dallas Crusade in September 1971. Richard went with his church group on Sunday night, September 19, 1971, and couldn't get in the stadium because of the crowd. We attended as a family Friday night, September 25, 1971. As member or Chairman of the Family Counseling Committee of Cliff Temple Baptist Church, I spent the next day in meetings at Brookside Inn, Waxahachie led by our new pastor, Dr. Doug Watterson where he outlined his vision for Cliff Temple.

Beth wrote her Grandmother September 29, 1971.

". . . We're all very busy. Jay goes to classes Monday through Thursday [nights at UTA]. I go Monday, Wed., Fri. [at TWU]. I think I may get a job as a teacher aide on Tuesday. Lisa is busy growing up.

We love you,
Beth, Jay and Lisa"

Whitaker - Tilton

Clyde Tilton, Chief of Medical Illustration at Shreveport VA Hospital was a close friend of our new Hospital Director. The two shared a mutual love of automobiles, Mr. Whitaker as master mechanic and Clyde as artist in automobile restoration. Clyde also served as an unofficial PR representative for his Dallas brother-in-law, the result being Psychology Service received special attention from the new Director.

Clyde and Margaret and Kathy and Bolin Higgs visited Dallas the first weekend of October. The Whitakers invited the Tiltons and Jernigans to their new home for dinner on Saturday night, October 2, 1971. The next day the Tiltons returned to Shreveport. The Fains and Higgs had Sunday lunch with us.

Jernigan Bell

During our brief stay at White House, Tennessee in August 1971, we visited Mr. and Mrs. John T. Hale, owners of the house built by James P. Jernigan, youngest brother of Grandpa Jernigan. The prominent dinner bell erected on the north side of "the Colonel's" house was greatly admired, and we asked the Hales to inform us if they ever decided to sell the bell. Mrs. Hale wrote they would sell the Jernigan bell for $50. Jean opened the letter, wanted to make it a surprise birthday gift, but did not have time to arrange shipment.

We mailed Mr. Hale the $50 check in October 1971. Austin and I drove to Tennessee to bring home the bell. That story appears in the next Chapter.

My fiftieth birthday fell on Sunday as noted in a letter to Mother, October 18, 1971, "I thought maybe either Friday or Saturday I might eat a bite with you since Sunday is my 50th and you started it all. I have to be at church on Sunday."

The Psychology Staff had a small party, and George Haven wrote a comical-spoof about my advancing age.

THIS IS THE DAY WE CELEBRATE
(ALBEIT SOME FOUR DAYS LATE)
PROGRESS OF HALF A CENTURY
MADE BY OUR FAVORITE PH.D.

HAPPY BIRTHDAY TO YOU, JACK
FIFTY CANDLES OUR CAKE DOES LACK
BUT FIFTY WISHES FOR YEARS MORE
GO TO OUR CHIEF WHO KNOWS THE SCORE.

TO LEAD PSYCHOLOGISTS IS QUITE A CHORE
BUT YOU'VE SURVIVED WITHOUT TOO MUCH GORE
DALLAS IS LUCKY AND WE ARE TOO
TO HAVE A CHIEF, A. J., LIKE YOU.

WE KNOW WE SOMETIMES GET IN YOUR HAIR
THIS PARTY'S TO SHOW WE REALLY CARE
BESIDES - IT GIVES US A CHANCE TO SHIRK
AND LEGALLY GET OUT OF WORK.

Writ by George Haven, Ph. D.
October 27, 1971

A Little Genealogy

Earlier Civil War Centennial research stimulated interest in discovering more about family heritage. Mother came for a visit and was encouraged to research the Jernigan-Fields connection through Anna Lou (Fields) Brown of Westminster. She and I attended James Whitmore's portrayal of Will Rogers at McFarland Auditorium November 1, 1971. She later spoke as if she saw Will Rogers, himself. James Whitmore's version was that authentic.

Mother's primary interest in genealogy at that time was to locate Great-grandma Elizabeth Stewart's date of birth, and have it recorded on her tombstone in the Jernigan cemetery at the Standridge place.

The 1850 census rolls gave Great-grandma Elizabeth Stewart's year of birth. The census recorded Elizabeth as "28 years of age Sept. 1850", thus born in 1822. An oil painting of her husband, Samuel H. Stewart that hung in our Sedalia dining room when I was a boy, recorded his birth at 1815. Great-grandpa Stewart died before 1849, and his name was not listed in the census. A six-page packet of research data re Jernigan - Stewart genealogy was mailed to relatives. 3

To Mother November 12, 1971:

"Thanks for the letters and contacting Annie Lou. We will have to go some other route to figure it out. James A. Jernigan's sister [Celia Jernigan Fields] was grandpa's aunt. Beth and Jay go on a church retreat to Tyler this weekend. We will keep Lisa for them. . . Hope you are feeling well. We are all busy."

Aunt Pansy Jernigan McDougal was interviewed about family history, and especially her knowledge of the Albert Jernigan family. She had an Austin address for Mary Belle Searight, whom Aunt Pansy mistakenly recalled as Albert's daughter. I wrote Mary Belle November 27, 1971.

"Mrs. Mary Belle Searight
410 East Monroe Street
Austin, TX 78204

"Dear Mrs. Searight:

"My Aunt, Mrs. Elmer McDougal of 237 Brooklyn, Dallas, Texas gave me your name and address. I am the nephew of Mrs. McDougal, son of Austin W. Jernigan, deceased, grandson of Andrew Jackson Jernigan who was a brother of your father, Albert J. Jernigan. I am attempting to bring together all of data on the family tree of James A. Jernigan, father of Albert and Andrew (and also Elizabeth J., Nancy A., and James P.)

"I would appreciate all the information you can give regarding the children of Albert J. Jernigan, their birthdates, (and date of any deaths), who they married, names of their children, who they married, etc. on up to the present date. I had the pleasure of meeting your brother Kenneth when I was a boy, and recall his beautiful singing voice.

"Another Jernigan, Bob Jernigan, a lawyer in Oklahoma City is working on the Elisha Jernigan branch (a brother of James A. and uncle to Albert J.). I would welcome information on that family group or of other siblings of James A. I believe a sister [Celia] married a man named [Green] Fields, but I have no other facts.

"I would also appreciate information about the off spring of Nan A. Jernigan Durrett, (sister of Albert J.). My information is that she lived in Paducah, Ky. I also have evidence that she married again to a man named Cole.

"About myself: I am 50 years of age, the youngest of three boys. My oldest brother, Stewart, is Professor of English at Texas A&M. My middle brother, Jim, is President of Texas A&I. I have three children, Beth Fain (20), Austin Jack, Jr. (17), and Richard (15). I married Jean Gibson of Melissa, Texas. I am Chief Psychologist for the V.A. Hospital, Dallas.

"I hope this letter finds you in good health and you are not overwhelmed by my request. I enclose a self addressed, stamped envelope for your convenience in answering."

The letter was the beginning of wonderful relationship with a charming lady that led to the biography of her Grandfather and my Great Uncle, Albert Jernigan.

Church Fund Drive.

Jean wrote her mother-in-law Thursday, November 18, 1971.

"Dear Mother J -

"Beth and I went to hear Natalie talk at our Pre-school Parent's Meeting at Cliff Temple Tuesday night. We were proud of her and she told about growing up at Cliff Temple.

"Richard is going to a church retreat at Wills Point this weekend. . . . Hope you are well. Love, Jean"

Natalie inquired about the Westminster church fund drive. The church voted to abandon the old Westminster Baptist Academy that had served as the church building for fifty years, and construct a new church sanctuary. Mother was an active leader in the fund drive. We gave $100 to the drive and most all of Blanche's numerous contacts made generous contributions.

Texas Psychological Association

My name received the largest number of mail in votes by the TPA membership for President-elect in the fall of 1971. The Nominating Committee requested permission to place my name on the ballot. The 1971 election procedure authorized the Nominating Committee to pair the person receiving the highest votes with another TPA member. By mail ballot the membership selected one of the two candidates for President-elect.

TPA members extended an honor with a great responsibility. It was a three year commitment and required many trips to Austin. I recall sitting in the balcony of Cliff Temple Baptist Church on a Sunday morning reflecting and praying about the ballot request. (When the children were small we sat as a family in the balcony so as to be less disturbing to older members, and continued the seating pattern.)

Jean knew it would place added burdens on both of us, but she graciously said to do what I thought best. The committee was notified to place my name on the ballot, the winner to be announced at the December Texas Psychological Association's annual meeting in Corpus. And so it was that I became President elect, and the 25th President of TPA.

A birthday greeting to Mother, December 5, 1971 told of visiting Jamie and Frances in Kingsville during the TPA meeting.

"I had a most pleasant visit with Jamie. I don't believe anyone ever had a more gracious host. We visited late each night and he either took me or loaned a car to go to the meetings in Corpus. Then, he cooked several excellent meals - he is a most versatile brother.

"We bought your [85th] birthday card a week ago so you would have it on Monday, and then forgot to send it. If I didn't have such a full schedule at the office tomorrow would come visit you. I'm hoping it will be so that I can take off Thursday or Friday and come up. I have annual leave to lose if I don't use it."

We held open house for the VA Psychology Staff Saturday night, December 11, 1971. As part of the entertainment, Austin presented some of his films past and present. Thirty individuals were present, and everyone seemed to enjoy the evening. Tom Toland was especially complimentary of Austin's creative films.

Christmas 1971

Mother had her Christmas Sunday, December 26. Stewart and Mary did not attend the dinner. I had the flu and stayed in Dallas. Everyone called and sent too much food. I wrote later, "Jamie was over about the time we got up yesterday [Tuesday] to have breakfast with us. (They spent the night at a Motel). Then a little later, the rest came and had breakfast. They left for Kingsville just before noon."

I took annual leave the last week of December. Clyde and Margaret invited us to Shreveport. We considered visiting Stewart and Mary in Bryan, and thought a bit about driving to Tennessee to get the bell. All possibilities were postponed until sometime in 1972.

Chapter 15 - 1972

We attended church January 2. Jean wrote her Mother-in-law two days later to thank her for Christmas gifts, and reported, ". . . the streets are bad. Guess the boys will be out of school tomorrow."

Dedication of New Church

We received an invitation: *"Dedication and Homecoming - First Baptist Church Westminster - Sunday, Jan. 16th 1972 - Morning service in old building - Lunch at Noon - Dedication service 2:30 PM."*

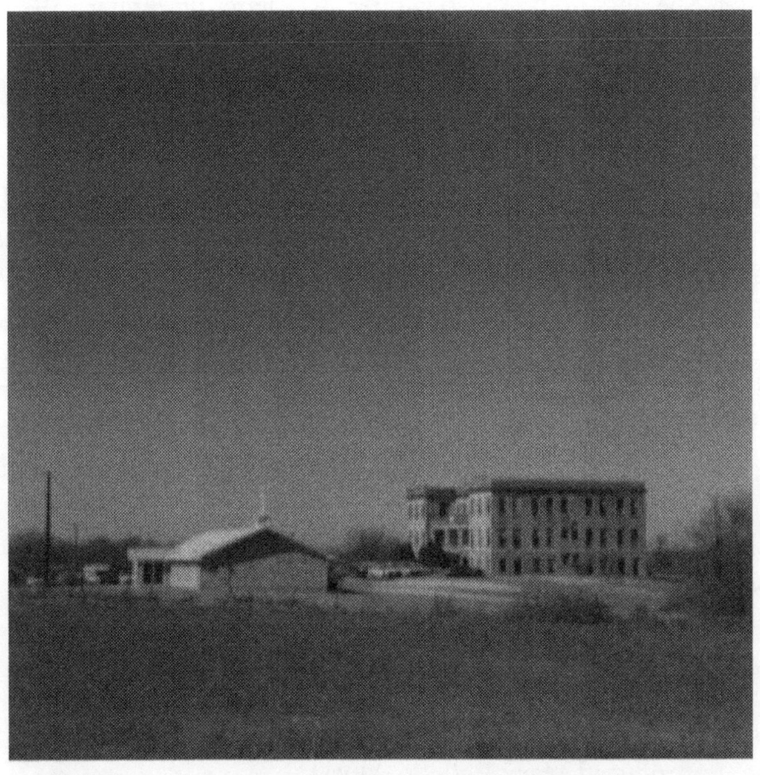

Westminster Baptist Academy Closed in 1916, building donated to Westminster Baptist Church – New Building, foreground

Jean and I attended the homecoming-service. Jean took a cake and one other dish. I took photos of guests at the old and the new church building. An exterior photograph of the two buildings in parallel was of such quality that many people requested a copy.

Data Processing and Mary Belle Searight

I visited the Veterans Administration Data Processing Center in Austin January 24, 1972 to discuss processing psychological research data. The Center housed an impressive bank of computers.

Mary Belle Searight lived near the VA Data Processing Center. She answered my November 1971 letter on January 19, 1972 (Chapter 14), and extended an invitation. Two days later I met a most gracious lady, then in her late 60's, never married. Mary Belle's house contained multiple artifacts of her grandfather, Albert Jernigan: His bed, bookcase, books, old files, but of most significance, seven lengthy letters by great uncle Albert written in the spring and summer of 1872 to his parents, James and Deborah Jernigan of Baggettsville, Tennessee, my great-grandparents.

Mary Belle shared one letter she had previously read. Later she wrote, "Will send you some zerox copies of those other letters I told you I had never read. They are sequels to the one you read and are very interesting. I got them out after your visit and read them. He wrote one to his parents - (Taking up the story where he left off) - about every two weeks. I wish I could write like he did. You almost feel you are there with him."

Those seven letters outlined salient segments of Albert's Civil War experiences including the tragic loss of his right arm on Missionary Ridge. Mary Belle introduced me to Albert's letters; in time, I introduced Mary Belle to Albert.

Many professional trips were made during the period 1972-1975 to attend Texas Psychological Association Executive Committee meetings in Austin as President-elect, President, and past President of TPA. After that first visit with Mary Belle in January 1972, the search for the "hidden Albert" was always a part of the Austin itinerary, and either a call or visit with Mary Belle was a must. She in turn graciously shared all content and listened with interest to my research efforts, and often gave new search leads.

We all received a great gift in meeting Mary Belle.

A Trip to Hawaii

The 80th annual convention of the American Psychological Association was scheduled to be held in Honolulu, Hawaii, September 1-September 8, 1972. Walter Penk encouraged the formation and presentation of a Hawaiian symposium on group psychological assessment, and suggested possible participants.

I wrote Dr. Paul McReynolds, Professor of Psychology, University of Nevada, at Reno, Nevada, formerly WWII Aviation Psychologist, T/Sgt. Paul W. McReynolds. Paul and I served together in 1942-1944 at San Antonio Aviation Cadet Center Psychological Research Center #2, and Medical and Psychological Center #5, at Miami Beach, Florida.

"Dear Paul,

It was a pleasure to talk with you this past week and renew an old friendship. I am honored that you graciously consented to be a discussant of the symposium on group assessment. I have verbal commitment from three of four participants.

I am attaching a copy of a paper on group assessment presented at the 1969 VA Cooperative Studies in Psychiatry held in Houston, Texas. I also include a summary of a symposium on the 1966 Texas State Survey given in Houston, Texas in 1967. These two documents will give you some idea of the kind of work we have been doing here at the Dallas VA Hospital these past few years.

. . . I am open to any suggestion you or the other three confirmed participants, Wayne Holtzman, Walter Penk and Matthew Buttiglieri have concerning the organization and presentation of the symposium.

Best wishes for the Holiday Season, and I look forward to seeing you in 1972.

Cordially,
Jack"

A January 13, 1972 letter to symposium participants asked each to respond to the "Call for Programs, Eightieth Annual Convention of the American Psychological Association - Honolulu, Hawaii, September 1-September 8, 1972." The deadline for submission was February 15. Following are excerpts from the letter to Walter Penk, an example of the letters sent to each presenter.

"Dear Walter:

We now have four confirmed members of the Symposium: you, Matt Buttiglieri, Wayne Holtzman, and Luciano L'Abate with Paul McReynolds as discussant. Although Dr. L'Abate had not intended to go to the APA convention, after reviewing the idea of the Symposium and hearing of the confirmed participants he stated he would be unable to turn down such an opportunity. He is currently working with assessment of family groups and proposes that his paper be on some of his current research and work in this area.

. . . I am suggesting that each member make January 31st the deadline for getting material to me. Although I have attempted to draft a Summary (copy enclosed), time is needed to rewrite the Summary after receiving a response from each participant."

Family Connections

I continued to explore the Fields Family connection. Mrs. Linvle Anderson gave some information and referred me to Nina Sparks Clinton.

I located great-great Aunt Celia (Jernigan) Fields grave in Elm Grove Cemetery, Grandpa Jernigan's aunt with whom he lived for a short time when he came to Texas after the Civil War. 1

Vietnam Veteran Interest

I wrote Mother February 10 about a talk to be delivered to the Physical Therapy Association of Dallas on the Vietnam Veteran. The presentation included notes from a talk given to Hospital Volunteers in November of 1970, "The Volunteer and the Vietnam Veteran" amplified with information Ron Kidd and I gathered in the interviews with more than 200 veterans in 1971.

The audience was encouraged to respond to the Vietnam Veteran with the same attitude, respect and service given to veterans of all previous wars. The "losing of a war" situation in Vietnam did not elicit the acclaim given to other returning veterans of the 20th Century. It was not a comfortable time for the veteran or the public. The Veterans Administration searched for new treatment as well as educational approaches.

Family Notes

We drove to Commerce, Texas one Sunday in mid-February as Austin had some interest in East Texas State College for the fall of 1972. The Fains found a cute dog. I wrote, "Jean is keeping up with two babies."

Jamie was in Dallas on a professional mission and shared Richard's 15th birthday dinner. Jay located a Coca Cola Machine along his route on Illinois Avenue at an African-American Beauty Parlor. We paid "Pauline Rolland $25" for the machine, now a collector's item.

A visitor from Central Office occupied much time one week, concluding with a Veterans Administration meeting in downtown Dallas on Friday. The next day was spent at the church as a committee member recommending goals for Cliff Temple Baptist Church.

St. Louis Meeting

The Veterans Administration agenda for the St. Louis meeting is no longer extant. (I stayed at the Park Plaza Hotel). This may have been the occasion Cecil Peck, as Chief, VACO, was invited to attend a very confidential meeting led by Masters and Johnson in St. Louis re Masters and Johnson's Sex Therapy Treatment. Cecil relayed his amazement about the content.

A postcard to Mother Monday, March 13, 1972 referred to the St. Louis trip.

"I delayed my trip by one day . . . sprained my knee and rested it yesterday. It is still sore but nothing serious. I'm looking forward to the meeting, will return Wednesday. We had a good visit with Jim and Marian [Wysong] on Sunday. . . Jackie showed them a number of films. The boys brought in some good grades Friday and we had fine reports on Richard at his school's open house. Hope you are feeling well. "

Before leaving St. Louis I visited sites viewed in 1904 by my Dad and Uncle Jim. A picture postcard mailed March 15, 1972 gave a bit of St. Louis history: "Statue of St. Louis - Art Hill, Forest Park, St. Louis. Louis IX of France, for whom the city was named is depicted as a crusader, clad in armor of the 13th century, holding his sword inverted to form a cross. The statue was donated to the city by the Louisiana Purchase Exposition in 1903."

"I have had a good visit to St. Louis. My knee is sore but much improved . . . visited the Museum and learned more facts about 1904 Fair. Please save this card for me."

Lamplighter Dedication

Jean, Beth and I attended the dedication of the Lamplighter School new building, March 17, 1972. Mayor Jonsson spoke as did a number of prominent educators. Wayne Holtzman was one of the guests. Natalie and Sandy Swain's special school stimulated much interest in academic circles. I took 8 mm movie film and also recorded the speeches. Later, Natalie asked if she could have the audio tape because the recorder gave a clear participation of my singing.

Mother responded to Natalie's 1972 invitation to the dedication. Sandy sent us the letter in February 1987 after the death of Natalie.

"Dearest Natalie and Sandy,

What a lovely day for your great coming out Affair!

How I thank you for my invitation and how I would love to be there but Jack would have had to come for me and bring me home and you know he has more than he can do.

I wish it would be on T. V. Wouldn't that be great! [It was.]

I am so proud of you two wonderful young ladies and the great work you have done and are doing.

May our Heavenly Father ever watch over you and may each of you give Him first place in your lives.

Love and always best wishes, Aunt Blanche"

I wrote Mother the details about the dedication, and added I had to work the next day, a Saturday. The Professional Log indicated, "March 18, conducted a psychological evaluation of a physician for Dr. Warren Johnson." I examined and conducted psychotherapy with a number of patients on Saturdays in 1972 at Dr. Johnson's Oak Cliff psychiatric office. Warren was our next door neighbor.

Easter

Beth, Jay, and Lisa mailed Grandma Blanche an Easter Card, titled, "HIS GIFT OF PEACE - An Inspirational Easter Message by Billy Graham."

On the riverse side of card, Beth wrote:

"Dear Grandma Blanche -

It has been so long since we have seen you - but that doesn't mean that you are not often in our thoughts. Just today Lisa asked about you.

. . . Jay and I get to vote in our first election this weekend and are really excited. Lisa has a new dress <u>with a hat</u> (which she loves) that Mother bought for her to wear this Easter Sunday.

Hope you are feeling well and have a peaceful Easter.

Love - The Fains"

All were at Cliff Temple's morning Easter Service when the early sun rays drifted through the beautiful stained glass windows. Beth, Jay, and Lisa had Sunday lunch with us and stayed most of the afternoon. The weekend of worship and rest made me ". . . ready for another week of work."

Film Festival

The 1972 Texas Student Film Festival was presented at St. Stephen's School in Austin, April 7-9, 1972. Skyline instructor, Mr. Collier took Austin's class to the Festival.

The Executive Committee of the Texas Psychological Association held its first 1972 quarterly meeting that same weekend in Austin. Jean and I drove to Austin for the TPA meeting. We visited the Film Festival and also visited Mary Belle Searight. It was the weekend Mary Belle gave us photocopies of Albert's seven letters. We stayed up late that Saturday night at the Chariot Inn reading Albert's remarkable letters that told of his Civil War and post Civil War experiences.

The letters precipitated a chain of events that extends to the present, even to the assembly of these autobiographical memories with the aide of letters preserved by my Mother. Following is the letter written to her that summarized our weekend trip:

"Dear Mother:

"We had a busy weekend. Jean and I went to Austin Friday, returned this afternoon. Jack [Austin] left Friday morning and returned tonight. Richard spent the weekend with the Fains and took care of Lisa while Jay worked and Beth took her National Teacher's exam. All had a successful weekend. Jack placed in 2 of 3 films - for one he won second place and the other honorable mention. After yesterdays meeting, Jean and I visited Mary Belle and she had copies waiting of a number of Uncle Albert's letters. Today we visited the LBJ Library. I want you to go see it sometime.

"We are all well and pleased with our accomplishments. Will look forward to hearing from you.

Love,
Jack"

Austin and Beth began developing a film for her TWU research project. All three Fains came by for breakfast one Saturday morning when a rain canceled an outdoor event in one of Beth's classes. We were scheduled to keep Lisa, so all three came for pancakes. That evening we met with our "42" Group.

Graduation Time

Jean submitted a $30 check May 1, 1972 to North Texas State University for Austin's "Room deposit."

Austin began to receive high school graduation gifts and made the only "A" given by his film course instructor at Skyline High School. We were very proud of him. His grandmother promised to come to the graduation, and did. Austin graduated from high school and looked for a second part-time job.

Jay and Beth took a three day trip to New Orleans. Lisa stayed with us.

Richard began a summer course in driver education and Austin enrolled for a course in typing at Mountain View Junior College. I received an invitation from the owner of the Stewart-Young ancestral land in Tennessee to visit and review ancestor's grave markers.

The 1972 Presidential primaries were in full swing when an attempt was made on the life of Governor George Wallace.

Meantime at the VA Hospital

I have very few 1972 Veterans Administration records. Donald Minnick was a summer trainee for 1971-1972, but there is no 1972 evaluation report. Don wrote an undated, two page Proposal for a Theraputic Film Program, and correspondence told of search for equipment to implement the project. Don Minnick wrote: "It is felt that this type of program may appeal to a younger, more acutely disturbed patient who is open to creative experiences in exploring himself. For this reason the Day Hospital might be an appropriate setting for such a program." Funds were found to bring Mr. Lawrence Becker of the Texas Film Festival to Dallas VAH to discuss and advise. The project did not reach fruition.

Mr. H. Les Jankey was recommended for assignment as a Level I Counseling Psychology Trainee by Dr. Royal Embree of Department of Educational Psychology, University of Texas. Within a few weeks Dr. Tucker and I found it necessary to explain to the talented student that his progress was not meeting expectations. He was given a new part-time assignment in Research Psychology with Dr. Penk. It was rare instance of finding it necessary to redirect an incorrect trainee placement.

A copy of the letter to the University recommending training alternatives was mailed to Mr. Jankey, and Dr. Joe Rickard, Secretary of the Regional Training Committee.

Walter Penk's Research Grant and Psychology Service's research in Group Assessment made it possible to hire clerical assistance. Tom Van Hoose was Walter's first research assistant. Tom left in September to take another position, and later received his Ph.D. He was replaced by a single male who subsequently married and moved to San Antonio.

Kathy Meyer, an ambitious young college graduate with great ability became a part of the staff. Kathy made many contributions to the statistical evaluation of the group assessment program. Another delightful addition hired in 1972 under a special research grant was Mrs. Ellen Harris, wife of Dallas Baptist's Dr. Cliff Harris. It may have been 1972 that we added Dr. Bob Strong to the staff, a psychologist who came from an educational setting. He entered the Civil Service register on a probationary status.

Drug Addiction

At the end of World War II there was need for only two Public Health Hospitals for treating drug addicts (Lexington and New Orleans). Out of the Vietnam War came a host of veterans addicted to a variety of drugs. VACO directed the establishment of a series of treatment programs at VA Hospitals.

Hospital Director Earl Whittaker appointed me Chairman of a joint Medical School -VA Committee to study and recommend a plan for the development of a drug treatment program. The Committee Chairman position made it possible to lead the committee to conclude a psychologist was the best trained and logical professional discipline to direct the Dallas VAH Drug Treatment Program. The Committee recommended that Dr. Ralph Robinowitz be appointed Chief, Drug Treatment Program. The Hospital Administration agreed. Time confirmed that Ralph Robinowitz was a wise choice for a very difficult and responsible job.

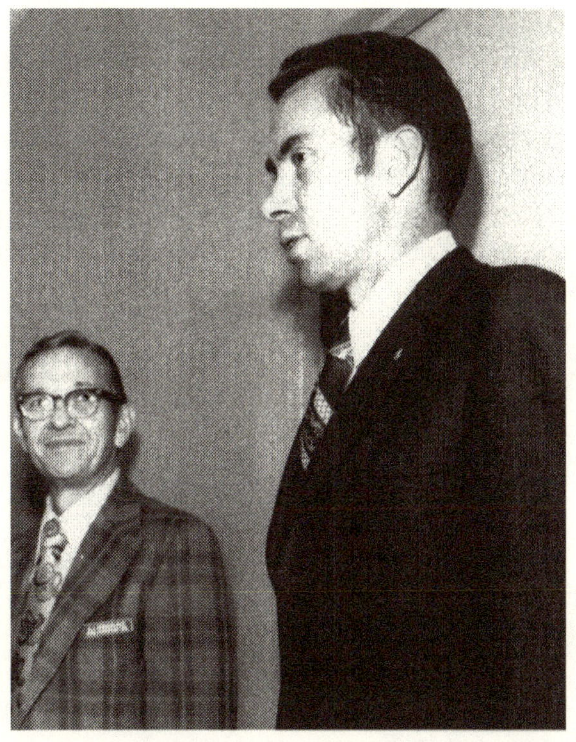

Jack Jernigan – Ed Nixon at Drug Treatment Center

The work of the Committee occurred in the summer of 1972, at the time the presidential campaigns were in hot pursuit. President Nixon's interest in the rehabilitation of the returning Vietnam Veterans with drug problems gave him reason to appoint his brother, Ed Nixon, to a leadership role in drug treatment. Mr. Ed Nixon came for the opening of our Drug Treatment Center in the fall of 1972.

Family Happenings

Jean received a letter from Edsel Martin, Swannanoa, North Carolina, postmarked June 2, 1972.

Mrs. Jernigan:

I'm slow, but I will be mailing your Dulcimer and Mockingbird around the 5th. I carved hawk's head on the Dulcimer, its curly Maple and Walnut wood, the Mockingbird this one I painted probably in a different position than the other. The dulcimer is 95.00 and the Mockingbird is 10.00. You can pay me when you receive it if you like. I'm sending it united parcels, UPS. Hope you all like them.

Many thanks,
Edsel

On reverse: "I packing it in plywood Box."

The mockingbird was not included with the shipment. The beautiful dulcimer continues to hang on the wall, yet to be played, unfortunately.

Austin accepted a forty hour a week job as a stock clerk with the VA Hospital Canteen, and occasionally served behind the counter. He and I rode together to work each day, a nice opportunity for both of us.

A note to Mother July 10, 1972 stated, "The Fains bought a new Plymouth Saturday, they had 63,000 on the Ford and it was giving them trouble. We had a good sermon yesterday by our new Assistant Pastor, Bill Entzminger. This is a busy week with all kinds of meetings and visitors. Hope you are feeling well.

Love, Jack"

We hosted a three hour Cliff Temple Counseling Committee meeting at our house July 27, 1972. The committee became acquainted with the counseling goals of Assistant Pastor Bill Entzminger. Bill was in the final stages of completing his doctorate in counseling, and outlined his plan for establishing a special center at the church.

TPA Executive Committee Meeting

We planned a mini-vacation to coincide with the July TPA Executive Committee Meeting. The four of us drove to Austin for a weekend of fun. I mailed a note to Mother and gave our locations during the coming weekend.

"We will be at the Ramada Gondolier Motel in Austin Friday night till Saturday after noon (512) 446-3611 and at the Sundown Motel in Burnet, Texas Saturday night until sometime Sunday (512) 756-2171."

On back of envelope, "Beth and Austin were asked to show their film to an Education class at TWU yesterday. The Dean of Education came in to see it. They both received a lot of compliments on the work." The film title: "Book Rider" encouraging children to read. Lisa was a member of the cast.

The trip to Burnet gave the boys an opportunity to be a part of a country musical festival of fiddle contests, dancing, eating, filming, etc. It was a nice experience.

A follow-up note Sunday, August 6, 1972, gave other details:

"We had a delightful weekend. The boys took their bikes and drove around Austin while I was in the meeting. Later, they met Jean at the LBJ Library, had lunch and then picked me up. We got to Burnet in time for the Old Fiddler's Contest - which we all enjoyed. Today we visited Ink's Lake and Glen Rose State Park - got back in about 5 PM."

The Fains took a late August vacation in Houston. They stayed with Jay's dad and step-mother. It was the weekend of Austin's 18th birthday, and he requested barbecued turkey for the celebration.

To Denton - On to Hawaii

Austin awaited his first day at college at Denton; we awaited our first trip to Hawaii. Cataracts diminished Mother's vision and arteriosclerosis brought cognitive changes in her writing skills. We communicated with her often, kept her informed, as in the note of Sunday, August 27, 1972.

". . . We are trying to get our plans completed for the trip - still have a good bit of work to do. We leave Friday, September 1 at 1:00 PM and get there about 3:45 (we follow the sun). Then coming back, we leave Hawaii Thursday, Sept. 7 at 6:00 PM and get back Friday at 6:00 AM (we go against the sun - so we take actually 7 hrs.).

"I hope everyone stays well while we are away. Richard will stay with Beth and Jay after Monday when Austin leaves.

"We sure did enjoy the Tilton's visit Friday night.

Love, Jack"

Jean, Austin, and I drove to Denton to take some of Austin's belongings, and check out his dormitory room at North Texas State University. To our surprise, his assigned roommate Daryl Arita, a handsome, personable young man from Hawaii arrived several days earlier. We told Daryl we were leaving the following day for Hawaii and was there anything we might do for him. He thought it would be nice if we called his mother and sister. Daryl gave us their address and telephone number.

Austin took us to the airport the next day. I carried the 8mm Bolex movie camera and the Rollicord. The recently purchased 35mm Nikkromat was left with Austin as there had not been sufficient time to learn how to use the camera.

Freshman Austin Jernigan wrote his grandmother before he left for college.

"September 1, 1972

Dear Grandma,

I certainly am grateful for the gift you sent me for my birthday. I used the money to buy a copy of The New American Bible, which is an English translation taken directly from the original language.

I was very sorry not to have gotten to visit you before leaving for college, but with all the activity around here lately it would have been very difficult to find any time. Mother and Dad got off for Hawaii today - where I'm sure they'll have a good time. It's sort of coincidental that my roommate at NTSU just got over here from Hawaii, his home place. I'm really looking forward to going to college. I've already taken some things up there, but I'll move in this Monday, and classes begin the following day.

Take care, and I hope to see you soon.

Love, Austin"

80th Annual Convention of the American Psychological Association

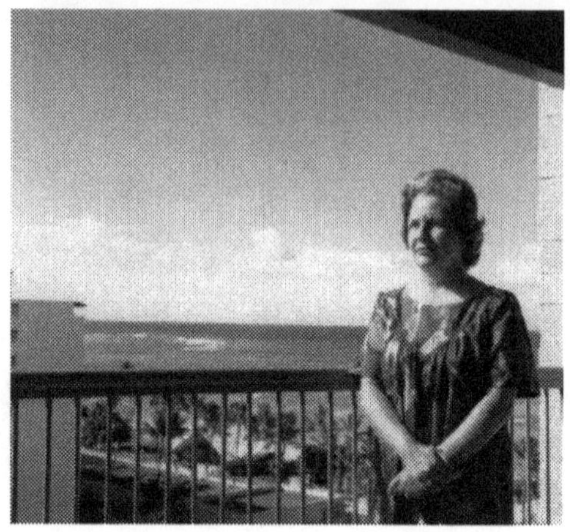

Jean and I registered at the hotel September 1, 1972.

"Honolulu Hawaii, September 2, 1972
Princess Kaiulani Hotel
Honolulu, Hawaii

Dear Mother:

We arrived last evening at 5:00 PM (10 PM Dallas time). We have a lovely room overlooking the beach and the mountains. We have had breakfast on our balcony. The weather is mild, but humid. Austin took us to the airport, where we had lunch with him as our plane was 1 1/2 hours late. Love, Jack"

And to the VA Hospital staff, September 2, 1972:

"Dear Friends:

". . . Honolulu reminds me of Manila - New Orleans - Miami and San Antonio. We have a nice ocean view and a Diamond Head view from our balcony.

The surfers were out before dawn. The storms out in the area are causing the weather to be atypically humid, so the cab driver said. Plan to register this morning and get to Ralph's paper. Keep up the good work, says I as I view this scenery. Jack"

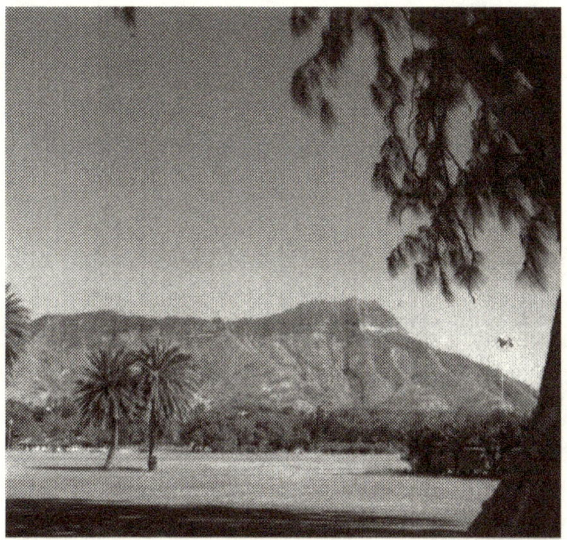

Diamond Head

And to Beth, Jay, Lisa, and Richard on September 2, 1972, a postcard scene of "Moonlight Over Waikiki:"

"We arrived at 10 P.M. (Dallas), and didn't know where our 'children were.' We have a nice beach and a mountain view. Sat on "our" balcony at dawn, ate breakfast and watched the surfers. Needless to say, we wish each of you could be here with us. Love, Daddy

A telephone call was placed to the mother of Daryl Arita soon after we arrived in Honolulu. The lady was overjoyed when told of the visit with her son the previous day! Mrs. Arita had received no communication from Daryl, and wondered if he arrived safely. I later told someone her exuberance was as if she had received a heavenly message. Mrs. Arita insisted we meet for dinner. Later, she gave us a partial tour of the island, and drove us to their home across the mountain from Honolulu. According to custom, we removed our shoes before entering.

Symposium

Matthew W. Buttiglierei, Walter Penk, Luciano L'Abate, Wayne Holtzman, and Paul W. McReynolds, and I presented the symposium, "Group Assessment Approaches," September 3, 1972 from 10:00 AM until noon. I introduced the subject and the participants:

"Psychologists, by training and experience, think of clinical assessment as a function which occurs only on a one-to-one, patient-psychologist basis. Schools, the Armed Forces, and industry have tested people in groups for many decades but psychodiagnostic testing of patients in groups first began approximately 25 years ago. There has been a significant upsurge of group testing of physically ill and emotionally disturbed patients within the last few years.

"In this Symposium, an attempt will be made to review the breadth and scope of group psychological assessment and discuss its implications for the future. Participants will explore into some of the major techniques tried and found most useful in the group method and survey the effectiveness of group testing programs. Some of the current research in the field of group testing will be discussed--research which involves the development of group test instruments and their application. Rapid accumulation of psychodiagnostic data requires innovation from the initial input to the final output and necessitates a review of such basic concepts as who should administer, score, and interpret psychological tests. The role of automation in psychological testing becomes an important variable when we begin to think of assessing patients in groups.

Group assessment may well become therapeutic for the field of Clinical Psychology in that it has the potential for improving the status of psychodiagnosis. It has been shown that group testing helps resolve immediate service problems in clinical settings and assist in upgrading research programs in that the method refines standardization of the assessment function. It is proposed that the group method of testing may give a more accurate evaluation of individuals than the traditional individual test method."

A picture postcard to Mother mailed the day after the symposium:

"We are having a wonderful time. Had dinner last evening with Austin's roommate's mother and sister. They are charming people. We are seeing a number of old friends. This is a beautiful place and the people are most friendly. Hope you are feeling well.

Love, Jack"

Among the "old friends" was the Frank Horner family from Alabama whom we discovered on the boat tour of Pearl Harbor. The Robinowitz family was also in Hawaii for the convention. And of course, seeing Paul McReynolds again was a highlight. He wrote before the convention, "It will be good to see you again, and to renew our acquaintances of some years back. It is amazing--and each year grows more amazing--how rapidly the years pass." 2

Back in Texas

Soon after returning to duty at the VA Hospital, Assistant Hospital Director, Paul Banks presented me a 30 year Certificate of Federal Service pin with proclamation.

We drove to Denton and had supper with Austin and Daryl. A note to Mother, Sunday, September 10, 1972 told of the visit.

"The two of them had gone to church this morning. When we arrived Austin was at the washateria, and soon came in puffing with a bag of washed clothes and his shirts on a hanger. He says he is having to study hard and seems to like his schedule. We were so glad we went. . . We enjoyed our visit with you yesterday."

And, Friday, September 15, 1972:

". . . I go to Austin Sunday and Monday for meetings. Don't know yet if Austin will be home this weekend. Tomorrow I'm in a church conference so I won't get to see much of him. Lisa and Beth had supper with us Wed. Jay goes to school every night. Hope you are well.

Love, Jack"

I attended the TPA Executive Committee Meeting in Austin September 17-18. An educational question about Texas' school system arose during the meeting, and the Committee suggested a consultation call to the President of Texas A & I. Jamie had an answer.

Aunt Ella Johnsey died September 19, 1972. We brought Mother to the funeral, and since she did not feel like attending, Jean stayed with her at our house. Stewart, Jamie and I served as pallbearers at the funeral.

Beth and Jay's Sunday School class met each week in the home of one of the members. Beth hosted the meeting at our house September 29. The class invited the Pastor, Dr. Watterson to visit with them.

Daryl came home with Austin the weekend of October 10. We hosted the "42" Club that Saturday night, and thoroughly enjoyed it all. Jean was on jury duty the next week

I attended a TPA Executive Committee Meeting October 21. Jean and Richard intended to go but all the motels were sold out because of the Arkansas-Texas game.

I thanked Mother for a letter she wrote on my 51st birthday:

"Thank you for your lovely note even though I don't begin to deserve all the nice things you say about me. Of course if they are true, then you are bragging, because it is due to your good training . . . I had a pleasant birthday - worked hard - but Jean had a lovely supper - with Beth and Lisa over for dessert."

I attended another TPA meeting in Austin on November 3, 1972. Clyde and Margaret Tilton moved from Shreveport to Plano that week. We were pleased they returned to Texas.

As these notes indicate, there were frequent trips to Austin in the fall of 1972, all related, to TPA executive committee meetings. The Committee met in Houston November 10 at the request of TPA President Jack Wheeler. The December TPA convention was to be held in his home city.

Thanksgiving

Austin invited Daryl home for the Thanksgiving Holidays. We drove to Sedalia for a turkey dinner Thursday, and stopped before arriving at Grandmother's House so Daryl could observe an armadillo, and pick native persimmons.

Mother sent the following squib for "News and Views of Van Alstyne" in the Leader's November 30th issue:

"Mrs. A. W. Jernigan was made very happy Thanksgiving Day when her son Jack and wife brought their prepared Thanksgiving dinner to the old farm home. All she had to do was to have the table long enough to find places for all the delicious food. Those present were: Dr. and Mrs. A. J. Jernigan, their sons Austin and Richard; Mr. and Mrs. Jay Fain and little daughter Lisa and Mrs. Florence Giles, Westminster. A special guest that was very welcome was Daryl S. Arita, Austin's roommate at North Texas, Denton. Dr. J. C. Jernigan of Kingsville spent a day and night with his mother this past week."

Lisa began attending a nursery school in the fall. Jean volunteered to tutor reading at Adamson High School. Beth was in her final semester at TWU. A concluding paragraph in a letter to Mother, November 26, 1972:

". . . I will be in Houston until Saturday. Jean may try to come down on Friday and be there when I officially take over as president. Beth called tonight. She has been sick with an upset stomach and won't go to school tomorrow. Jay will bring Lisa by for Jean to take to nursery school. Then she goes to her school, then to pick up Austin's film, and will carry it to him in Denton. She will try to get back in time to be here when the T. V. repairman comes. I'm glad I just have to go to work."

The 24th Annual Meeting, Texas Psychological Association

I drove to the TPA annual meeting at the Sheraton Hotel in Houston, November 30- December 2, 1972. The retiring President, Jack Wheeler arranged for a Business Meeting luncheon, gave a prepared address, and introduced me as the in-coming President - George Kramer, the new President-Elect.

The Dallas Morning News published a "VA Information Service News Release" December 19, 1972 announcing my installation as the incoming president of the Texas Psychological Association with photograph. The Van Alstyne Leader took notice, and under its byline, "News Around Van Alstyne" by Claude McKinney, reported:

"Dr. A. J. Jernigan, chief of psychology service at Dallas Veterans Hospital and a native of Van Alstyne, has been installed as president of the Texas Psychological Association. He succeeds Dr. John I. Wheeler, Jr. of Houston. Dr. Jernigan has been at the Dallas VA Hospital since 1956. An Air Force veteran he also participates in three doctoral level training programs in psychology with the University of Texas at Austin, the University of Houston, and Texas Tech University. He is also a faculty member of the University of Texas Southwestern Medical School in Dallas. He received his doctorate of philosophy from University of Kentucky. His mother is Mrs. A. W. Jernigan of Van Alstyne."

December 1972

Beth wrote her Grandmother December 8, 1972.

"Dear Grandma Blanche,

This is a happy birthday letter to you. Sorry we cannot be there with you.

We are all fine. Only another week of student teaching - and I'm through. These next few weeks are going to be really hectic. It seems like we haven't gotten any Christmas shopping done and I don't think I'll ever finish the Christmas cards.

Lisa is really enjoying nursery school. She told me her version of the Christmas story. I wish you could have heard it. She is excited about Christmas, choosing toys from the catalog. She thinks Santa Claus is living in Grandmother's chimney.

I've started doing needle point. It's very relaxing for me and I enjoy seeing the finished product.

Love,
The J. L. Fains"

"P.S. Did Mother tell you that I am playing the piano for the school Christmas program? Happy Birthday Young Lady!"

Beth did her student teaching at Carroll, a Dallas school for handicapped students. A poignant scene at the program was the actress playing Mary entering the stage in her wheelchair.

Staff Luncheon

Jean prepared a lunch for the Psychology Staff on a work day noon hour in early December 1972. Seated in the den were: Kathy Meyer, John Geers, Mrs. Susan Gallo, George Haven, Ellen Harris, Mary Louise Toland, Bob Strong and in the dining area: Ralph Robinowitz, Walter Penk and his new assistant. The efficient hostess was not photographed as she was busy in the kitchen.

Icy weather closed school for a day the second week of December. Later in the month Richard, Jim Tilton and I transplanted a cluster of oaks from Grady Niblo's farm to the Tilton's front yard. Clyde watched (and supervised) as his heart had begun to give problems. Blanche had a Christmas Dinner December 24 for her children and grandchildren.

Beth wrote her grandmother about Christmas gifts and future plans.

". . . Unfortunately, our vacation is about over. Jay registers for school Thursday night and begins classes a week from Monday. Lisa and I certainly have enjoyed having him home. This weekend we may go to Austin. The following week Jay will be a groomsman in a wedding. And of course, I start teaching the 18th January 1973 at Grand Prairie! This vacation is being followed by a busy time . . . I really cannot wait to begin teaching!

". . . The Bijou, Austin and Richard's theatre, opened today. We really enjoy the old Gary Cooper movie, 'Mr. Deeds Goes to Town Washington.' They were very organized.

Hope to see you soon
Love, Beth"

The Fain Family accomplished in three years: Beth completed a BS in Special Education and secured a teaching position. Jay, well on the way toward achieving a college degree, held down a full time job. Delightful Lisa was in kindergarten.

Chapter 16 - 1973

New Professional Role

I became Chairman of the Texas Psychological Association's Executive Committee (EC) January 1, 1973 as its 25th President. The Committee established the 1973 agenda, and outlined the Association's goals for the year. Good friend, Past President Jack Wheeler was a most helpful member of the Executive Committee.

In the latter half of 1972 Dr. Wheeler and I jointly interviewed Mrs. Naomi Meadows of Austin, and selected this remarkable young woman to be the Association's paid Secretary. Presidents for the subsequent twenty five years praised our choice.

A generous Veterans Administration made it possible to integrate the necessary weekday management of this added professional responsibility with the administrative demands of the Psychology Service. Many telephone calls were received and made during the year and Secretary of Psychology Service, Mrs. Susan Gallo became a valuable assistant. 1

I maintained a TPA log of all contacts and decisions, filling three books before the year ended. The inside cover of extant Logbook #3 listed the following index of names and telephone numbers:

"Naomi Meadows; Judge Bell; Betty Cleland; Ira Iscoe; Dr. Montgomery (Texas Education Agency); Wayne Holtzman; Carl Hereford; George Kramer; Jack Wheeler; Joan Anderson; Larry Abrams; Emily Sutter; Dick Slater; Joe Rickard; Mac Sterling; Al Burstein; Wayne Gill; Luis Laossa; Larry Smith; Dave Lipsher; Harry Parker; Ruby Morris; Martin Gluck; Dan Logan; Al North; Joy Anderson; Jane Halebian; Cliff Jones." These and many others were called for advice and counsel.

Walter Penk and Ralph Robinowitz of the Dallas VAH Staff were immediately available for consultation. Each gave valuable service to TPA throughout the year. Walter accepted the editorship of TPA publications and Ralph served as program director for the annual meeting.

A Family Log

January 4, 1973, Austin Jernigan, Jr., James Tilton, Clyde Tilton, and A. J. Jernigan, Sr. took a clothes line Clyde removed from his Plano backyard to Sedalia, but did not install it that cold winter day. Mother served lunch.

A Christmas gift from Richard was a copy of the 1904 St. Louis World's Fair Official Souvenir Book that he discovered at a used bookstore. Mother gave me the 1904 St. Louis World Fair photographs taken by Daddy and Uncle Jim. One of Daddy's photographs was identical to one in the souvenir book. That was an exciting piece of research.

Austin drove the Tempest to Denton to register for the second semester while I drove south toward Austin for the first Executive Committee meeting held at Sheraton Inn.

Jean wrote her 86 year-old mother-in-law January 16, 1973:

"Jack and Richard took Austin back to school Sunday. I had planned to go but by the time he got packed there wasn't room! He went up Friday and registered. Had a flat, but in the parking lot so had no trouble. Daryl got back Saturday.

"Jack had a good meeting in Austin and was glad not to have to postpone it [because of icy roads]. He will have another in April, I think.

"The boys had about 25 in to see their film Sat. night, then got up and went to S. S. - guess they have lots of energy.

"Thank you so much for the nice gifts - the waffle iron is the first one we've had that didn't stick, and the nice skillet is a real help.

". . . The Fains are well and Beth is about ready to start her teaching job.

"Take care of yourself. We are proud of how well you manage everything.

Love, Jean"

Richard Nixon was sworn in as President of the United States January 20, 1973 the day I pruned trees and set the clothes line poles at Sedalia. A note to Mother the next day:

"I hope you suffered no ill effects from all your outside work. I enjoyed the visit with you, the good lunch and getting to watch the inauguration. The weather has been sort of miserable here today. We went to church, and this afternoon Jean collected for the March of Dimes. . . We had a nice long letter from Austin; he seems to be settling down to school."

Beth reported she enjoyed teaching in Grand Prairie.

Austin sent a flier from Denton indicating he would be home on the weekend. He typed an advertisement "Bijou Motion Picture Palace" and wrote at the bottom of the page:

"Have the chairs been ordered? What about picking up the film Friday? As to the '42' showing, it would be fine.

We were the scheduled hosts of the "42" Club that weekend and had asked if the adults could attend the Bijou movies. The feature film was David O. Selznick's 1947 production "Duel in the Sun" plus many shorts, Charley Chaplin, Popeye, etc.

I wrote Mother February 13, 1973: "We have watched Vietnam POWs landing. What a joy! We enjoyed Austin's visit home. All of us had lunch together yesterday. Love, Jack"

Again, February 25, 1973: "I'm in Dr. Darold Morgan's class at Cliff Temple discussing the theology of Karl Barth. It's way over my head, but I'm enjoying it. Maybe you'd like to read the book when we are through."

The Albert Research Saga

Trips to Austin in 1971-1973 and visits to Dallas Public Library provided brief opportunities to collect information about Albert Jernigan. Discovery of the Austin Statesman account of Uncle Albert's suicide in 1896 was startling, and more so for Mary Belle Searight. Gradually, a series of 8 x 10 spiral ring notebooks were filled with the gathered facts about the life and times of Albert Jernigan. 2

In May 1972, Mary Belle introduced Laura Jernigan Congdon, Albert's only surviving child (twin). We corresponded (Ft. Pierce, Florida). Cousin Laura concluded one of her letters with, "When I addressed your letter, felt like I was writing to my father." (Same initials: AJJ.)

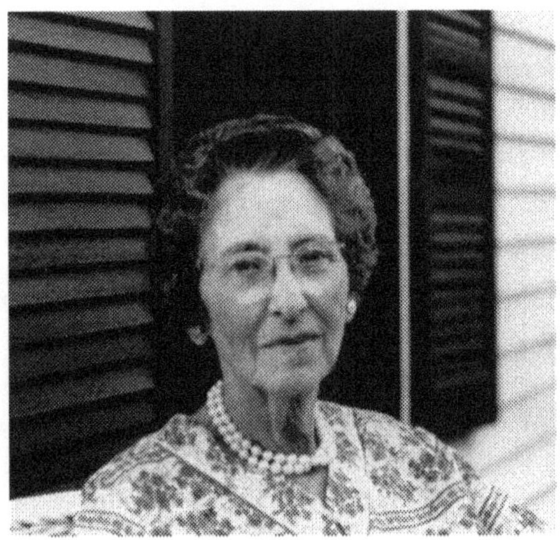

Laura Jernigan Congdon

Excerpts from a letter to Mary Belle in 1972:

". . . visited the Austin Library . . . reviewed the file on Uncle Albert and other early settlers of Austin. . . Mr. Crow, County Treasurer told me of some stored files at 5th and Pleasant Valley Road. There I found 3 Registers from Uncle Albert's tenure, 1873, 1894, and 1896, with much of the content in Uncle Albert's handwriting. I wish these could be stored at the Library for I fear they will be ruined or destroyed in time if not better preserved."

The attic where the Registers were stored was over run with rats. Soon after the visit the building and all content burned to the ground. Fortunately, I took a few photographs of one Register.

Veterans Administration - New Orleans

The Veterans Administration reserved the Jung Hotel for Regional meetings held in New Orleans during the 1960's and 1970's. The employee paid for food, hotel, and travel to and from the airport, and was later reimbursed by a per diem allowance. The travel section of the VAH Dallas procured my airplane ticket.

There are no extant agenda documents for the Veterans Administration March 1973 meeting. As usual on my New Orleans trips, an evening was spent at Preservation Hall listening to jazz renditions from elderly, talented black musicians, (an occasional white musician), mostly male.

An April 1, 1973 note: "I had a good trip to New Orleans. . . We are going to Estes Park, Colorado this year, the first week in July."

We four drove to Kingsville Friday, April 13, 1972, took a tour of the King Ranch Saturday, and returned home Sunday after attending early morning Easter Services at the A&I football stadium. Jamie was named Chancellor of A&I in 1972. He and the family moved to a home once owned by a member of the King Family designated as the Chancellor's residence.

VA - SWPA - Cecil Peck - Film Festival - TPA

I returned from Kingsville for two weeks of concentrated professional work.

Cecil Peck came the third week of April to review Dallas VA Hospital's Psychology and Psychiatry programs. He stayed with us Tuesday through Friday. Cecil delivered a major address to the Southwestern Psychological Association at its annual meeting in Dallas that week.

We drove to Austin April 29, 1973, to view Richard's Film Festival entry, and respond to a TPA Executive Committee need. Richard's entry did not place, but we all had a good time.

Jernigan Bell

Austin and I drove 678 miles to Springfield, Tennessee Monday, May 14, 1973 to bring to Texas the "Colonel" Jernigan bell stored in Mr. John T. Hale's barn.

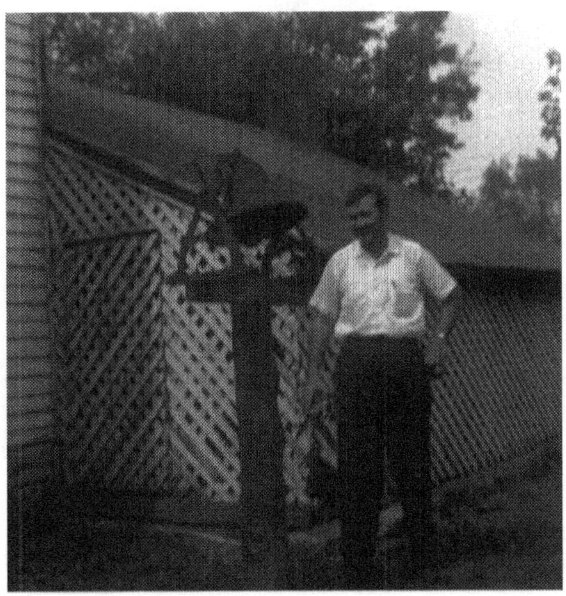

Jack beside bell at Colonel's home in 1961

We worked out of the Key Motel in Springfield, stayed three nights, visited and cleaned family gravesites. Mr. Ben Robertson of Portland, Tennessee knew the location of the displaced Stewart gravestones, removed when the national highway overran the cemetery. He led us to two tombstones hidden at the edge of a wooded area. Of great concern: How to preserve Great Grandfather Samuel Stewart's tombstone. Daddy's cousin, Nannie Wright suggested they be brought to her family cemetery, and regret we did not accept her offer.

Another highlight of the trip was Mrs. Hale's gift of Civil War "Morning Report of the Sick and Wounded" discovered in J. P. (the Colonel) Jernigan's office in 1950. There were no "Civil War type" notations, but the huge leather covered book contained financial entries by Great-grandfather James Jernigan and his three sons (Albert J., Andrew J. and James P. {Colonel}), each of whom had distinct hand writing. The book carried a price mark of $3.00. Was it purchased from a Civil War type Army Surplus Store?

We left with the bell and the book Thursday morning at 7:30 A. M., went through West Memphis at noon, and arrived home at 6:30 P.M., 677 miles. We drove 191 miles in and around Robertson County. It was a fast and memorable trip.

Graduation - Employment

The entire family, and Jay's mother, Jeanne Fain attended Beth's outdoor graduation from TWU, a lovely night in May, 1973. As Beth needed to be in Denton early in the evening, Lisa and Grandmother Fain rode with the four of us to the graduation. We were all so proud of Beth, and Jay, for it had taken sacrifice and teamwork to achieve their goal.

Austin located a summer job with the City of Dallas surveying commercial signs to insure that signs complied with the city's new sign code ordinance. Richard found work at one of the local movie theaters.

I spent the weekend of June 1 in Austin attending a TPA Executive Committee meeting. Blanche's "Guest Book" recorded I trimmed the hedges at Sedalia on Saturday, June 23, 1973.

National Wildlife Conservation Summit

We departed June 30, 1973 for our third National Wildlife Summit, the second at Estes Park, Colorado. I sat up late each night during the week before we left listening to a replay of that day's Watergate hearings.

Jean mailed her Mother-in-law a picture postcard Sunday, July 1, 1973 with the caption: "Approaching Estes Park village on the Big Thompson Highway (U.S. 34) with the peaks of the Continental Divide in the distance."

"Dear Mother J.,

"We had a very nice trip up here, stayed at Hays, Kansas, last night. All feeling well and in good humor. The boys brought their bikes and are having fun.

Love, Jean" 3

Austin and Richard continued their film-making interests at the Summit. Austin's cinematography interest received his undivided attention. He took several rolls of 8 mm film with the Bolex movie camera, producing a 1973 Summit document of excellent quality.

A picture postcard of "Peak to Peak Highway south of Estes Park, Colorado" written on our 26th wedding anniversary, July 5, 1973:

"Dear Mother:

"This is a nice place to celebrate a 4th and a 26th. All four of us are quite pleased with our vacation. We are meeting some fine people and learning a few things as we go thru the week. Hope this finds you well. We will be in Sunday night if the gas holds out. Love, Jack"

There was a gasoline shortage that summer. We stayed at the XIT Hotel in Dalhart, Texas July 7, 1973, detoured through Archer City so the boys could visit the filming site of the recently released movie, "The Last Picture Show." It was a very good vacation!

Beth and Lisa visited Grandma Blanche the Saturday we left for Colorado. Beth mailed a card to her grandmother postmarked 5 Jul 1973.

"Dear Grandma,

"Lisa and I had a fine time Saturday. The squash, green beans, and beets were really good. I shared some of the beets and beans with Jay's mother and she's still raving about them!

We love you,
Lisa and Beth and Jay"

Back Home

A one page letter July 15, 1973 after a visit to Blanche's corn field:

"What beautiful corn! We had it in the freezer by 5 o'clock and a mess for supper and Sunday lunch. I didn't find a single worm.

". . . I go to Austin Saturday for a meeting. I will leave Friday and make a talk at noon to the Central Texas Psychological Association. The boys will be working."

The noon presentation to the Central Texas Psychological Association at Temple, Texas was hosted by the Association's President, Dr. Tom Herod, father of former Trainee Joy Herod.

One item discussed at the luncheon was the TPA School Psychology Task Force's charge to explore interests of the School Psychology Division of TPA. An especially sensitive issue was Texas Education Agency's failure to recognize the need for doctoral level training for School Psychologists. The Task Force charged to study the issue, chaired by Dr. Al Burstein, and funded by the Hogg Foundation met at the University of Texas Health Sciences Center in San Antonio. I made two or more trips to San Antonio in 1973 as a member of the Task Force. 5

Austin joined me on the July return trip after making dorm arrangement for his transfer to the University of Texas as a Sophomore, as documented in a letter to Mother dated July 23, 1973.

". . . I had a good two days on my trip. Austin met me down there and got his dorm situation all straight; he will stay at Jester Hall. Then he helped me drive back which was restful.

". . . . We heard a good sermon this morning, Bro. Estrada, of the Language Mission of Texas. He was born in Mexico and gave a number of facts about his life. He has had a very fruitful life.

"We are having all the Psychology Staff and their children (about 35 people if they come), for ice cream Friday night. The boys are going to show some of their films for entertainment.

Love, Jack"

The weekend of the Friday night staff party was a busy one: Examined a private patient Saturday; Jean gave a shower that afternoon for Dell and Dottie Burrell's son, Douglas. Late Saturday afternoon we drove to Sedalia to visit Jamie and family as recorded in Blanche's "Guest Book" July 28, 1973.

Veterans Administration

Total air conditioning came to the Dallas VAH in the summer of 1973. Window air conditioners were scattered here and there in some offices during the preceding years, but very few patient areas had the luxury of a single window unit. The lack of funding for total air conditioning was attributed to Dallas Republican Congressman Bruce Alger who was in disfavor with the Democratic led Congress. Whatever the cause for the long delay, hospital employees and patients were very happy when air conditioning finally arrived, as exclaimed in a letter July 26, 1973, "I'm enjoying working in an air conditioned office."

Only brief content is here presented about the firing of Dr. George Haven in the fall of 1973. A patient made the complaint of a sexual impropriety and was planning to sue.

Dr. Haven admitted the accuracy of the charges. Senior staff and I met with George on a Saturday, advised him to inform the Texas State Board of Psychological Examiners, and to seek psychological help. It was a very unpleasant experience. Once again it was necessary to terminate a psychologist.

One other staff change occurred in 1973. In this case, the question was definitely not morality. Dr. Bob Strong's training and experience did not blend with the requirements of the staff position to which assigned. As he was still in probationary appointment status, the contract was terminated.

Dr. Strong appealed to the Civil Service Commission and later located a position with another Federal agency. The role of Service Chief sometimes demanded unpleasant decisions.

New Trainees - New Staff

Two new trainees were accepted in 1973: Donald Carver, Level III, Counseling from the University of Texas and Earl Patterson, Level III, Counseling from Texas Tech. Donald Carver had interest in the writings of ---- Cayce and Donald shared Cayce's autobiography that told of an untrained individual's experiences in healing, even surgery.

Earl Patterson came with strong interests in behavior modification. Earl completed his doctoral work while at Dallas and joined the staff.

Three Ph.D. psychologists joined our staff in 1973. David Johnson a University of Kentucky graduate, with years of VA experience was assigned to the Mental Hygiene Clinic. Jack Fudge, a University of Texas Ph.D., joined Ralph Robinowitz in the Drug

Treatment Program. And former trainee Ron Kidd returned to Dallas VAH after a year of teaching at University of Texas at El Paso. Two research assistants, Verle Childers and Coy Craig joined Dr. Walter Penk in his expanding Research Program.

Excerpts – August Correspondence

August 2, 1973: ". . . The boys' work keeps them on a schedule that doesn't permit much flexibility. I go to San Antonio Sunday for a meeting . . . will fly down and back the same day."

August 19, 1973: "Tuesday is Austin's birthday and we have a camera for him. He will continue to work through Friday and leave for Austin the following Wednesday. I'll be in Montreal so guess Jean will take him down. I leave next Sunday morning and come back on Friday. Richard starts school tomorrow, 11th grade and Beth begins her 1st full year of teaching tomorrow. Jay winds up his summer work with a final on Tuesday night. So, everybody is preparing for school one way or another."

APA - Montreal, Canada

I attended the 81st Annual Convention, American Psychological Association in Montreal, Quebec, Canada, August 27-31, 1973. I submitted two papers: "Group Assessment: A Procedural Review" and "Clinical Data As a Resource for Population Study." The former paper was rejected but the latter was published in Proceedings: APA 1973, 8lst Annual Convention, Vol. 8, Part 1, 491-492.

The study was an outgrowth of an interest in family planning:

"For some time this author has observed that certain psychological instruments pull information relative to an individual's attitude toward children. This study deals with some of the affective components of memories of patients concerning children as elicited by structured and semi-structured instruments from the standard group assessment battery at the Dallas Veterans Administration Hospital (Jernigan, Penk & Tucker, 1969)."

Mailed picture postcards gave a sketch of the Canadian experience.

Sunday, August 26, 1973 to Jean, Austin, and Richard, "An impressive view of the skyline of downtown Montreal."

"The trip up was nice except it was noisy and busy at New York. The people are friendly and pleasant and the city at dusk looks quite attractive. So far I've seen no one I know. I was pleased I had some food with me when I arrived for convenience and cost. I have a small but comfortable hotel room. Wish each of you was here. Love, Jack and Dad."

Sunday, August 26, 1973 to Mother:

". . . Montreal is a nice pleasant city with friendly folks. . . I will represent Texas in a number of meetings as President of the Texas Association.

Love, Jack"

Monday, August 27, 1973, to: "Dear Folks,"

"John Geers, Bill Rigby and I ate dinner together; a most pleasant evening. I've had a full day of good papers. . . I plan now to come back on Friday . . . miss each of you, and love you.

Jack and Dad."

Wednesday, August 29, 1973 to Jean and Richard:

"I assume Austin is at the University. Cecil wants us to come to Washington next month and spend the weekend with them at their beach home and go from there (30 miles) to Baltimore for the Cooperative Research meeting. Love, Jack"

Two TPA Logbook # 3 entries: "8-29-73 @ APA attended meeting on PSRC Professional Standards Review Committee. Cliff Jones was also present." 8-30-73 "Sat in for Ira Iscoe on the Counsel of Representatives meeting with Dr. Leona Tyler, Chairman."

Ira Iscoe, the TPA Representative to the APA Counsel was unable to attend a meeting and asked me as TPA President, to substitute. It was a nice learning experience to sit in and see and hear first hand the executive deliberations of APA.

Montreal's 1967 World Fair, Expo '67 was held on an island adjacent to the city. Much of the original fair structure and some exhibits were still intact, including the magnificent Geodesic Dome, United States' Pavilion at the Fair, a "vaulted structure of lightweight straight elements that form interlocking polygons." The Dome could be seen from the city long before one reached the island. Numerous slides of its interior were taken while riding the multiple floor escalators. A few years later the dome burned to the ground in a matter of minutes.

University of Texas

Austin wrote his grandmother September 6, 1973. "Room M 533 - Jester Center, University of Texas."

"Dear Grandma,

". . . So far, things are going well down here. The living accommodations are very nice, and there is always plenty going on. I just hope I'll be able to find time to study. I'm taking English, Spanish, Astronomy, History and a Communications course.

"My address is on the envelope, so write whenever you have a chance. Hopefully I'll see you again Thanksgiving. Take care.

Love, Austin"

VA Baltimore Meeting

I was appointed Dallas VAH Principal Investigator in the VA Nationwide Cooperative Research Project to collect research data from the nation's VA Day Treatment Centers. It was a first visit to Baltimore, a flight up on Sunday and back to Dallas the next day.

A picture postcard to Mother from Baltimore: "Fort McHenry National Monument and Historic Shrine, Baltimore, Maryland - Authentic replica of the flag which inspired Francis Scott Key to write 'The Star Spangled Banner.'"

"Sunday, September 23, 1973

"I spent a couple of hours this afternoon visiting Ft. McHenry. This is a most interesting place. The weather is mild and I am enjoying the trip. Love, Jack"

Numerous slides documented the Sunday afternoon visit to Ft. McHenry and the city of Baltimore. Dr. Scarborough, Principal Investigator from Waco VAH and I flew back together.

The Young Teacher

Beth thanked Grandma for her 22nd birthday check.

"Dear Grandma,

". . . I'm really enjoying school this year. So far I've only got 8, but I'm supposed to get some new students next week. My class maximum is 12, but I had 13 last year. My class is made up of a really good bunch of kids. There are 5 other Special Ed. teachers in our school, all in their early 20's, and we're all good friends. In fact, one teacher and I switch out on driving which really helps.

"You'll be pleased to know that the other 2 MBI teachers & I have got a pretty good music program going. Of course, I play the piano. We've done folk dances, rhythm band, and singing.

"I'm taking one Master's course thru TWU in kindergarten so I can get my Early Childhood Spec. Ed. certificate & of course, it counts toward my M.E.D. as an Educational Diagnostician. Jay is taking 13 hours this fall and working himself to death! I worry about him. He's enjoying his promotion & that helps.

"Lisa's taking ballet to help her turned in toes. She seems to enjoy it.

"They've started building our house. Our loan has gone through. By the 1st of the year, we'll be much nearer to you with a 3rd bedroom for you to <u>spend some time with us</u>!

Love, Beth"

Beth and Jay contracted for a Fox & Jacobs home in Richardson in the summer of 1973, and placed a down payment of $500. They later canceled the contract and forfeited the down payment.

Texas Psychological Association Annual Meeting Preparation

The Texas Psychological Association annual convention was scheduled for Dallas in 1973. Ralph Robinowitz, Harry Parker, and I visited local hotels in the summer, and chose the Sheraton as the Convention Hotel to celebrate, "Twenty-five Years of Texas Psychology, 1948-1973."

TPA Logbook #3, 8-14-73, "The program committee plan group met - Ralph, Harry Parker, Martin Gluck, and A. J. Devoted most of time to workshops (spoke of 12). We touched on criteria of leader, qualifications for participants, etc. No known principal speaker."

The Program Committee developed a rough draft of program subjects:

Harry Goolishian	6 hrs. 50 people
Betty Pehl	Diagnostic Interv. School Psy. 3 1/2
Dan Logan	Adult: Behavior Mod.
Marian Yeager	Marital Couples Therapy
Stephen (?)	Innovations in Community Mental Health
Blair Justice	Battered Child - Focus on parents.
Vincent [no name]	Organization of Clinics
Jack Tractor	Hypnosis
Bob Anderson	Learning Disorder
Don Whaley	Behavior Mod. in Children
Mary Moore	Program Evaluation - MHMR
Don Giller	Private Practice (?)
Ralph Robinowitz	Drug Treatment"

The logbook identified a multitude of individuals who contributed to the development of the convention. Because it was the Association's 25th anniversary, an attempt was made to have all living past presidents in attendance. A September 28, 1973 entry, "Joan Anderson - Be glad to take responsibility on suitable scroll for past presidents."

Emily Sutter followed up on a professional genealogy idea gleaned from the 1972 Hawaii APA convention. She developed a presidential questionnaire to solicit data on such topics as: "Changes in the organization over the preceding twenty-five years, what kind of people were selected, how is the future perceived, etc." All past presidents responded and Emily presented the findings at the convention.

Fourth Quarterly Executive Committee Meeting

Jean and Richard accompanied me to Austin October 19-20, 1973. Austin presented a birthday gift he purchased from a University of Texas artist of a Sailing Ship outlined by silver nails on a black wooden background.

In the Twenty-Fifth Anniversary Issue of The Texas Psychologist, Vol. 25, No. 4, December 1973, Editor, Walter Penk reported "Highlight's" of the TPA Fourth Quarterly Meeting of 1973:

"TPA Executive Committee, committee chairmen, and division directors met in Austin on October 20th for the fourth quarterly meeting of 1973. . . For a broader view of what transpired at the meeting, TPA members are encouraged to review reports by TPA officers presented elsewhere. Following are names of those attending quarterly meetings:

"TPA Officers: President, A. Jack Jernigan; President - Elect, George H. Kramer, Jr.; John I. Wheeler, Jr., Past-President; Treasurer, Joan S. Anderson; Parliamentarian, Joseph C. Rickard; APA Council Representative, Ira Iscoe.

"Committee Chairmen: Laurence Abrams, Council of Area Societies; Joseph C. Rickard, Ethics; David Lipsher, Legislation; Wayne Gill, Insurance; Mac Sterling, Membership; Laurence C. Smith, Elections; Walter Penk, Publications; Ralph Robinowitz and Harry Parker, Convention; Alvin G. Burstein, Committee on State Agencies; J. Ralston Kennett, Constitution.

"Division Directors: George H. Kramer, Jr., Applied Psychology; Richard D. Slater, School Psychology; Joy Anderson, Psychological Associates."

Editor Penk concluded his article re the Association's good financial status:

"Participants in the TPA governing body volunteer not only time but money. For example, TPA did not pay any expenses for Judge Bell, Cliff Jones, Jack Jernigan, and Ira Iscoe when they attended APA's Annual Convention in Montreal and conducted TPA's business. The state association is solvent not only because members pay "adequate" dues, but also because elected officers pay much of their own expenses when they accept an office or a duty."

Significant Loss of Vision

Because of a sudden loss of vision in one eye, Mother saved only one other 1973 AJJ family letter (October 14, 1973). "Dear Mother:

". . . I've been busy on the paper these past few days. I know you are concerned about your eyes but I have confidence in Dr. Truett.

"We were proud of Richard. He made straight A's for the first 6 weeks. . . We are looking forward to our visit with Austin this Friday and Saturday. All three of us will go down in the afternoon and come back Saturday afternoon.

". . . I'm sure we will be talking with you soon.

Love, Jack"

The reference to "paper" may have been a report for the TPA Newsletter. 4

Jean and I took Mother to the Ophthalmologist in McKinney October 2. Dr. Truett suggested she return six months later. Within three weeks she became essentially blind in one eye and vision in the other eye was quite limited by a well developed cataract. It was uncertain what happened to the "good eye" but it was suspected Mother may have experienced a small stroke.

TPA Trip & 1973 Annual Convention

Tax return for 1973 documented a trip to Houston on November 30, 1973, to represent TPA at a Texas Legislative hearing or seminar held on the campus of the University of Houston. Congresswoman Barbara Jordon spoke and I had the privilege of meeting and taking her photograph. I met with Joan Anderson and Emily Sutter in Houston to discuss final convention plans.

It was traditional to award the TPA President a VIP Suite at the annual convention hotel. The 1973 suite was on the top floor of the Dallas Sheraton. Officers, Committee members, the Press and those members wishing to identify with the "VIP's" visited throughout the three day meeting, December 6, 7, and 8, 1973. Jean joined me at the hotel suite from time to time during the convention, as did Richard.

John Geers assisted in the social hour with buffet. The twenty-three living past presidents were presented a "special scroll of recognition for service rendered." Richard served as one of the photographers. Emily Sutter gave her historical findings. It was a memorable evening.

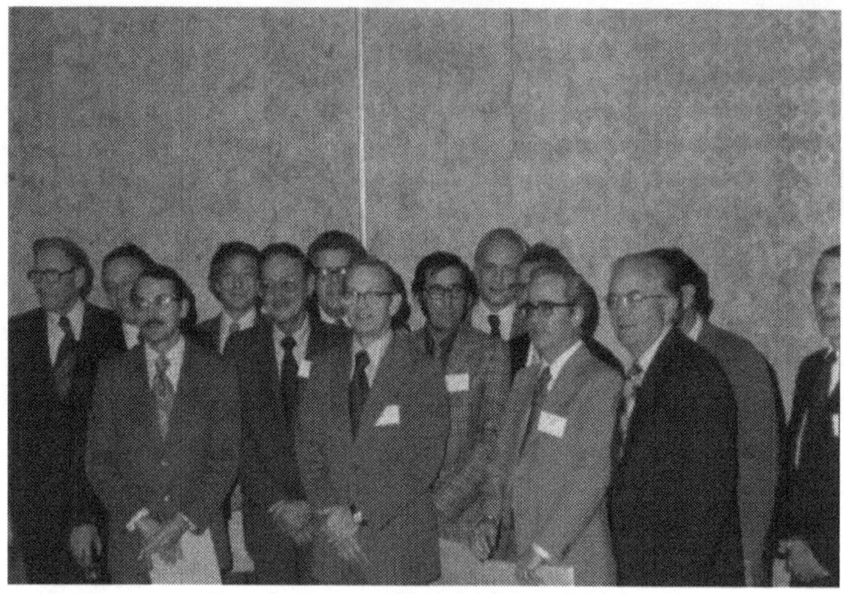

Anderson, Calicutt, Phillips, Iscoe, Hereford, Kramer, AJJ, Goolishian, Foster, ( ), Wheeler, Sartain, ( ) Smith

Naomi Meadows reported that 415 individuals registered for the convention. The figure did not include those who came on Saturday, December 8.

VA Staff Luncheon

The VA Psychology Staff and the Director of Professional Services, Dr. George Edwards came to our home for a noon-break luncheon in mid-December. Those present in photographs: Verle Childers, Kathy Meyer, Donald Carver, Mary Louise Toland, George Edwards, Buzz Tucker, Ron Kidd, Earl Patterson, Jack Fudge, David Johnson, Sue Gallo, Coy Craig, and of course, Jean Jernigan who made the luncheon possible. Those absent or not photographed: John Geers, Walter Penk, and Ralph Robinowitz. The Psychology staff increased significantly in 1973 as new programs were added at Dallas VAH.

Year's End

When Mother's vision declined, it became necessary to take care of all her business interests. A Guest Book entry indicated we drove to Sedalia the day after the TPA convention: "Guests - 12-9-73 - A. Jack Jernigan - Sent Christmas checks (to children and grandchildren)."

All the families visited at Sedalia during Christmas week. Twenty five photographic slides documented a sunshiny day, mild temperature as all outside scenes were of people wearing light sweaters or jackets. Good food and opening of presents highlighted the day as well as a photograph of the "three sons" at the west side of the house, and indoor photos of all the guests surrounding Grandma. David and Pat were in Germany and Susan and family in Georgia.

Chapter 17 - 1974

Austin, Richard and I attended the Cotton Bowl game Tuesday, January 1, 1974. Four days later I met with the TPA Executive Committee in Austin. 1

We brought Mother to Dallas January 8, 1974 for consultation with our Ophthalmologist, Dr. F. Gene Braun. Dr. Braun recommended cataract surgery and she was admitted to Dallas Methodist Hospital.

There is an amusing anecdote concerning Mother's post-op behavior. Dr. Braun gave specific instructions that she be very quiet for the first few days, as cataract surgery was a delicate and risky procedure in 1974. Mother, a life-long advocate of "morning exercises," arose the day following surgery, lay on the floor and, "did her exercises." At that moment, the astonished ophthalmologist entered the room.

Afterwards he told the family, "I gave her careful instructions about every movement, never thinking it was necessary to tell an eighty-seven year-old woman not to do limbering-up exercises." Mother responded to his criticism with, "You didn't say I was not to do my morning exercises."

Jean nursed her mother-in-law during rehabilitation. Our first floor south west bedroom where Mother recovered was filled with flowers from relatives and friends. Jean served as the hostess-greeter for the many who came to visit. Blanche returned to her "much-loved" home in Sedalia February 9, 1974.

Professional

Al Burstein scheduled a School Psychology Task Force meeting in San Antonio for February 10, 1974. Those present were: A.J.J., Joy Anderson, Ruby Morris, Gene Walker, Larry Abrams,

Tom Pollard, Jim Tucker, Al Burstein; absent: Mel Sikes, Ruth Turner, Bob Burdine, L. Lasso.

A February 1974 Veterans Administration Psychiatric Conference meeting in New Orleans included representatives from psychiatry, psychology, social work, physical medicine, and administration. Psychiatrists Drs. Musser and Caffey and Cecil Peck were present to represent Central Office. Those from Dallas VAH including myself were H. Burnine, Administration, Dr. George Edwards, Chief of Staff, and Jack Gaston, Physical Medicine.

Photographs were taken of many friends and associates from the past: John McKelvain - Social Work at Waco; Arnold and Marion Krugman – Psychologist at Kentucky; Tom Frank – Psychiatrist at Waco; Bob Ferguson – Psychologist at Kentucky; Mike Williams – WW II, Aviation Psychologist.

Management Seminar

We purchased a 1974 Plymouth Duster for $4,000 from Gene Hays of McKinney February 23, 1974 and began making $98.20 monthly "repayments to savings." The automobile's first 20 miles was a drive to Sedalia. Mother was thankful to be home with improved vision.

Two weeks later I drove the new Duster to San Antonio to attend a two-week VA Management Seminar conducted by the faculty of Trinity University. There was a brief stop in Austin to visit Mary Belle Searight, her niece, and a grand-niece.

It remains a mystery why the Dallas VAH assigned me to attend a seminar oriented toward the development of hospital administrators. Trinity University was one of the first universities to offer training in hospital administration. Dallas VAH subsequently selected one or more Trinity graduates for its expanding hospital management section.

Among the interesting lectures at Trinity were those presented by Philosophy Professor, Dr. Leonard Duce. He invited participants to his home one afternoon to view museum quality wood carvings he produced as a hobby. Dr. Paul Golliher was another talented lecturer from the Trinity staff.

We stayed at La Quinta Motel near the airport, and bused from there each morning to the Trinity University Campus. A variety of administrative services such as personnel and registrar divisions were present for the Veterans Administration seminar. Two other psychologists were in the group, Dr. Joe Schenkel from New Mexico, and Dr. Earl Guyer, Chief Psychologist, Little Rock VAH. Fifty photographic slides taken during the two weeks concluded with a group photograph of the Veterans Administration participants. 2

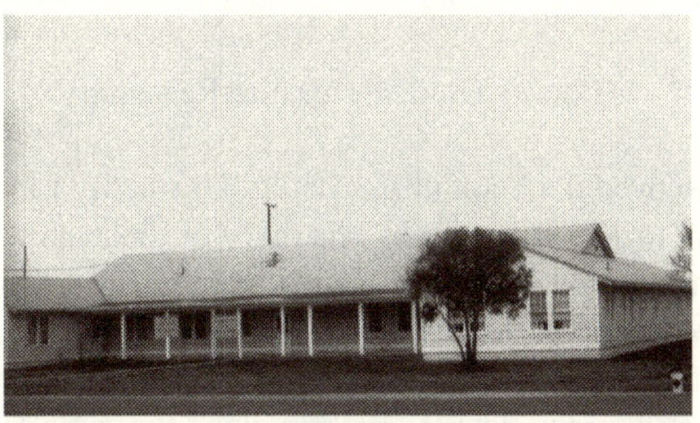

1942-45 Group and Psychomotor Test Building
San Antonio Aviation Cadet Center seen in 1974

Many old WWII sites were visited that first weekend in San Antonio. I attended early Chapel Service at Randolph Field, and afterwards toured the field, including a drive by the School of Aviation Medicine and the barracks where I was quartered. Then across San Antonio to the Aviation Cadet Center haunts. To my surprise, the two buildings where we tested 500 cadets each day, our mess hall, barracks, day room and supply room buildings were (from the outside) much as we left them in 1945.

Visits were made that Sunday afternoon, to all the Missions surrounding the city. It was a pleasant time to be in San Antonio. Delightful odors from the blooming lilacs and hursache trees permeated the atmosphere.

We had opportunities to visit other attractive San Antonio sites: Alamo, San Antonio River walk, San Antonio Zoo, and attend University literary productions.

A picture postcard to Richard March 18, 1974 stated, "Mission Concepcion - It was here that the 'Battle of Concepcion' was fought on October 29, 1835."

"I found an excellent zipper brief case at Trinity book store for you (1950). I bought the last one and would like one also. I toured this and the other 3 missions Sunday – should have some good slides. Will see you and your Mother Friday."

Albert's Hidden Treasure Research

I discovered a book in the Trinity University Library that was relevant to Albert research: The diary of Lieutenant Colonel Arthur James Lynon Tremantle, Coldstream Guards, a British officer who described in great detail his trip across Texas from Bagdad to San Antonio during America's Civil War. In reverse order, Albert Jernigan detailed his trip along the same route from San Antonio to Bagdad, dated a few months after Tremantle made his journey. The language and descriptions by the British Officer and the Confederate Officer were remarkably similar. 3

Allied Health Coordinator

Hospital Director Whitaker was in search of an appropriate candidate for a new hospital position, titled "Allied Health Coordinator." The search for a candidate was discussed at San Antonio with participant Marie Saunders, Ph.D., Coordinator, Allied Health Education at Temple VAH. Dr. Saunders wrote, "If

I can help you in any way in the development of health sciences, please do not hesitate to call."

Soon after receiving Dr. Sanders' letter, Dr. Delores Little a charming young widow of a Texas A&M Professor of Chemistry, mother of four small children, inquired about a psychology position. Delores began her graduate work at the University of Kentucky as a VA Psychology Trainee with the Lexington VA Hospital, and completed academic training at Texas A & M.

Psychology did not have a vacant position, but I introduced Delores to Mr. Whitaker as a possible candidate for the Allied Health Coordinator position. Mr. Whitaker readily agreed that Delores Little was the person to develop the new program. Years later, Dr. Little became Mrs. Walter Penk.

Letters from a Cousin

The exchange of letters with Douglas Brady began in April 1974. Doug, great-grandson of Aunt Jessie Williams had completed most of his doctoral work at Oklahoma, was considering an internship at Austin State Hospital, and asked if he could visit at Dallas VAH. I wrote him April 23, 1974:

". . . From April 30 to May 2, 1974, I will be attending a meeting in El Paso, Texas, but otherwise during the next two to four weeks should be generally available."

Doug wrote June 5, 1974 that his plans changed and he would do his internship with the "Oklahoma State Department, Guidance Center Division, at Bethany, Oklahoma." He concluded with, "I hope that you enjoyed SWPA, I plan to attend the next meeting, and present a paper I am now completing."

Doug completed his doctoral work in clinical psychology, entered private practice, became professionally active, and was elected President of the Oklahoma Psychological Association. We were never able to visit in person, only by telephone.

El Paso Workshop

Dr. Charles Stenger from Central Office led the Psychology Training Workshop at El Paso meeting held April 30 to May 2. Dr. Charles Stenger, Associate to Cecil Peck, was a pleasant, modest, former POW of the Korean Conflict. The meeting included Directors of Clinical Training from many Universities and representatives from VA Training Committees. Ron Kidd and I represented Dallas VAH.

A San Antonio Visit with Jean

Jean began tutoring students with reading problems at Adamson High School in 1973. She took a reading tutoring course through Texas Woman's University, and completed the course June 20, 1974, the day I drove to San Antonio to attend a TPA Task Force meeting. To celebrate, Jean flew to San Antonio to join me the next day.

We attended an afternoon event on the San Antonio River, and visited the enormous mural by the artist, Peter Hurd depicting a cattle roundup and branding. One could "smell the dust and hear the shouting of the cowboys."

Psychology Trainees

The following excerpts from a June 6, 1974 letter to Dr. Victor H. Appel, Department of Educational Psychology University of Texas at Austin tell of subtle modifications in the VA Psychology Training Program.

"Attached is completed Intern Evaluation Form on psychology trainee Don Carver. Mr. Carver will continue on our internship rolls through June. . . Level III contract will be completed. . . Under the old VA training plan of a couple years back, recommendations would have been made to promote Mr. Carver to Level IV . . . under our current stipend plan we maintain only a one year contractual arrangement with a trainee."

However, the VA Training Program retained flexibility as reflected in excerpts from Earl Patterson's evaluation dated September 4, 1974.

"Earl Patterson, Level III trainee from Texas Tech University, began an internship at the Dallas VA Hospital September 4, 1973, and completed the internship August 30, 1974. . . Dr. Mary Louise Toland was his assigned coordinator of training. He was also supervised by Drs. Fudge, Johnson and Tucker."

Dr. Toland gave specific recommendations to enhance Earl's experience at the fourth year level. In my summary statement, remarked: "Mr. Patterson has shown growth and development during this year and has accomplished all academic goals except dissertation research. Following a number of contacts with Central Office, officials at Texas Tech University, and review by the Station Psychology Training Committee, it was decided to offer Mr. Patterson fourth year level training at Dallas VA Hospital. His coordinator . . . will be Dr. David T. Johnson, and his primary assignment . . . the Mental Hygiene Clinic."

The evaluation summaries for the next two trainees do not identify their Universities, but believe they were graduate students at the University of Texas.

Robert E. Rein, appointed Level II Clinical Psychology Trainee effective September 1, 1973, began his training experience on May 28, 1974. He was assigned to the GM&S Consultation Unit under the supervision of Ron Kidd. He had learning opportunities in consultation to physicians and nurses on psychological aspects of patients requiring medical and surgical treatment, and vocational counseling. Mr. Rein was promoted to Level III in September to complete an Internship at Dallas VAH in 1974-1975.

Timothy C. Wiedel, appointed as a second year level Clinical Psychology Trainee September 1, 1973, entered active training status at Dallas VA on June 1, 1974. He was promoted to Level III in September 1974 with Dr. Walter Penk as coordinator during both levels of training. In the summer of 1974 Tim received training experience in the Drug Dependence Treatment Center, Inpatient Psychiatry, and an opportunity to experience work with Dr. Penk in an ongoing Central Office approved research project.

John W. Craighead was appointed as a Level II Counseling Psychology Trainee January 12, 1974. He entered the program in his final academic year, having fulfilled all requirements, including dissertation, for a degree in Educational Psychology. University of Texas Professor, Dr. Carl Hereford recommended John be permitted to shift to Counseling Psychology, complete the necessary course work to qualify academically, and not be required to develop a second dissertation.

Mr. Craighead arrived for duty July 1, 1974, and completed 500 hours of training by September 30, 1974 under the supervision of Dr. Jack Fudge in the Drug Dependent Treatment Unit. Although not eligible for promotion to Level III until January 1975, he was permitted to begin his Internship year with the concurrence of Dr. Elton Ash of VA Central Office, Dr. Royal Embree of the University of Texas, and the Dallas VA Psychology Training Committee.

Joyce G. Allen, appointed as a Level IV Trainee September 1, 1974, with an annual stipend of $6,790, became the first trainee to receive traineeship in the joint VA-University of Texas Health Science Center program. Her time was divided 3/5 VA, 2/5 UTHSC, with Buzz Tucker coordinator at VA, and Martin Gluck, coordinator at UTHSC. Miss Allen was our first African American trainee. She had an earlier appointment as a Level II trainee at Pittsburgh VAH in 1971-1972.

Family Matters

Austin was home for 1974 Spring Break, and began filming "Better Basketball for Boys." Richard and friends of Austin and Richard assisted in the production. The crew included me in their cast of characters. One of the "cast members" wore my Whitewright High School, black and gold letter sweater with the prominent gold "W."

Mother resumed preservation of correspondence in March 1974 following her recovery from cataract surgery. She returned to her daily habit of letter writing. I responded:

"Your good letter again makes me thankful for your renewed vision. We are well. I must work Saturday so may try to come up one afternoon to see you and go to the grocery store."

Almost every week one, both or all of us went to Sedalia to take Mother for groceries at Bill Barrett's store in Van Alstyne. We frequently ate lunch at Bill's cafeteria within the store, and Bill often joined us. Jean included Mother's sheets when she washed ours, and returned them on the next visit to Sedalia according to a comment Mother made in a later letter: "Jean - I just can't help thinking those sheets should not be put on you. I appreciate so much all both of you do for me. But some things I must not put on either of you. When I think how you all are managing your own family - putting them through high school and college it is wonderful!"

Aunt Pansy Jernigan McDougal died May 7, 1974 and was buried in Laurel Land Memorial Park Dallas, Texas in Space #10, Lot 94, Section 41. Jean and I assisted Mozelle select a minister for her Mother's funeral service. Neither mother nor daughter was an active member of a church at the time of Aunt Pansy's death. She was the last of my father's siblings to die.

I interviewed Aunt Pansy on April 4, 1972 - two years before she died - and invited her to share memories about her early life at Sedalia.

Mother's letters gave evidence of the corrective effect of the cataract surgery. Eighty-seven years of age, yet she wrote with bold, secure pen strokes. Excerpts from a letter:

"My dear Ones,

"What would I do without you two?. . .The Youth Rally was at Sedalia last night and I went. Russell Presley came for me. I enjoyed it. Yesterday morning I made a cake - not knowing about the affair [youth rally]. I thought I'd make one and give Edgar some for his supper. He had asked how to make one. . . I had such good luck and just about the time I took it out I heard of the affair. I was so glad I had it to take, have Edgar's for today.

". . . I will be glad when it is time to go back to see Dr. Braun [5-31-74]. The sight of my eye is fine.

". . . . Jack - you won't have to come this week, will you? So I hope you and your children can have a happy Mothers Day with Jean Sunday. Instead of waiting on me- this weekend - take Jean and your family out for dinner on me. She surely does deserve it. There is nothing I want for Mothers Day that I do not have. Have the best family any where. I know the Lord and where I'm going when I die, and have had more - many more blessing always than I ever deserved. How truly thankful I am of our children and grandchildren. O how thankful I am that I can read my Bible each day. I wish every one would do that. Much love to all."

"Lamplighter Founders Retiring"

That was the headline in Dallas Morning News, Section 7C for Wednesday, June 5, 1974. Some excerpts: "The changing of the guard at Dallas' Lamplighter School is at hand, and the two women who built the nationally known school are finding it as hard to leave as to stay. . . Carmel, on the California seacoast south of San Francisco, is the idyllic retreat the two women will retire to June 11. Their departure will close 21 years of work and worry at Lamplighter, the once-modest school they've built into one of the nation's showcases for innovative early childhood education. Natalie admitted to 'shedding a tear or two. . . Still when we get to Carmel, it'll be hard to get us back to Dallas.'"

Natalie and Sandy were remarkable teachers and administrators. Beth later compared her approach to teaching with "Aunt Natalie's" teaching technique, a model to be followed. We visited Natalie in her home on Churchill Way June 8, 1974. All of the Dallas cousins came to say goodbye to Natalie and Sandy.

TPA - VA

I flew to Austin in July to attend a TPA meeting. Every Austin trip gave an opportunity for additional Albert Jernigan research: "Notebook #3, p. 24-25, July 27, 1974, visited State Archives."

Note documented discovery of, The Campaigns of Walker's Texas Division; The Official Atlas of the Civil War, by Tomas Yoseloff, 1958, and The War of the Rebellion - A Compilation of the Official Records of the Union and Confederate Armies. Photocopies of the latter were requested from the State Archives. The State Archives staff mailed the data a few days later.

The VA Staff gave a goodbye party in the 9th floor conference room for Research Technician Coy Craig and his new bride. Those present in the photos were: Kathy Meyer, Earl Patterson, Buzz Tucker, Mary Louise Toland, Dave Johnson, and Steve Wroten, a summer student from Kimball High School who assisted in clerical assignments.

I drove to Austin on August 16, returned the following day, Saturday, August 17 after attending a TPA Executive Committee Meeting, chaired by President George Kramer of Corpus Christi. There was a typical rest stop on the return trip at the Village Bakery in West for a dozen apricot kaloches.

And there was the usual visit with Mary Belle Searight while in Austin. She loaned a box of letters of a Spanish War soldier to Arabelle (Alberts's daughter); all letters of Belle to Albert and their son, Moore; letters of Albert to Moore; Rebecca Moore to her grandson; and Belle to Albert from Tennessee."

All the data were photocopied before their return to Mary Belle many months later. The photocopies were donated to the Barker Texas History Center in 2000.

Family - School - Task Force

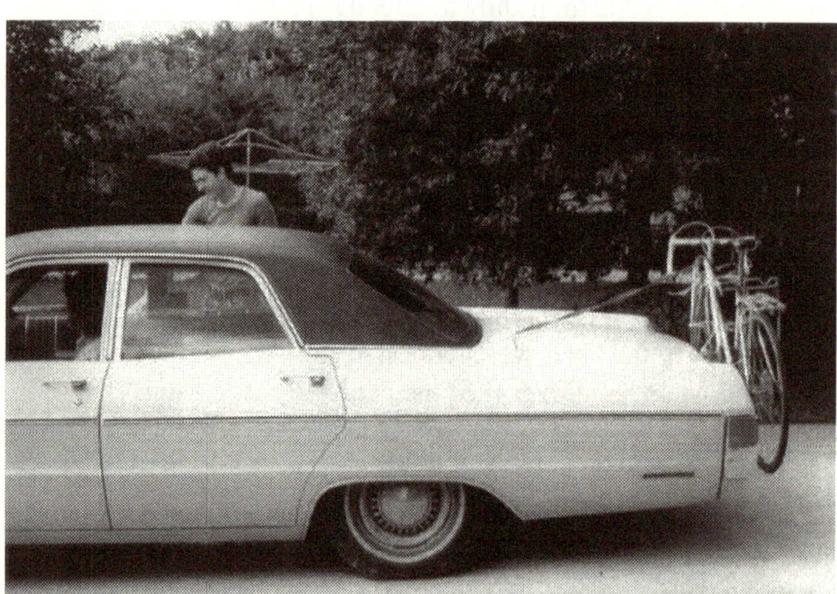

Austin began his junior year of college at University of Texas in the fall of 1974. Austin and Richard were photographed as they departed with bicycle on rack. Richard returned to begin his senior year at Kimball High School that included a second year of media training at Skyline High School. He rode the bus to Skyline from Kimball.

One wet weekend evening in September, Richard and his girlfriend drove the Tempest to attend an event at SMU. The car hydroplaned on North Central Expressway, but thankfully, no one was injured!

Two shaken-teenagers were comforted by a nice African American family that lived just off North Central, and from whose home they telephoned about the accident. I drove over and brought them back to Oak Cliff and arranged for the Tempest to be towed to our driveway. With much regret by all, it was necessary to declare the Tempest "totaled" as the cost of repair was prohibitive.

I drove to San Antonio on October 4, 1974 for a TPA Task Force meeting, and on the way, stopped to visit with Austin in his comfortable apartment north of the campus. In San Antonio, I visited with Ira Iscoe, Cliff Jones, and former Waco trainee, Buzz O'Connell.

Nine days later, the Nikkromat camera recorded my presence in Washington. D. C., with scenes of October foliage between D. C. and Baltimore, the bus route toward another VA Cooperative Research meeting. Among the Baltimore scenes was one at the harbor of the docked Frigate Constellation, "World's Oldest Ship Continuously afloat, launched on September 7, 1779."

We docked our sailboat in the barn at Sedalia on Saturday, October 19, 1974, and the next day drove to east Texas to visit former Fountainhead neighbors, the Mac McDonalds, at their lake home. Saturday night, October 26, 1974, Richard entertained a number of his friends in the upstairs "Casbah Theater."

Mother wrote at the approach of my 53rd birthday. She resumed the communication of social-spiritual experiences in her letters, but with some mild cognitive loss. Excerpts:

"I had quite a crowd part of yesterday. I went to church with Maggie and Clarence but Mrs. Brown brought me home. Arthur Giles called to see if I were going to be at home. So he and Bertha and Florence came up and while they were here Anita and Swain came. [All signed Guest Book 10-20-74.] Later Anita and Swain and I went down to Mrs. Standridge's. I went in to see Mr. Standridge I think he knew me but he dies [lies] about as well as I do. I had just heard from Pansy's daughter and I did not know Swain, so I got them mixed up at first. We all went out to the cemetery. I enjoyed seeing all of them.

". . . Jack - I hope you have a truly good birthday. You deserve it. I am so proud of you and your family and most thankful by far, that you are all Christians. May you ever give God His rightful place in your hearts and life. You bring much happiness to me.

Love Mother"

A VA Conference

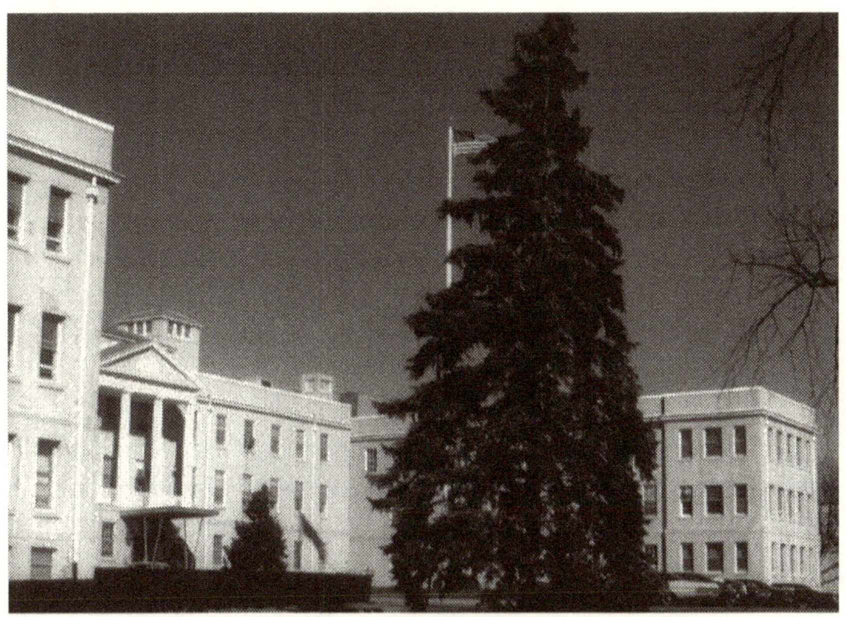

Jefferson Barracks VAH

I attended a Veterans Administration Conference at the Jefferson Barracks Missouri VA Hospital, Wednesday, November 20, 1974. During a break four of us walked over the historic hospital grounds that included a National Cemetery. The mighty Mississippi River could be seen through the trees. Three VA Service Chiefs stood for a group photo: Roy Brenner, Fred Royer, and Phil Laughlin.

A Photographic Diary

I was back in Texas by Saturday, November 23, 1974, and at Sedalia to photograph fall scenes around the farm. The next week we celebrated Thanksgiving. Our typical Thanksgiving trip pattern included dinners at both ancestral homes.

I flew to Corpus Christi to attend the 26th annual meeting of the Texas Psychological Association on Friday, December 6, 1974. Photographic slides included scenes of Dallas and Corpus from the air, a sea gull at Padre Island (site of the meeting), a early morning breakfast during TPA with photos of Wayne Gill, Naomi Meadows and her husband. Later in the day, there was a visit with Laura and Frances in the A & I Chancellor's home, and a football game in the afternoon.

I recall how warmly the people responded to Jamie, many seeming to want to reach out and touch him as he walked among his people. Later, Jamie prepared a steak for us on the outside grill. The next morning he drove me to Corpus Christi Airport for a sunrise flight back to Dallas, with a brief stop at Houston Intercontinental.

In mid-December I photographed little Wendy Seaman holding her dog, a photo that was entered in the 1975 State Fair photo contest. (It didn't win, but Wendy liked the photo.)

During the week of December 15, 1974 the Dallas VA Psychology Staff held a going away party in the 9th floor conference room for Dr. Dave Johnson. Among those present were: Kathy Meyers, a wife of a trainee or staff, Dave Johnson and wife, Buzz Tucker, Tim Wiedel, a young American Indian, then on duty as a clerk, Ron Kidd, John Craighead, Jean and possibly Richard (back turned, taking photo), Ralph Robinowitz, and Dr. George Edwards.

Dr. Pamela Profant a new 1974 staff member for the Drug Treatment Unit was also present at the party. With the hiring of Pam Profant, Jack Fudge moved to the Mental Hygiene Clinic. 4

Jay Graduated

Jay graduated with distinction from University of Texas at Arlington. He was interviewed on campus by Proctor & Gamble, and began training as a Proctor and Gamble salesman. Beth, a special education teacher at Carrollton was taking graduate courses at TWU. Lisa was in kindergarten.

The last 1974 extant correspondence that Mother saved was a letter from Beth at their new address, 2311 Valleywood, Carrollton, TX 75006, postmarked 15 November 1974.

"Dear Grandma,

Everything is super here. Lisa has had a cough but is doing better. My classes are going well. One of them, Theories of Learning is really hard but at this time I have A's in both courses. I love my teaching this year. Not only is Carrollton- Farmer's Branch an excellent school system, my school, Woodlake, is outstanding. It is very similar to Lamplighter.

This is Jay's week to go to Abilene. He really doesn't enjoy going there but really loves working for Proctor & Gamble. His boss is very considerate and says that Jay's the best trainee he's ever had.

Mother and Daddy came over for supper Friday night. We really enjoyed them. Lisa spent the day with Mother while I went to the TSTA Convention. Enclosed is a picture of me made at school. We love you -

Beth"

Enclosed with the letter was a very mature five-year-old drawing of birds, trees, blue sky, green grass and a little girl. (Signed)

"Love
Lisa "

Christmas 1974 at Sedalia was celebrated on Christmas Eve. Eleven family members signed the Guest Book on 12-24-74, and also S. W. (Weldon) Lane and his daughter, Bookie. Grace Lane died on June 29, 1974.

In early January 1975, Mother wrote her friend Mary Lance about Christmas 1974:

"We had a good Christmas. Jamie and Frances wanted to take all of us to McKinney Christmas Eve and did all but Stewart and Mary. They went to Ala. to see their daughter and family. (Susan is finishing her college work and both children are in school now.) Stewart's son and wife are still in Service over seas. I had a nice letter from them and a box of fine soap. We hope we get to see them this summer. We had a wonderful dinner and it was service not to have dishes etc. to work with. Jamie took me and Laura (his daughter) by the [Highland] cemetery on the way home."

The Fains came Christmas Day to join in the opening of gifts, and afterwards the annual photo of Lisa and me in the front yard beside the "Christmas" cedar, then in its fifth year of growth. Two days later we visited Clyde Tilton in his room at Baylor hospital where he was recovering from open heart surgery.

Chapter 18 - 1975

We visited Jay, Beth and Lisa in their Carrollton home New Year's Day 1975. Jean and I made trips to Sedalia January 4, 18, and 21, the latter to attend the funeral of Cousin Jim Coffey. He died at age 93.

Investigation at Little Rock

I was invited (detailed) to Little Rock VA Hospital February 3 - 6, 1975, a one week assignment, ". . . to investigate and evaluate recent happenings at the Little Rock VA Hospital (Fort Roots)." Psychologist Jack Davis was a key team leader.

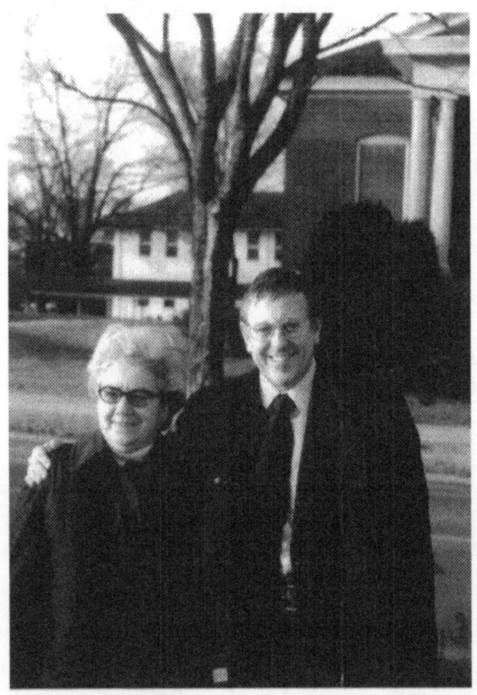

Chief Nurse, VA Central Office and Dr. Jack Davis

I do not recall the gravity of the incidents. Central Office sent personnel from Psychiatry, Psychology, Nursing, and Social Work from Washington, D. C. to investigate.

I flew to Little Rock on Monday and returned Friday. All investigators and the Central Office staff stayed at Ramada Inn near the VA Hospital. We had lunch in the VA Canteen, but in the evening sampled one or more of the Little Rock "name" restaurants. The evening fellowship was relaxing after a hard day of investigative interviews and record reviews.

There were opportunities during the week to explore the historic grounds and old buildings that dated back to the Civil War when the place was called Ft. Roots Army Post. The father of General Douglas MacArthur was Commandant at Fort Roots when Gen. MacArthur was a small lad.

There were also opportunities to visit Little Rock Psychology Staff. Former Waco trainee, later staff member at Dallas, Earl Wilkinson was a member of the Little Rock Psychology Staff. Long time friend, Earl Guyer was the Chief Psychologist. The review report was not critical of the Psychology Service.

Family

I returned in time Friday, February 7, 1975 to attend the Kimball High School senior play. Richard played the role of a "Mad Russian" with "false hair" on his chest. One of our couches was borrowed for the set.

Stewart came by the next day for a visit, on his way to Sedalia. Two weeks later a beautiful snow covered the landscape, an amateur photographer's paradise.

Austin wrote his grandmother from his apartment at 1020 E. 45 #15D, Austin, TX, February 12, 1975: "It has been a busy semester so far, but a very good one because I am finally getting to take courses in film."

Beth mailed her grandmother a lovely card, postmarked 11 Mar 1975. "We are Busy, Busy! Last weekend we put in our garden. . . Jay still loves his job and got a raise. Lisa is staying in a new place - a mother and 2 kindergarten boys. . . I can't wait to tell you about my Masters paper."

Jean mailed a room deposit check ($50) for Richard to University of Texas for the fall semester of 1975, and a brief letter to her Mother-in-law, in large script for easier reading.

Richard wrote his grandmother March 24: "Being eighteen years old doesn't seem any different but then again I didn't expect any great wall to fall on me March 4 proclaiming my manhood and that I would have to on that day step out into the world and begin my living. . . I hope you'll be able to come down for my graduation this May."

Joe Gallo, son of Psychology Secretary, Susan Gallo, and another student from Dallas Baptist drove to Sedalia Saturday, April 5, 1975 in search of wildflowers. Along the way we stopped at Westminster to photograph the partially dismantled Westminster Baptist Academy. All five of us went to the Bill Barrett store for groceries and food, and brought Mother back home where she served a cake she baked that morning. The two students found many samples of wildflowers to exhibit to their Dallas Baptist class including the Star of Bethlehem.

Chicago - A Telephone Call

I flew to Chicago the week of April 7, 1975 to attend the annual Veterans Administration Research Meeting.

One of the meetings presented by Les Robbins reported drug research related to Vietnam Era Veterans. Almost all the 1400 veterans examined in the research study reported first time experience with a drug began in Vietnam.

Roy Brenner and Hugh Creeden discussed the benefits of Family Therapy. The subject was of special interest as Dallas VA planned to establish a Family Therapy Program. Our new staff member, Royce Scrivner subsequently developed the Family Therapy Program.

Thursday morning, Dr. Theodore Cole talked on the subject, "Sexuality, the Practitioner, and the Patient." Other topics were "Ethical Treatment of Patients by Drugs" and a "Right to Treatment" by a James Robitschen, lawyer and M.D. Jack Baker and Charles Stenger brought "reports" from Central Office.

I was in a meeting Friday morning when a telephone call came from Jean that her father had died. I caught the next plane to Dallas.

William Marvin (Jake) Gibson, born March 29, 1884 died Thursday night, April 10, 1975. He arose from his chair when the baseball game ended and fell to the floor. Mr. Gibson's Masonic Lodge was meeting in downtown Melissa and Mrs. Gibson called the Lodge. Lodge member, Dr. Scott Wysong came immediately to the house to pronounce the death of my good father-in-law.

Jean talked with her Dad that morning and told him of her secretarial position to begin the following Monday with Social Rehabilitation Service at the downtown Regional Office of Health Education and Welfare. She received the news of his death that evening.

The funeral services were held at Melissa Baptist Church on Saturday, April 12, 1975. During the service, one of Mr. Gibson's sheep birthed a lamb in the pasture south of the house. Richard took a poignant photo of Jake Gibson's teenage great-granddaughter, Nancy Stewart on her knees cuddling the newborn lamb after the funeral. Jake would have loved the lamb. Mr. Gibson was a very good man! 1

One weekend in the fall of 1975, all the buildings, trailers, barns, gates, etc. were photographed as Mr. Gibson left them when he passed on to Heaven. He could have told a story about each building. Mr. Gibson was a detailed story teller, and fortunately over the years I tape recorded some of his tales as the two of us sat together on his wrap-around front porch and talked.

Richard and Lisa

Richard responded to a Skyline Media Course assignment with a film script that included Lisa as the central character. Either Richard or his instructor arranged the use of an abandoned downtown Dallas hotel for the film site.

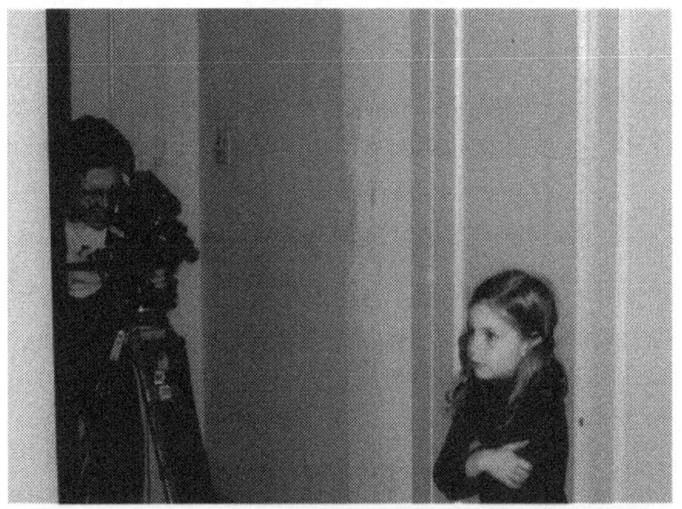

Lisa Fain – Richard Jernigan at camera

Jean was uncomfortable with the isolated location and asked me to monitor Lisa (and Richard). I took photographs of Richard filming the patient little actress in the old hotel.

Professional Publications

Jossey-Bass published Paul McReynolds' Advances in Psychological Assessment:, Vol 3, in the spring of 1975. Luciano

L'Abate, Ph.D., one of the participants in the 1972 Hawaii Symposium, requested ". . . A reprint of your chapter 'Use of Group Tests In Clinical Settings' that appeared in Advances in Psychological Assessment: Vol. 3."

I wrote Luciano on April 25, 1975, "Attached is a xeroxed copy of the chapter. . . The second edition will carry some minor changes but the content is essentially the same as in this copy. . . It was good to hear from you again."

Alexander Tolor, Ph.D. wrote from Fairfield University, Fairfield, Connecticut on April 29, 1975, "I am planning to prepare a comprehensive review of the Bender-Gestalt Test literature in order to update the information that had been presented in the book: An Evaluation of the Bender Gestalt Test, by A. Tolor and H. C. Schulberg. . . Therefore, I would very much appreciate receiving a reprint of your paper entitled: Rotation Style on the Bender-Gestalt Test, Journal of Clinical Psychology, 1967, 23, 176-179. 2

Staff Changes

John Geers emphatically requested there be no staff party or "going away" dinner when he retired, and the time of his departure is undated. He silently faded from the scene, but his input to the Dallas VA Hospital continued, especially in the rehabilitation area of Patient Work Therapy.

Royce Scrivner became a member of the Psychology Staff in January 1975. He was on duty when Reagan H. Andrews, Jr. joined the staff in March 1975. John Geers departed before Reagan's arrival. 3

Royce served as a member of the Counseling Psychology faculty, the University of Texas, Austin before joining Dallas VAH Psychology Service as a Counseling Psychologist. He subsequently qualified on the Civil Service Register as a Clinical Psychologist.

Dr. Scrivner made immediate contributions to the Medical Service Unit. He saw a need for a service for the dying patient, those primarily diseased with cancer, and worked in that and other areas of service on the general medical wards until we opened the Family Therapy Program.

Royce was single when he came to Dallas for interview. He spoke of a marriage to a Social Worker in Austin, but gave no details of why or how the marriage ended. Royce did not announce he was gay until after my retirement. He became positively active as a professional leader in the psychological understanding of Gays and Lesbians at State and National Psychological Association levels, and later was elected President of the Texas Psychological Association.

Reagan Andrews was one of the first graduates from the Southwestern Medical School Psychology Ph.D. program. He had a background in journalism in addition to psychology and quickly made valuable contributions to the VA Hospital Psychiatric Service.

Buzz Tucker retired in May 1975. Unlike John Geers, Buzz welcomed a "going away" dinner and most all the staff gathered May 22, 1975 at Dallas' downtown Spaghetti Warehouse to wish Buzz a fond farewell. Dr. R. B. Tucker left a void when he retired from the Veterans Administration.

Family

Chancellor James C. Jernigan's long tenure at Texas A&I (1946-1975) came to an unexpected end. Frances wrote on Thursday, May 15, 1975 and included a copy of Corpus Christi Caller for Wednesday May 14, 1975. The paper carried a front page article with photograph of Jamie, titled: "Jernigan submits his resignation on date still unsettled."

"Dear Jack and Jean,

". . . Jim had a press conference Tuesday afternoon at which time he released his letter to the board, with the approval of the board president. The TV coverage that night was not too good. Representatives of the two stations arrived late, disturbing Jim's presentation, as he was determined to start on time. However, he did get a good opportunity later to talk to the reporter who had 'broken' this story originally

". . . Laura and I still hope to get off on our trip to Europe the 27th of this month, although I am reluctant to leave under the circumstances. If Jim is to leave August 31, this year, he wants to take his accumulated 3 months vacation prior to that, which would mean his vacating the office in June, but who knows."

Excerpts from Beth's "school teacher" letter to Grandma Blanche May, 1975:

"Well, it's the last week of school. It seems the year has just slipped by - I have really loved my job this year. . . You would love my school, Woodlake. It is bright-yellows, oranges and whites, and is a very happy place - there's always something going on.

". . . . Now I'll tell you about my professional paper. To get a Master's in Education at TWU you have to submit a professional product showing your competency. All semester I've been working on a <u>prospectus</u> which gives background information about a topic which you are interested in and a plan for your project. It is submitted to your advisor, and if he thinks your idea is all right, based on what you said in your prospectus, he approves and you do your project. My project is to make a training film for the teachers about eye tracking. Eye tracking is how well you have control over the muscles in your eyes. This year I have found many children who have trouble reading and one of the problems is that they can't adequately control small movements with their eyes. The result is that they may lose their place when reading or words or letters may skip around on the page, etc. It's easy to check and remediate, but many teachers do not know how. My film will show children's eyes moving improperly, how to check for it, and what to do about it.

"Jay seems to be traveling around more lately. A man in his unit quit, so Jay has his territory and this man's to take care of. This week he has to go to Abilene, Oklahoma, and Wichita Falls. I hope it doesn't last for long (the extra traveling).

"Lisa is finishing up her kindergarten year. Tomorrow she is going to the zoo and she gets to take a Sack Lunch! She is really excited. A week from Sunday is her dance recital and she'll be glad to get dancing over with, I believe

"My hand is getting tired. You are so often in my thoughts, and I miss your chatter and love."

Richard graduated from Kimball High School May 28, 1975. All his immediate family was present for the graduation. However, grandmothers, Mary Gibson and Blanche Jernigan were unable to attend.

Mother wrote her friend Mary Lance on June 2, 1975, "Jack is helping me so much these days about the farm business. Bill Barrett has a big store at Fan [Van] Alstyne and that is where we go to get groceries. He has such a nice place to serve meals there too. We go there and get us a nice hot dinner too. I can't do much cooking but of course I cand [can] all that I need."

Mother's limitations were becoming more obvious. She did not want to leave her home of almost seventy years.

We mailed a check to University of Texas June 16th "For orientation for Richard." A $120 deposit check was mailed July 6 to the University for "Room for Richard."

Dr. Driggs, Orthopedic Surgeon, examined my back on July 18th. When he reviewed the x-rays, Dr. Driggs remarked it was the arthritic back of a 70 year old man. It is assumed the back was that of an 86 year old when I turned 70.

TIGER

Mr. E. P. Whitaker, Hospital Director announced the TIGER program in a Hospital Memorandum dated July 24, 1975 to: "Coordinator, Allied Health Education (152), Dr. Delores Little with copies to all Service Chiefs." Mr. Whitaker "Authorized absence for three dozen employees to attend the 'TIGER' Workshop, July 29, 30, and 31, 1975, to be held at the Holiday Inn, Duncanville, Texas." My name and that of Ron Kidd were among those designated to attend.

TIGER, an acronym for "Training In Group Effectiveness and Resourcefulness" was a program that dealt with human interactions and the dynamics of group behavior. Houston VA Hospital was a developmental leader. Many of the handouts to workshop participants came through Houston Psychologist, Philip G. Hanson, Ph.D., Director, Human Interaction Training Laboratory, VA Hospital, Houston, Texas. Opening excerpts are quoted from a Hanson handout titled, "What to look for in Groups."

"In all human interaction there are two major ingredients: content and process. The first deals with subject matter or the task upon which the group is working. In most interactions, the focus of attention of all persons is on the content. The second ingredient, process, is concerned with what is happening between and to group members while the group is working. Group process, or dynamics, deals with such items as morale, feeling tone, atmosphere, influence, participation, styles of influence, leadership struggles, conflict, competition, cooperation, etc. . . Since these processes are present in all groups, awareness of them will enhance a person's worth to a group and make him a more effective group participant."

The Houston VA Hospital Training Laboratory received nationwide recognition. Members of the Psychology staff developed a program to assist the Houston Police Force improve their relationships with the public, and promote meaningful group experience within the Police Force.

Ron Kidd and I became members of the Station TIGER Committee. However, mine was a supporting role, encouraging other Psychology staff to become active leaders in the program. The program remained active at Dallas VAH through 1979, and possibly beyond.

St. Louis Conference

The Veterans Administration presented a Training Conference for Chiefs of Psychology the week of August 17, 1975. But before leaving for St. Louis I took Austin and Richard to University of Texas at Austin for the 1975 fall term. Junior, Austin Jernigan moved to a garage apartment near the campus. Freshman, Richard Jernigan was required to room at Moore Hall. As soon as Richard was settled in his room, he was photographed bicycling off to explore the campus.

I stayed at the downtown Holiday Inn, St. Louis. Many slides were taken at the St. Louis Zoo, and I again visited the site of the 1904 St. Louis Worlds Fair.

Back at the Hospital

Former trainee, Dr. Earl Patterson joined the Psychology Staff at the Day Hospital Unit in late 1974 or early 1975. Dr. Mary Louise Toland wrote a summary of Earl's training in September 1974. "Mr. Patterson's professional competence has developed satisfactorily in most areas. One significant area has been his role in interdisciplinary settings. During his time in the Day Hospital, he was able to achieve quite rapidly a close working relationship with each staff member and to enjoy a mutual exchange of respect and cooperation in handling the daily activities of the program."

The August 1975 summary evaluation of the training experience for Trainee, Joyce G. Allen is the first extant documented reference to Earl Patterson as a staff member. Miss Allen completed her Internship August 30, 1975. Her assignments at the University of Texas Health Science Center included rotations at the Child Psychiatry Outpatient Clinic and the Juvenile Department. At the VA Hospital she had assignments on Psychiatry (supervised by Dr. R. B. Tucker), the Medical and Surgical Service (supervised by Dr. Ronald Kidd), the Day Hospital and the Mental Hygiene Clinic (supervised by Dr. Mary Louise Toland), and the Drug Dependence Treatment Center (supervised by Dr. Pam Profant). Dr. Royce Scrivner and Dr. Earl Patterson also participated in her supervision. Such a variety of settings enabled Miss Allen to have contact with most all the unit psychologists. (Drs. Robinowitz, Penk, and Fudge indirectly contributed to her training.) 4

John Craighead was promoted to Level III training status on January 11, 1975 and continued in training until June 21, 1975. His last day at the VA Hospital was May 16, 1975. As previously mentioned, John was an atypical Counseling Psychology trainee. He was assigned to the Drug Dependence Treatment Unit with Dr. Jack Fudge as coordinating supervisor. John left the VAH to accept a post-doctoral position with the Fort Worth State School.

Level III Trainee Robert E. Rein completed his internship in May 1975. His 1975 training experience included the following: Psychiatry, January to March; Drug Dependence Treatment Center, March through May 1975. He was given an opportunity to devote one day a week at the Dallas Child Guidance Clinic. He did not choose to develop a dissertation research topic. However, he completed two very informative research studies of benefit to the hospital, one involving a survey of group psychotherapy practices and the other a review of admission procedures on the Psychiatric Service.

Level III Trainee Timothy C. Wiedel completed his internship in June 1975. He was assigned part-time to the Mental Hygiene Clinic through April 1975, Inpatient Psychiatry from January 1975 through May 1975 part-time, and the General Medical and Surgical Consultation service in April and June 1975. He also returned to the Drug Dependence Treatment Center for more advanced experience in May and June of 1975. His station research project involving the Word Association Test gave him an opportunity to observe the Day Treatment Center during the period October 1974 through April 1975.

As noted by the schedule, Mr. Wiedel was an unusually energetic trainee who took full advantage of every training opportunity. From November 1974 through March 1975, Mr. Wiedel had an extra-station assignment with the Dallas County Juvenile Department, accumulating approximately 180 hours of experience under the supervision of Dr. John Price. The Chief of Psychology and the Chairman of the Department of Psychology at Southwestern Medical School expressed an interest in the young man as a future staff member.

Jack Gold served a joint psychology internship at Dallas VAH and at UTHSC-Dallas beginning in September. Dr. Kidd was assigned as his VA coordinator of training during the internship year, 1975 to August 1976. Jack began his training on the GM&S Consultation Unit from September 1975 to January 1976 under the supervision of Drs. Kidd and Scrivner.

Doctoral candidate Stephen Close, Oklahoma State University began an internship in September 1975, finishing in August 1976. He spent three days a week at Dallas VA Hospital and two days a week at University of Texas Health Science Center (Supervisor - Dr. Frank Trimboli). Dr. Walter Penk was the coordinating supervisor. His 1975 assignment began on Inpatient Psychiatry Unit under the supervision of Dr. Reagan Andrews.

Burt Brodnitzky, South Carolina State began an internship in September 1975 and was assigned to the Day Hospital and Mental Hygiene Clinic under the supervision of Dr. Toland. He conducted a weekly goals group with Dr. Patterson and a weekly couples group led by Delbert Hughes, M.D. He was assigned individual therapy patients at the Mental Hygiene Clinic and was co-therapist with Dr. Toland in an evening group.

Family Happenings

Photographs were submitted to the State Fair Creative Arts Department for the first time in 1975 (check-book entry, August 27, 1975, "State Fair of Texas $4.00.") One of the entries was of Wendy Seaman holding her dog. None of the entries won a prize.

Jamie retired in August 1975. Mother wrote her friend Mary Lance August 28, 1975:

"Jamie has resigned from his place in the school at Kingsville, Texas. They will be moving some where this fall - I do not know just where as yet. They are having <u>two</u> nice affairs for him and Frances and I have invitations but will <u>not</u> try to go."

Jay, Beth, Lisa, Jean and I, the Seaman family and others from the "42" group visited Lake Texoma, with an overnight stay at Eisenhower State Park.

I attended an Executive Committee meeting of TPA in Austin on Saturday, September 13, 1975. Mileage for the one day round trip was 385 miles.

Our dentist, Dr. Burnett fitted a crowned tooth October 1, as noted by checkbook entry, "Jack - crown, $140.00."

Beth responded to a gift from her grandmother in a letter postmarked 7 Oct 1975. ". . . Lisa and I are off for the Fair today. We're enjoying being together. I'm going to try to work on some stuff for school; in particular, the script for the film I'm making for my Master's project."

Land Heritage

The Jernigan farm, 1875-1975, qualified for the Texas Family Land Heritage Program. I completed all the necessary paper work. John C. White, Commissioner, Texas Department of Agriculture announced in a letter to Mother, ". . . your land has qualified for recognition in the 1975 Family Land Heritage Program." 5

Family Land Heritage
Certificate of Honor
to
Jernigan Farm
founded
1875

Jamie and Frances came from their temporary apartment in Austin to attend the ceremony. He and I received the scroll from Commissioner White at the 1975 State Fair of Texas as representatives of the "Jernigan Family Farm."

Beth wrote me a note, postmarked October 24, 1975.

"Dear Daddy,

"Happy birthday! I'm afraid if I stop after school today to get you a card it won't get to you on your birthday. I really wanted you to receive a thought from me on your birthday.

"Daddy, if I could have chosen my father, I couldn't have picked a better, more perfect father than you. You have always been kind, understanding, a good listener, forgiving, patient always saying and doing the right thing at the right time. I've run out of room, but I guess you get the idea how super special I think you are. Love, Beth"

Wow! I'd like to meet that man. Beth and Jay prepared a lovely birthday dinner. Lisa read to us. She had advanced well beyond the first grade level.

Fall 1975

The three Jernigan brothers, their wives, their mother, and five grandchildren gathered at 4012 Fountainhead for Thanksgiving 1975. Numerous photographic slides documented the individuals and the table filled with food.

Jean wrote her mother-in-law:

"Dearest Mother Jernigan,

"We were very honored to have you with us at Thanksgiving. I thought everyone had a good time. Tell Mrs. Sarah Wallen how much we enjoyed the cake. Thank you for the beans and turkey.

"It will be lonesome without the boys. We have enjoyed them.

Love, Jean"

I flew to San Antonio to attend the 1975 annual meeting of the Texas Psychological Association held at the St. Anthony Hotel on December 5-6, 1975. TPA legal counselor and friend, Judge Bell, died on the lobby floor of the St. Anthony Hotel during the convention. Many psychology friends stood at the mezzanine perimeter transfixed as we looked down helplessly as paramedics administered shock treatments. It was a sad, memorable scene, the day that the jovial Presbyterian Judge passed to his reward.

The Veterans Administration held a regional meeting in Dallas, titled "Mental Health Practices," December 8-10, 1975. Income Tax Return documented "6 trips to Sheraton Hotel to attend VA meeting, 132 miles." Dr. Pat Kuekes, Chief of Psychology, Oklahoma City VA Hospital was one of the participants.

Christmas 1975

I took a poignant photograph of Mother playing her piano Christmas day 1974. The photograph became center theme in her 1975 Christmas cards to family and relatives.

Beth referred to the photo in her 1975 Christmas greeting to her grandmother, "Your Christmas card is the most special one received. The picture is one of our treasures."

Mother wrote the Van Alstyne Leader an after Christmas letter, published under the by-line, "Sedalia Lady, 89 Reaps Joys of Christmas:"

"Mrs. A. W. Jernigan of Sedalia is 89 years old and it is her philosophy that one never gets too old to enjoy Christmas with family and friends. - So she entertained dinner guests at her country home and they all gathered around the piano to sing Christmas carols after dinner. - Guess who played the piano? Mrs. Jernigan of course.

"But that wasn't all. She had a barrage of Christmas cards, gifts, visits and telephone calls during the Christmas season. The kind one loves to get to make the Yuletide complete.

"Those attending the Christmas repast on Christmas Day included Jack and Jean Jernigan, of Dallas, Austin and Richard

Jernigan, both students at the University of Texas in Austin; Beth, Jay and Lisa Fain of Carrollton, and Julie and Jill Fain of Dallas."

Chapter 19 - 1976

Jamie and Frances were "settled in" at their new Richardson address, 300 Meadowlark Drive by January 1, 1976. Son, Jim married Denise Lydon in California December 26, 1975. Laura transferred from A&I to Stephen F. Austin University in January 1976.

Austin was a junior and Richard a freshman at the University of Texas at Austin. Beth and Jay lived in Carrollton. Beth was a Special Education teacher in the Carrollton Public Schools, and continued her work toward a Masters degree at TWU. Lisa was in the first grade.

Jay made great strides as a sales representative for Proctor and Gamble. Jean was a secretary in downtown Dallas at the Department of Health Education and Welfare. She elected to ride the bus each day to her office rather than take a car. I was in my 20th year as Chief of Psychology Service at Dallas VAH.

Letters

Austin wrote his grandmother January 7, 1976. She in turn wrote on the front of the envelope, "A letter to keep."

"Dear Grandma,

"I certainly do thank you for the generous Christmas check. I used it to buy two records that I have already enjoyed a lot, both of which happen to be mainly piano music. I really came to an appreciation of how kind and generous you have been all these years this morning. I used the cookbook you loaned me to make something, I drank out of the glass you gave me; and although I didn't smoke the pipe of Grandpa's you gave me I enjoy looking at it on the shelf. You've certainly been a wonderful Grandmother to us all.

"I've been doing quite well here in Austin since getting back, and hope the same is true of you. I only work half time at the Campus Mail Service, picking up and delivering mail to the different buildings, and since school is out now the work has been pretty light. And not having to go to class or anything makes it real nice.

"Well, write soon, and I hope to get to see you again before too long.

Your loving Grandson,
Austin"

"Grandpa's pipe" was an artifact from the 1904 St. Louis Worlds Fair purchased by my Dad, and "passed on' to his grandson, Austin. Austin (the third) was introduced to the Campus Mail Service job by an Albert Jernigan descendant, a staff member of the University's Mail Service.

Jamie and Frances' move to Richardson was timely because of Mother's increased deterioration. Jamie, a dedicated educator, made a valiant effort to rehabilitate his mother. Following is an excerpt from one of Mother's 1976 letters that Jamie saved.

"Friday night - I think - [Friday, January 9, 1976]

"My dear Ones,

". . . I meant to write as soon as I knew your address but misplaced your letter. You will have so much to tell me - I'm surely looking forward to it. I know the wedding was so sweet and then I want to here [hear] all about your new home. It's wonderful that you will be so near me. You can't imagine how much that means but I do not want to be any more trouble to any of you than I can help. See I'm writing bottom side up - I'll just wait until in the morning. [The gold embossed top-border of sheet interfered with the last sentence.]

". . . I guess Jack will come tomorrow. There is one or two things I need to see about but it can wait.

"I am so sorry I have gotten to where I forget names more than I like but I try not to let a lot of things such as that bother me too much. Just count my blessings and when I do so, I realize how very fortunate I am. How truly thankful I am of all of you dear children and O how thankful I am that I can stay here where I have been so happy these many years and what wonderful children all of you are. I just hope I can take care of my self partly ha. All of you do so much for me."

Freshman Richard Jernigan typed a letter to his grandmother from his dormitory room at 329 Moore-Hill, Austin 78705.

Monday
April 8, 1976

"Dear Grandma,

"I hope you can read this, I probably should write it out in longhand, but my handwriting is pretty illegible so I thought it would be better to type.

"It's about 6:15 right now. I had supper about thirty minutes ago at the cafeteria. It's been raining off and on all day, and I had four classes to go to. I have an umbrella, though, so I didn't get very wet.

"I'm doing pretty well in school. In English, no matter what I turn in, I end up getting an A on whatever I write. I'm just doing average work in my other courses, though. I'm studying French, American History, Astronomy, Art History, and of course, English. I work at a used book store here in Austin - Half-Price Books. I go in about three afternoons each week. I've bought about seventy-five books since coming down this fall from that one book store, and no doubt I'll buy more before the semester is over.

"I see Austin several times a week. I had breakfast with him the other morning, and last night he came by my room. He was trying to decide on someplace for supper. It was raining outside and he was on his bike and didn't want to go riding all over town to get something to eat. He ended up going home and making cornbread and beans.

"It's beginning to get dark now. The street outside my window is wet, and the sky is overcast. Occasionally cars and buses pass by. Some of the boys in the dorm are yelling in the hallway. I have only one roommate by the way. His name is Doug Holmes and came from Rockdale, Texas. I get along with him real well, which is fortunate compared to what many of my friends have said about their roommates. He studies music.

"I don't know what else to say. I usually write on spur of the moment, and I was just sitting here with my typewriter in front of me, so I decided to write you a note.

"Anyway, I do hope you're doing all right. I like it down here pretty much, although I don't believe I'll return here next fall.

"But, until I write again or come up to Sedalia,

Love, Richard"

An Albert Discovery

A brief visit to the Travis County Court House led to the discovery of a microfilm of the trial of a Courthouse Janitor. The trial gave detailed facts about the circumstances that led to the suicide of Albert Jernigan. I received a copy of the proceedings on 16mm film March 24, 1976. The following day was spent in the library reviewing Austin Statesman files.

Death of a Neighbor

Mother's neighbor Lester T. Standridge died in April 1976. The burial was in Restland Cemetery, Richardson, Texas. He was a good friend of our children, and owner of the land that surrounded the Jernigan Cemetery. 1

Mother wrote Jamie and Frances April 27, 1976, soon after the death of Lester Standridge.

"My Dear One:

"So glad you call[ed] this morning. I'm feeling alright and am glad I have been up here this week. Mrs. Standridge still calls me each ~~morng~~ morning and she is doing real well. She went to church Sunday and they were all so glad to have her, it did her much good. They have belonged there all the time. She is going to live in her home, too.

"She and her husband have belonged to this church all these years. His pastor held the funeal [funeral] the other day she told me he said it was his first. I did not know it. Jack and I were there and we thought it was all so nice."

Professional

Clyde Tilton became a certified Nursing Home Administrator and secured an administrative position in Denton after he retired from the Veterans Administration. Clyde invited me to confer on the care of a mentally retarded adult at the Denton Nursing Home.

I drove to University of Texas at Austin April 24, 1956 for a VA Psychological Training conference and returned April 25, 1976. Trips to Austin were an added pleasure for it gave an opportunity to visit with Austin and Richard, take them to dinner, and help with grocery shopping.

I attended a Hogg Foundation for Mental Health Symposium May 2 --3, 1976 at the LBJ Library, Austin. A return trip was made to Austin May 17, 1976, "To interview VA Psychology trainee candidates at the University of Texas."

Psychology Trainees

We had eight Psychology graduate students in training assignments at Dallas VAH during 1976.

Burt Grodnitzky continued internship training with assignments in Psychiatry and GM&S under the supervision of Drs. Andrews and Kidd. His experiences included assessments, psychotherapy (group and individual), consultation, staff meetings, and an Epilepsy Education Group. Dr. Kidd observed that "Mr. Grodnitzky's sensitivity and concern with individual patients to be perhaps his most outstanding asset as a clinician." Burt completed his internship in August 1976.

Jack Gold continued his internship in January with Dr. Scrivner, and from February to May under the supervision of Earl Patterson in the Day Hospital. He developed an interdisciplinary therapy team of special social skills learning at the Day Hospital. He served as a co-therapist with Dr. Patterson in a "behaviorally-oriented approach to therapy." From May to August he was supervised by Dr. Pam Profant in the Drug Dependence Treatment Center where he assisted in psychiatric admission screening interviews. "His experiences at DDTC consisted of assessment of specified individual patients, interpreted those test results with patient and staff alike, participated in staff treatment planning conferences, followed individual patients during treatment, employed behavior modification techniques in some individual cases, and participated in a progressive patient group therapy program." Mr. Gold was seen as a productive intern who maximized the outcome of his training experience.

Steve Close continued his internship into 1976 under the supervision of Dr. Walter Penk. He worked three days a week at VAH and two days at the University of Texas Health Science Center under the supervision of Dr. Frank Trimboli. He was also supervised by Drs. Andrews, Scrivner and Kidd at the VAH. "His experiences included diagnostic assessment, individual and group psychotherapy. Steve designed an educational, didactic group to explain behavior pathology for student nurses. He followed several veterans in individual therapy on an outpatient basis under auspices of the Mental Hygiene Clinic. His last major effort was to assist in the training of second year Psychology students. Steve assumed responsibility for reviewing the Exner scoring system of the Rorschach. He presented at two psychology staff meetings: First, his dissertation and at the second his analysis of Rorschach protocols obtained from veterans with heart attacks. Steve also worked briefly in consultation with Neurology Service." Dr. Penk summarized, "He completed all objectives usually considered necessary in third and fourth year level training experience."

John Ubersax, Level II Clinical Trainee from University of Texas, Austin was appointed July 1, 1976 and completed 320 hours of training before resuming academic studies August 28, 1976. He was given training assignments under the supervision of Drs. Kidd and Scrivner, administering a variety of psychological tests, and participated in a rehabilitation therapy program, and under the supervision of intern Steve Close, assessed cardiac patients. He was supervised by intern Burt Grodnitzky in the assessment of psychiatric patients.

Marvin D. Abney, Level II Counseling Trainee from University of Texas, Austin began a 40 hour-week tour of duty on July 1, 1976. His training was interrupted August 27, 1976 when the academic year resumed. He assisted Dr. Reagan Andrews in pre-vocational counseling of a number of psychiatric patients on the Psychiatric Unit. Mr. Abney designed a procedure for sampling patients in the admission area with the assistance of Dr. Kidd, inquiring systematically of the vocational needs of that population, interviewing in excess of 100 patients. His summary was used as a part of a justification for development of a job clinic at Dallas VAH.

Gary Pettigrew was appointed as a Level III intern at the Dallas VA Hospital effective September 1, 1976 under the joint VA-University of Texas Health Science Center Program. He was assigned full time to the General Medical Consultation Program under the supervision of Drs. Kidd and Scrivner. He rotated to the Day Hospital/Mental Hygiene Clinic under the supervision of Drs. Patterson and Toland in December. He also served as a co-therapist with Dr. Toland in a night group that continued during his second six month rotation at UTHSC.

Ruth K. Morehouse was appointed a Level IV intern effective September 1, 1976 under the joint VA-University of Texas Health Science Center Program.

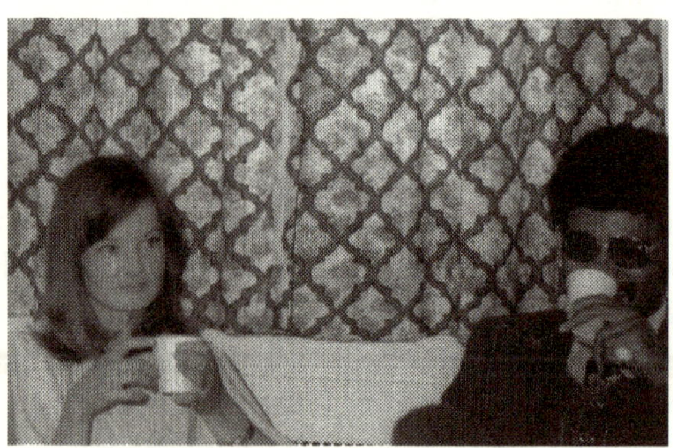

Ruth Morehouse and Marvin Abney

Ruth was unique for the 1970's in that she progressed through four years of VA training at New Orleans and Dallas. Her VA block assignment was within the Day Hospital/Mental Hygiene

Clinic programs under the supervision of Drs. Patterson and Toland.

Ardith M. Zander was appointed a Level IV intern under the joint VA-UTHSC Program September 1, 1976. Her 1976 assignments were in the Drug Dependence Treatment Center and Day Hospital with four hours each week in the Mental Hygiene Clinic.

Family Happenings

Beth received a Master of Education in the Graduate School of Texas Woman's University May, 1976. The title of her professional paper: "Oculomotor Evaluation and Remediation - A Process Video Tape."

Beth wrote the following undated note after the occasion:

"Dear Mother and Daddy,

"I enjoyed the beautiful flowers so much. I'm pressing some of them to frame for a permanent remembrance. Thank you for all you did to help me get my Master's - taking care of Lisa, typing papers, teaching me about testing, etc. It's your degree, too.

Love, Beth"

Austin wrote his grandmother from a new address, 1216-B West 22, Austin 78705, June 14, 1976.

"Dear Grandma Blanche,

"Well I've done it again, gone and waited much too long to write you. Lately I've been pretty preoccupied with getting moved into my new house and buying a motorcycle. My new address, by the way is 1216-B West 22nd. Austin, TX 78705. The house is 100 years old, and I live on the second floor with four other guys. They are all quite congenial, and I like my room a lot - it has a whole wall of windows facing west, with a really nice view. I bought a motorcycle for cheap transportation, and am just learning to ride it, but having a great time with it.

"It was quite a surprise, and most pleasant one I assure you, when I got the letter from you with the check enclosed. Your great generosity never ceases to overwhelm me, and yes, I know it's been a good three weeks since you sent it, and that I should have thanked you immediately; but let's just say I was too overwhelmed even to write, but I guess you may have noticed by now that I wasn't too overwhelmed to cash the check. Well, I guess you knew how much I appreciated it and thank you now. It was a very timely gift, as, you may know, I'm on my own now financially; having decided, in all appreciation to my parents that it was high time I started to make my own way in the world.

"I'm sorry I couldn't get up that way when I was last in Dallas, but circumstances didn't allow it. Anyway, I promise to make a special effort to see you next time I'm up, which should be before long. Now that you know my new address, please write soon. Thank you again for the gift.

Love, Austin"

National Wildlife Conference

Jay, Beth, Lisa, and I attended the National Wildlife Conference in Estes Park, Colorado July 4-10, 1976. Jay and Beth traveled by car. Lisa and I flew to Denver, and took the bus from the airport to Estes Park. It was Lisa's first flying experience.

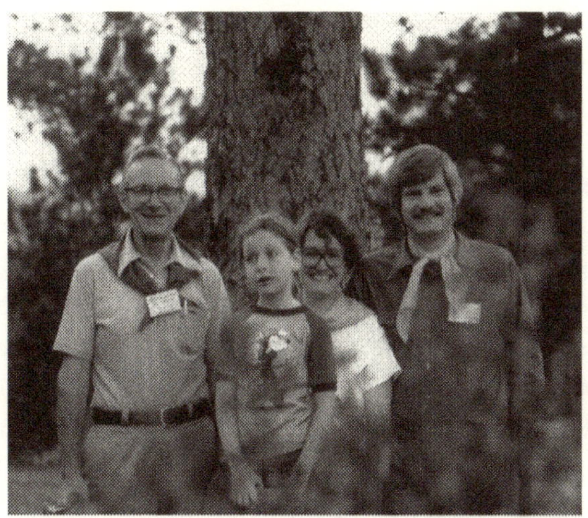

Jack - Lisa - Beth – Jay at 1976 Summit

Lisa and I had a great time together, documented by photographic slides of Lisa as she sat by the outside window coloring in the book supplied by the stewardess. Jean and Richard did not go to Colorado because of their work commitments. Austin stayed in Austin that summer.

The bus Lisa and I rode from Denver airport to Estes Park ran out of energy a few hundred feet before reaching the crest of the hill leading into Estes Park. Beth and Jay were anxiously waiting our arrival. It was a memorable week documented by several rolls of film.

It was my fourth National Wildlife Conference and as the Conference offered formal and informal courses in pollution, conservation, and family planning, the fees and transportation were declared on IRS statement. An example of its utility: a carousel of slides from the 1976 Summit was presented to Day Treatment patients to stimulate discussion on the preservation of nature and the people there in, with emphases on rehabilitation.

A picture postcard was mailed to Jean and Richard July 4, 1976 of "The Columbine" from "Rm. 223, Harvard Hall, YMCA, Rockies."

"Dear Jean & Richard: We arrived 'on foot' about 2:30 - Beth and Jay had arrived a few minutes earlier. About 25 miles out our bus would not shift out of second, stalled as we climbed the hill to camp. Everything is much greener than 3 years ago - also seems cooler, but so much different without you here. Am already missing you. Lisa was a pleasure coming up. Was a lovely ride and I took notes of her comments for Jay and Beth. We appear to have an enlightening schedule. Have introduced Lisa to Dr. Mulaik. Beth and I have similar and overlapping schedules. Hope your flower arrives on 5th [29th wedding anniversary]. They were sent with much love. Jack & Dad."

Richard took his Mother to dinner for our anniversary.

Back Home

Jamie, Frances and I attended a Whitewright High School reunion in early August. Former Superintendent, Mr. Harold Key and Mrs. Key were present along with many 1937-1938 classmates. Jamie and Mr. Key served together in Whitewright, and Mr. Key subsequently followed Jamie as Superintendent of the Pilot Point school system.

Austin rode his motorcycle home that summer. Soon after his arrival a photograph recorded his eager responsive bite into a delicious red watermelon.

A series of slides documented an August 1976 social gathering of VA Psychology Staff in the 9th floor conference room, possibly before two of the trainees Marvin Abney and John Ubersax returned to academic studies at University of Texas. Other trainees in the slide series were Burt Brodnitzky, Jack Gold and

Ruth Morehouse. Rutha Waters, Ivonne Widows, and Pam Profant of the Drug Center were also present.

Four photographs were submitted to the Creative Arts Department, State Fair of Texas in 1976. It was Creative Arts Department policy that all photo entries were taken within the previous year.

APA Meeting

In September Jean and I attended the 1976 American Psychological Association annual meeting in Washington, D. C. We flew American and stayed at the American Hotel.

The trip was well documented in slides of animals at the Washington Zoo, scenes of the Smithsonian, including photographs of Lindberg's Spirit of St. Louis, and a returned Capsule from the space age.

I retain one professional memory of APA 1976. We stayed in the hotel where Gay Psychologists were making their professional "coming out" in the APA organizational meetings. As one meeting broke, Jean and I waited for participants to fill the elevator, and rode with the group to the ground floor. We both commented later, with some reservation, about the new development.

The last extant 1976 correspondence retained by Mother was a picture postcard from the National Gallery of Art - Washington - View of the Rotunda - "Mercury" by Giovanni Bologna (Andrew Mellon Collection), dated 9-5-76.

"Dear Mother:

"We spent most of the day at Gallery, Smithsonian Archives, etc. We have had a very good time. The weather has been almost perfect. I'm planning to see you this Thursday when we go to the dentist.

Love, Jack"

Mother Entered Nursing Home

Excerpts from one of Mother's 1976 last undated letters reflect her struggle to maintain stability. The day before, I had taken her to Sherman for the dental appointment. Mother was tired, and fell asleep soon after we returned to Sedalia. I made the mistake of not waking her to inform her I was leaving.

"Dr. A. J. Jernigan,

"I come appoligising [apologizing] to you, my dear son, who does and hashem [?] so long done so much for me. I must have been more tiried [tired] than I thought yesterday. Just to think I went to sleep and did not know when you left. I just could not believe it. I did not here [hear] when you left the room [not legible] did I hear any sound of your buggy [car]. Just woke up and you were gone and O how it did hurt me. To think I could do such a think [thing] after all you do for me all the time. I guess the old lady was nearen [nearer worn] out than she realized. Just hope you never let that happend [happen] again. I was so very sorry. . .

"Because of you, I am so happy to stay here in the home that meant so much to me but I do not want to stay here in this home if it causets [causes] too much trouble to our children. (But O how I love it and get all the rest I need.)"

Hindsight suggests Mother should have been hospitalized, admitted to a nursing home, or other living arrangements made. The extent of deteoriation was quite evident to her sons, and her physical needs were reviewed by Dr. Charley Wysong. The family honored her request for independence, and made the decision that she continue to stay in her home a while longer.

Mother fell to the floor the night of October 19th and remained there. When the early morning telephone calls by faithful neighbors received no response, they came to the house, cut the screen wire to unlock the back door, and entered her bedroom. Mother was admitted to the Wysong Hospital in McKinney. 2

Change of Hospital Administrators

E. P. Whitaker, Hospital Director wrote September 10, 1976:

"TO: All Employees

1. This will be my last day on duty with the United States Government because I have elected to retire from the service after many exciting and inspiring years. One could never have had a more enjoyable or satisfying career than I have experienced. The VA is still one of the better Governmental agencies. VAH, Dallas is one of its better components. I leave with regret and sadness but with hope and admiration.

2. The VAH is fortunate in the Director who will follow me. He will build a greater and better hospital than we have today.

3. Effective September 12, 1976, please prepare all hospital documents, requiring the signature of the Director, as follows:

C. WAYNE HAWKINS
Hospital Director"

Duster for the Boys

Richard located a stored Volkswagen that he believed was a good buy. With some reservation we agreed to his using savings to purchase the car. It proved unreliable, and too costly to repair. Checkbook entry for September 19, 1976, "Gene Hays Motors

- $789.50" documented the purchase of a 1970 Green Duster for $1089.50, with a $300 trade-in value for the VW.

Richard began his sophomore year at UT and moved to 1216-B West 22nd., to the 100 year old house shared with Austin and three or four other guys. We believed the Duster would be very helpful to Austin and Richard in maintaining their work and study schedules.

Although the Duster "was very clean with low mileage" it soon became evident the motor needed maintenance. Our McKinney mechanic, James Culberson evaluated the car during the Thanksgiving Holiday, and reported the motor needed overhauling. We postponed the major repair decision because Gene Hays was at his winter home in Hawaii. We believed (hoped) he would repair the highly recommended automobile.

Photographs taken in the fall of 1976: Jamie and Frances' home in Richardson; Kimball Art Museum with Beth with her friend, Katherine Messina; Van Gogh's works on exhibit at the Kimball; the weathered south wall of the Sedalia car shed and wheelbarrow; Mr. Nance and son of Van Alstyne at Sedalia to make offer on the1940 Ford; Mother at the Wysong Nursing Home; the Nursing Home after an early winter snow; and Austin and Richard when they drove a large truck from Austin, loaded with books destined for Half Price Books' main Dallas store.

Thanksgiving at the J. C. Jernigans

Mother adapted to the drastic change of complete home freedom to the more structured Nursing Home environment. In our early visits, she occasionally commented she would like to go home, that she could take care of herself that Edgar Edwards would check in on her each day, etc. But in time she accepted the need to be cared for and soon charmed the staff.

Our family and Jamie's family gathered at Jamie and Frances' home for lunch at Thanksgiving. Jean and I drove to the Nursing Home and brought Mother back to their home in Richardson. In the afternoon, Austin and Richard took a number of posed outdoor shots of photogenic Lisa. Many photographs were taken of Mother with members of the families. Mother consistently misperceived Jamie as her husband.

Professional

Between Thanksgiving and December 6, 1976, the Veterans Administration broke ground for a Research Building at Dallas VAH. A number of individuals from Central Office came and spoke to the large group of employees gathered out side on a bright, mild, late fall afternoon. Mr. Hawkins was in charge of the program and Mr. Whitaker returned to sit in the distinguished guest section. I took photographs of the occasion and some close up shots included Ralph Robinowitz, Reagan Andrews, Dr. Edwards, Mrs. Edwards, Mr. Whitaker, Mr. Hawkins, and Delores Little.

Ninetieth Birthday Party

Jamie was hospitalized at Baylor University Hospital in Dallas for herniated disc surgery and unable to attend Mother's ninetieth birthday at the nursing home December 6, 1976. Stewart and Mary came from Bryan. They, Jean and Beth prepared for a small birthday party. Many Sedalia friends including their young pastor, Dennis Garner, of the Sedalia Baptist Church and his family also came to the party, and brought additional cake and refreshments. The children entertained with songs accompanied by the pastor on the guitar. All ambulatory residents were invited to the 90th birthday party held in the dining area. Family members present: Stewart, Mary, Jack, Jean, Beth and Lisa.

A Sedalia friend sent an article about the birthday party to the Van Alstyne Leader, along with a copy of the photograph taken the previous Christmas of Blanche at her piano. The December 9,

1976 article identified members of Mother's family and Sedalia guests. Guests were photographed as well as a member of the nursing staff, Laura Wilkinson, Sedalia native and former student. 3

Professional

I drove to Houston December 9, 1976 to attend the Texas Psychological Association's Annual Meeting and stayed at the Hyatt Regency. Hawaii's Senator Inouani was a guest speaker. The Program Committee purchased a large Texas Stetson to present to the Senator, and I was asked to be responsible for the hat. Ralph Robinowitz and I exchanged photographs wearing the Senator's overwhelming Stetson.

The Psychology Staff hosted a Christmas party in the VA Hospital's 9th floor conference room. Richard, home from UT for the holidays, assisted in the photography. The following are some of the individuals who came by that afternoon: Ardie Zander, Royce Scrivner, Richard Jernigan, Reagan Andrews, Dr. Edwards, Ralph Robinowitz, Earl Patterson, Mrs. Gallo, Kathy Myers, Dr. R. H. Rodriquez from Psychiatry, Ron Kidd, Pam Profant and one of the men from the mailroom.

Christmas 1976

Early Christmas scenes at 4012 Fountainhead were of Lisa assisting in the decoration of the tree. When Christmas Day arrived, there was a blue bicycle for Jean from her two sons prominently displayed before the Christmas tree, followed by a slide of Jean astride her new German-made bicycle.

Mother visited in the homes of both of her North Texas sons on Christmas day, 1976. She visited with Jamie, Frances and Laura and later the same day at our house. She continued to misidentify Jamie as her husband. The dinner table scene at our home included Jay, Beth, Blanche, Jack, Lisa, Jean, and Richard.

Mother returned to the Wysong Nursing Home late Christmas Day. Weeks later she fell from her bed and was hospitalized at Wysong Hospital with a broken hip.

The 1976 Holiday Season ended with the annual photograph of Lisa and her grandfather in front of the live cedar "Christmas tree." The tree line reached the roof of the house, and Lisa was an arm load. The tradition continued.

Chapter 20 - 1977

The Veterans Administration Regional Conference held in the downtown Dallas Sheraton Hotel January 5-7, 1977 was titled "Training in Chronic Care Concept of Long-Term Chronic Psychiatric Patients." Former Waco neighbor Social Worker John McKelvain attended along with many other old friends and were photographed at the VA Conference. Sid Cleveland, Chief Psychologist, Houston VAH was a member of a panel discussion group. 1

The boys came that weekend to drive the 1970 green Duster back to Austin. Ramey Repair Service of McKinney removed and replaced the Duster's "slant-six" motor with a "factory" overhaul equivalent." We began a $98.20 a month repayment schedule to savings.

Jean and I visited Ron Kidd and wife, and met their new daughter at Presbyterian Hospital Saturday afternoon, January 29, 1977. From there we drove to McKinney and visited Mother in the Nursing Home.

Early 1977 photographed activities and scenes: Neighborhood children snow sledding in the alley; VAH 9th floor reconstruction; VAH Day Treatment Center from 9th floor office; a Volunteer Lady at VA Hospital; snow in the woods at Sedalia; a visit with Mr. and Mrs. Robert L. Scrivner (Air Force buddy from Oregon) at 4012 Fountainhead; variety of snow scenes at 4012 Fountainhead and VA Hospital; Standridge barn and cows; Edgar Edwards's new Buick; house on fire on Fountainhead; Ron Kidd and son, "digging up" basketball goal; Wysong Hospital; Garden at Sedalia begun by Edgar; and----

And Then Came Death

There are only a few extant documents of visits to the Wysong Hospital during those final days of Mother's life. Jean and I made frequent trips together and alone. Mother began to refuse food and on more than one occasion I took annual leave at noontime, drove to the Hospital, and encouraged her to eat. I did not recognize that it was nature's way of shutting down. Jean recalled near the end Mother called out, "Come on girls lets go."

Around midnight March 23, 1977 the nursing staff encouraged us to ". . . go on home." In the early hours of March 24, 1977, Blanche Coffey Jernigan passed from life to LIFE. Dr. Charley Wysong was with her at death. When Stewart was informed of her passing, he stated, with a sob, "She died on my birthday (65th)."

The article, "Rites Set For Prominent Area Woman", published by the Dallas Morning News included a copy of the photograph I took of Mother on a fall afternoon as she left to attend a funeral. "Mother, you look so pretty - let me take your picture." Later, Miesels of Dallas turned an enlarged copy into an oil-type portrait that the family donated to the Westminster Baptist Church for the Blanche Coffey Jernigan Education Building.

The article concluded with: "On March 25, 1977, her body was laid to rest by the side of her late husband in Highland Cemetery." 2

Photographs documented those of us who gathered at the farm before the funeral service for lunch organized by Marian Wysong: The Jernigan farm house and buildings surrounded by cars (photo taken by the boys from the field to the west); Kermit Jack Rosser and Kermit; Richard, Laura and Lisa; Mary, Jean and Frances; Jay, David and Stewart; David and Stewart; Jay and David; the grandchildren; 3 sons and wives. Later in the afternoon many of the same people and additional relatives were photographed at Highland Cemetery.

Totaled

Austin and Richard kept their Green Duster parked in front of their house at 1216-B West 22nd., a dead end street. Late one evening a University student rear-ended their car, damaging it beyond cost to repair.

The two sons collected all necessary data and the identity of the person responsible for the wreck. The student's wealthy father had good insurance coverage. A problem arose with the insurance carrier who wanted to compensate by "book value."

I drove to Austin April 14, 1977, invited "Forrester Body Shop" to estimate cost of repair, and through the recommendation of Betty Cleland, contacted a young attorney, Alvis G. Schultze. The attorney attempted to negotiate for equitable value, the cost of the car and the price paid for the "new motor" in January, e.g. $1524, plus reasonable expenses.

We accepted a settlement of $1250, rather than engage in a court hassle. The body shop evaluation and attorney's fee were less than $50. I regret we did not attempt to replace the wrecked automobile.

Annual Meeting - Southwestern Psychological Association

The annual meeting of SWPA in April 1977 at the Sheraton Hotel in Fort Worth, Texas was a signal event. Thirty years after the end of World War II, five leaders of Aviation Psychology assembled to present the symposium, "A Reminiscent Evaluation of the Aviation Psychology Program of World War II."

It was this veteran's delight to listen to and interact with Frank A. Geldard, symposium chairman, and participants, John C. Flanagan, Glenn Finch, J. P. Guilford, and Robert L. Thorndike. It was a disappointment that Randolph Field mentor, Arthur W. Melton, listed as a participant, became ill and could not attend. I took a number of photographs of each presenter and tape recorded the symposium. 3

I also chaired a symposium at the convention titled, "Assessment of Patients: Some Current Trends. Participants were Kathy McElwain and Ron Kidd, Dallas VAH staff; John Overall, Research Psychologist at Galveston Medical School; and Jack Davis of VA Central Office.

After returning to Dallas, I learned that Dr. Melton was a patient at Parkland Hospital, visited with Colonel Melton at Parkland bedside, and later wrote him. He in turn, responded June 8, 1977 with a hand written letter on American Psychological Association stationery, with sub-title, "Office of the Chief Editorial Advisor, Arthur W. Melton." 4

Graduation Time

Austin graduated from University of Texas May 21, 1977. It was a beautiful spring day and the event was documented by numerous slides: Members of Austin's graduating class, Austin receiving his diploma, and Austin with parents, photograph taken by Richard. The series concluded with a slide of Ira Iscoe in gown, member of the faculty procession, long time professional ally and friend.

Austin rode his motorcycle to Dallas a few days after graduation. One of his activities while at home was to replace ridge row shingles on peak of roof. He soon returned to Austin.

Austin was in search of himself. In early June he wrote on picture postcard:

". . . After thinking it over and almost backing out and moving back to Dallas, I've decided to go ahead with my summer projects. I've got contacts in KUT FM, TX Union, Feature Film Svc., a local small media production Co. etc., and am going to investigate possible"

Continued on another picture postcard,

"... semi-internships. Also plan to take CATV Video Prod. Course. So if you're agreeable please deposit about $200 from my [college] account.

"I may come up Thursday.

Austin"

Pilot Grove Methodist Church

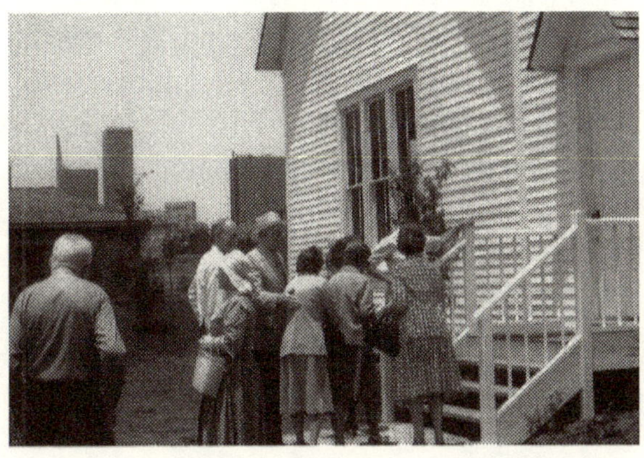

Rea Nunnallee – Billy Ray and Arthur Giles

The founders of Old Settlers Park near downtown Dallas selected Pilot Grove Methodist Church building as typical of early Texas church architecture.

The vacant building was moved from Pilot Grove to the Park and dedicated in early June 1977. Numerous Grayson County friends, white and black were present at the dedication that warm Sunday afternoon: Elford Lane, Dorthell Cowan, Rea Nunnallee, Fred Starr and Butch Kaiser's brother, Mrs. Kaiser, Arthur Giles, Billy Ray Giles, a "Graybill Webb" daughter, etc.

Naming of a Building

Soon after Mother's death, the Westminster Baptist Church voted to name the proposed Educational-Fellowship Wing, the "Blanche C. Jernigan Building."

Jamie wrote Bro. Joe Smith, Pastor Westminster Baptist Church a letter of "deep appreciation" and also told of the family's desire to establish a "Lottie Moon Christmas Fund" in Mother's memory, and donate her piano to the church. 5

European Trip

Beth and Richard flew to Amsterdam June 1977. They were met in Amsterdam by Richard's friend, Kelli Bennett, and Kelli's friend Sherryl. Beth's postcard was addressed to "Dr. A. J. Jernigan" since Beth, Kathryn, and I attended a Kimball Art Museum's presentation of a Van Gogh Exhibit in the spring. Her mention of "Starry Night" was reference to Jean's framed replica that hung at 4012 Fountainhead.

The picture postcard from Beth: "Vincent Van Gogh, 1853-1890."

"6-12-77 Amsterdam

"Dear Daddy, Guess where we went today? The Van Gogh Museum! Daddy, you must come here. I had one of my ever present sore throats and still a bit of jet lag, but it real[ly] perked me up. It was indescribable. I've seen just about everything he did plus preliminary drawings (except Starry Night). This says [postcard of "The Harvest"] is his best landscape! Yesterday we went to the Rijshmuseum which has many Flemish painting, especially Rembrandts - and best of all "The Night Watch!" Amsterdam is charming with the several hundred year old town houses. Our room is 4 flights up - everything is narrow but tall. Tomorrow night, Paris. Love, Beth"

That same day Beth mailed a picture postcard to Jean of Van Gogh, "Kitchen gardens on Montmatre."

"Dear Mother, the ride from Bangor to Amsterdam was very rocky and Richard and I both felt terrible. Kelli and Sherryl, her roommate, met us at the airport and have been fantastic guides. Just about every one here speaks English, so there is little culture shock. Our room comes with a huge breakfast. The food is delicious and fresh tasting but hardly any fruits and vegetables are served. We took a boat ride on the canals today. Amsterdam is still very much 'old world.' I lost my return plane ticket, but some most helpful people fixed it for me. Love, Beth"

Richard's first picture postcard was a Van Gogh's self portrait with a pipe in mouth. At top of card: "Hi from Beth, Hi from Kelli, Howdy from Sherry."

"June 13, 1977

"Dear Mother and Dad,

"I'm sitting on the floor in the reservation area of the Amsterdam R. A. terminal waiting behind about 100 people trying to get reservations for tonight's trip to Paris! Amsterdam is great. Looks like all the postcards. Really. This morning we went to Anne Frank's house. Yesterday Van Gogh museum. No problems. Everyone speaks English. Tomorrow I put French into practice. Give me a delayed wish of luck.

Love, Richard"

Beth wrote the next day, a picture postcard of "St. Peter's Square" with postmark "Vaticane."

"6-14-77 Dear Mother and Daddy, I am in the train station in Rome hoping my call to Jay will go through. I tried to call Jay from Paris - he wasn't home. I like Rome much better than Paris. Paris is very dirty and people were rude and cold. Rome is sunny, warm, with a ruin on just about every corner. Our pensione is very old with marble floors; the room is the largest and nicest we've had. It's across the street from Hadrian's Castle and down the street from Vatican City. Italy is much more beautiful than one can imagine - lots of greenery. This afternoon we'll tour the ruins. Love, Beth"

Richard wrote three days later - a picture postcard of Mona Lisa, June 17, 1977.

"Dear Mother and Dad,

"Yep, I saw this one, too. Also went to Shakespeare Co. Bookstore and spent the afternoon reading. It's run by one of Walt Whitman's kin. Today we see the Eiffel Tower and Arc du Triemphe. So far I've just seen the tip of Tour Eiffel. Then tonight to Rome. The whole trip is going backwards but it's lots of fun.

Love, Richard"

Richard concluded his series of postcards with Michelangelo's Moses.

"June 21, 1977

"Dear Mother and Dad,

"We saw this guy the other day. Kelli's sick right now and Beth and I are sitting on a train that doesn't seem to want to get moving. We are going to Florence for the day. Rome's beautiful. I take three or four rolls of film each day. I believe we're going to stay in Italy until the weekend, or maybe we'll go to Germany, or France, I don't know. We will be in London by Sunday. See you in 1 1/2 weeks. Love, Richard"

Beth's last (extant) postcard documented European tour concluded with a picture postcard of "Firenze - L. Ghiberti."

"6-23-77 Dijon, France

"Dear Mother and Daddy. We are spending the day and tonight in Dijon. We toured the wine country today. Tomorrow I imagine we'll start heading towards London. Tuesday Richard and I rode the train from Rome to Florence and spent the day. Do you know that Pizza is really good in Italy? David (by Michelangelo) was awesome, perfection and moving. I am enjoying this part of France - <u>much</u> better than Paris - it's more provincial and pleasant and Richard's and my French are holding up well. Richard bought a felt hat in Beune France that he wears everywhere. I will be glad to come home, though, because I miss my family. Love Beth"

Professional

A Management Personnel Inventory dated June 14, 1977 required that its accuracy be confirmed. Two Sections are quoted:

<u>Experience</u>

Description of Current Work: "As Chief Psychologist, I am responsible for the overall organization of the Psychology program at Dallas VAH. The Service has an FTP ceiling of 13 positions distributed as follows: a secretary, 3 psychology technicians, and 9 doctoral level psychologists, which includes the Chief of the Drug Dependence Treatment Center. A research psychologist, a research technician, and a part-time clerk are peripheral to the Service. There are 6 psychology trainees. There are eight Psychology Units with consultation services to Day Treatment Center."

<u>Training, Development and Awards</u>

"Attended VA Regional Conference for Chiefs of Psychology Service, Kansas City, Missouri, June 29, 1976. Attended VA Conference on Training in Chronic Care Concepts of Long-Term Chronic Psychiatric Patients, Dallas, TX, January 5-7,

1977. Attended VA Mental Health Practices, Dallas, TX, Dec. 8-10, 1975. Was Chairman and presenter of symposium, "Assessment of Patients, Some Current Trends," Southwestern Psychological Annual Meeting, April, 22, 1977. Total: 64 hours."

Psychology Trainees

John Ubersax, Level II clinical psychology trainee returned to Dallas VAH June 2, 1977 to complete 180 hours of training under the supervision of Dr. Reagan Andrews, Psychiatry Service. Dr. Andrews gave John psychiatric literature reading assignments, concentrated on John's administration and interpretation of the Rorschach, encouraged attendance at staff meetings, and introduced him to group psychotherapy.

Mr. Ubersax was a dedicated student, eager to learn. He was promoted to Level III July 1, 1977 with a 40 hour work week schedule until August 25, when he returned to the University of Texas for his third year of graduate study. He was scheduled to resume Level III training in January 1978.

Marvin Abney returned to Dallas in May 1977, and requested a 48-hour week schedule making it possible to achieve training experience in the Mental Hygiene Clinic and psychiatric wards. Under the supervision of Dr. Andrews, Marvin concentrated on psychodiagnostic testing, with special emphasis on the Rorschach. He participated in an evening couples group with Dr. Toland in the Mental Hygiene Clinic, and also evaluated three patients. Dr. Toland wrote: "In the group, Marvin appeared to be comfortable and participated freely at the encouragement of the co-therapist. His behavior was mature and appropriate in relating both to the patients and to the therapist. His observations and comments were of a quality beyond what would be expected of a student at his stage of training and I was most impressed by his sincere desire to have feedback regarding the appropriateness and the effectiveness of his group interactions."

Mr. Abney established an educational group of an intermediate care psychiatric population, focusing on job hunting and interviewing for jobs. The patients were so impressed with the help that they petitioned Psychology Service to continue this effective program.

Marvin was African-American. He and I occasionally ate our sack lunches together during the noon hour. One day, as I gathered up orange peelings for disposal, Marvin related that his eight year old son loved the peelings, but cared little for the fruit. I ate a bite of the peeling and agreed with his son.

We were unable to promote Marvin to Level III training because the University reported he was not progressing as rapidly academically as experientially. The summary evaluation paragraph submitted June 27, 1977:

"Mr. Abney demonstrated superior personality characteristics for work with a patient population. He is consistently pleasant and gracious in his relationships with patients and staff. He is respected by all who come in contact with him. His industry and willingness to serve as well as learn in a training setting sometimes lead to an over-extension but he always fulfills his obligations. He is highly motivated to achieve his goal of obtaining additional clinical knowledge and experience. All effort possible should be directed toward helping him achieve his goal of a Ph.D. in Counseling Psychology."

A few years later at a psychological meeting I asked Dr. Abney about his son's eating preference. "Still eating the peelings," he reported, and I confirmed a personal taste for good orange peelings.

Gary Pettigrew continued Level III internship until he completed 2,000 hours of experience equally distributed between assignments at the Medical School and VAH. His VAH joint assignment at Day Hospital/Mental Hygiene Clinic was under the supervision of Drs. Toland and Patterson. He accepted additional night training in group therapy as a co-therapist with Dr. Toland when he began the second six month rotation at UTHSC under the supervision of Drs. Gluck, Trimboli, Fougerousse, and Wolf.

All Medical School psychologists gave Gary complimentary evaluations. Dr. Royce Scrivner wrote, "He quite successfully met the myriad of challenges unique to the development of consultation services to medical wards." I added, "Mr. Pettigrew should develop into a most competent psychologist."

Ruth K. Morehouse, Level IV trainee from LSU, received a joint appointment in September 1976 and continued into 1977, completing 2,000 hours of training. Drs. Gluck, Gilbert and Ateek were her supervisors at UTHSC in the Child and Adolescent Psychiatric Clinic - Parkland Outpatient Psychiatry. Her VA block assignments were with Drs. Patterson and Toland in Day Hospital/ MHC. Dr. Patterson wrote in his summary evaluation:

"Ruth was able to achieve all of the experiences she set for herself at the beginning of the rotation. She has demonstrated competency in all of the goal areas consistent with a doctoral level. In addition, she has demonstrated that she can function both as a professional psychologist and as a member of a team. During her rotation at Day Hospital, she has added a new dimension to our program and has become a member of the team. Her leaving will leave a void in our program and our team, a void which will be difficult for anyone to fill."

Dr. Morehouse took a position with a non-federal agency in St. Louis.

Ardith M. Zander, Level IV intern from Ohio State University, received a joint UTHSC-VAH appointment in September 1976. In December she rotated to the Drug Dependence Treatment Center for a three month assignment. Her UTHSC assignments were with Child Adolescent Psychiatric Clinic and the Juvenile Department under the supervision of Drs. Gluck and Ateek, and she spent one day a week at the VA during the summer of 1977 on the GM&S Unit.

Mrs. Zander was supervised at the VA by Drs. Patterson, Toland, Profant, Kidd and Scrivner, in that order. Mrs. Zander was evaluated to be a very good student with strong therapeutic skills. Dr. Profant's summary: "Mrs. Zander has many strengths. She has insight and ability to respond to the manipulation of the DDTC patient. She seeks assistance from supervisors willingly and integrates the comments made with her own ideas. She is clearly goal-directed in therapeutic, one-to-one, treatment and takes treatment very seriously. She has completed written material quickly and efficiently without being reminded. She has taken this rotation seriously, placed her energies in a goal-directed manner within the setting, and has the respect, I believe, of all our staff and patients."

My summary: "Mrs. Zander should be quite effective as a staff psychologist in many clinical settings with children, juveniles or adults. She has been offered and has accepted a position as Staff Psychologist on the DDTC Inpatient Unit at the Dallas VA Hospital effective September 28, 1977."

Three new trainees were appointed September 1, 1977 to joint VA-University of Texas Health Science Center Psychology Training Program: Michael J. McGrath, Level III Intern, University of Texas; Thomas H. Harrell, Level IV Intern, University of Georgia; William C. Alexander, Level IV Intern, Bowling Green University, Ohio.

Michael McGrath rotated through the Parkland Outpatient Clinic and the Scottish Rite Hospital during the first six months of his appointment. Thomas Harrell began his first six months rotation at the VA Hospital under the supervision of Dr. Kidd and from December 1977 through March 1978 under the supervision of Dr. Patterson. William Alexander's initial assignment was at the Health Science Center under the supervision of Drs. Fougerousse and Roberts at the Children's Medical Center and the Routh Street MHMR Center respectively.

Rozen Patmon, a diminutive, personable African-American female Intern was a fourth 1977 appointment. The only extant record is the Roster of Trainees:

"Rozen Patmon, Okla. State U. Level III - IV '77 - '79."

Family Happenings

Lisa visited in the summer of 1977 and we spent some time at Sedalia. She was photographed in a straight-back chair on the century old front porch of Andrew Jackson Jernigan's parlor, her great-great grandfather.

Jean and I drove to Stage Coach Inn, Roundrock, Texas for our 30th wedding anniversary dinner, July 5, 1977.

A Broken Arm

Jean fell one weekend as she practiced riding her bicycle on Fountainhead. She experienced pain in her right arm, and the next day, a Sunday, the pain reached a threshold requiring emergency help at Methodist Hospital (August 7, 1977). The Emergency Room physician ordered an X-ray and diagnosed a broken right arm (her preferred hand).

There is no recollection that Jean complained about the inconvenience of having an arm in cast. Richard and I helped some with the housework and cooking. Jean continued to honor her downtown office schedule. She was - is - quite a trooper!

On August 16, 1977 Robin Ellis and Angharad Rees, stars of Masterpiece Theater Series, "Poldark" came to Dallas KRRV

Channel 13 studios. Richard and I attended and took a number of portrait shots of the two.

APA - San Francisco, California

Shortly before I attended the annual convention of the American Psychological Association in San Francisco, John Rhodes, Dallas Morning News photographer, advertised a 28mm Nikon 2.0 lens ($125) for sale. Jean and I drove to his East Dallas apartment, and purchased the lens. The lens made possible some fabulous slides of San Francisco including the Golden Gate Bridge. During the convention I flew to Carmel to visit with Natalie Murray and Sandy Swain.

Carmel was in the midst of a drought and there was barely sufficient water to flush a toilet. Late in the afternoon Natalie drove me around the resort area including Pebble Beach for a photograph of its famous 18th hole. The next morning I was up early to photograph daylight beach scenes including a poignant misty-beach photo of Natalie looking out to sea. Natalie and Sandy gave me royal treatment.

There are no documents from the convention. The Veterans Administration paid for the trip, probably to recruit staff. I stayed at the San Franciscan Hotel.

Austin, Texas

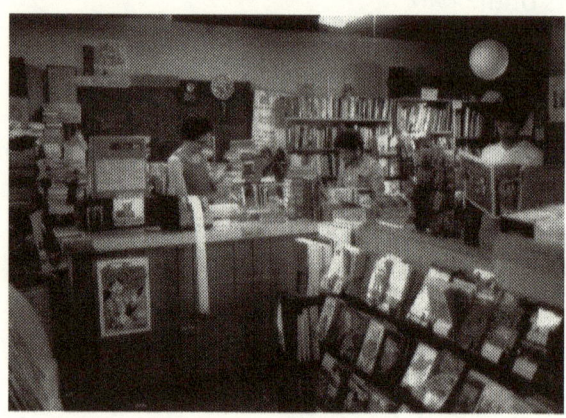

Richard – Austin – (?) Half Price Books

Richard returned to the University his Junior year, and continued to live with Austin. I visited them in early September.

Austin's handsome room filled with windows over-looked Shoals Creek and its cliffs to the west. Richard had a comfortable south room filled with the many books he purchased from Half Price Books where he worked part time.

VA Hospital

The Drug Treatment Center staff gave Dr. Pamela Profant a party when she and her husband moved to another state. I took photographs of Pamela receiving her gift, and of the staff who worked on the unit that included Psychology Technicians Ivoune Widows and Rutha Waters. Dr. Ardith Zander replaced Dr. Profant the latter part of September 1977.

Duncanville

Mrs. Sharon Bryan, Occupational Investigation Teacher of Byrd Junior High School, Duncanville invited me to speak to classes about the work of a psychologist on two occasions, May 4, 1977 and October 20, 1977. Mrs. Bryan wrote letters of appreciation after each visit. Following are excerpts from her October 21 letter:

"When education and the community merge to provide the very best learning possible, the students as a whole see a relationship between what they are doing in school and what they will be doing in the near future. Learning becomes relevant and interesting; therefore, the students are motivated to strive for their very best.

"Your presentation to the classes was most helpful. The students responded very enthusiastically to the information given. This was beneficial for a better understanding of the duties of your profession."

Professional & Personal Visit

I was in Austin from October 31 to November 3, 1977 to "Confer with Hogg Foundation and Department of Psychology on programs." One of many contacts made in Austin during the trip included a visit with Careen Phelan, Ph.D., Acting Deputy Commissioner, Mental Health, Box 12668 Capitol Station, Austin, Texas 78711. 6

One purpose for the visit with Dr. Phelan may have been to make a post Veterans Administration employment contact. Two paragraphs from a letter to Dr. Phelan on November 10, 1977 so suggests:

"Attached are three documents, two of which concern the Large Scale Assessment of State Mental Patients in 1966; also enclosed is a copy of my Curriculum Vitae.

"It was a pleasure to visit with you on Wednesday, November 2, 1977. Thank you for sharing information about the state hospital programs."

I also visited Warren G. Harding, State of Texas Treasurer. Warren and I lived at the same boarding house in Denton pre WWII, and worked for Mrs. Gross, the owner. We were good friends.

And there was a visit to the O. Henry Museum related to Albert Jernigan research.

Austin returned home for a brief visit and we contracted with him to paint the outside of the house. He efficiently reached the high gables that were difficult for me to paint.

I attended the Texas Psychological Association annual meeting, Thursday through Saturday, December 1-3, 1977. Dr. Joan Anderson, Houston, and Dr. Bob Anderson of Texas Tech were among those making presentations at the convention.

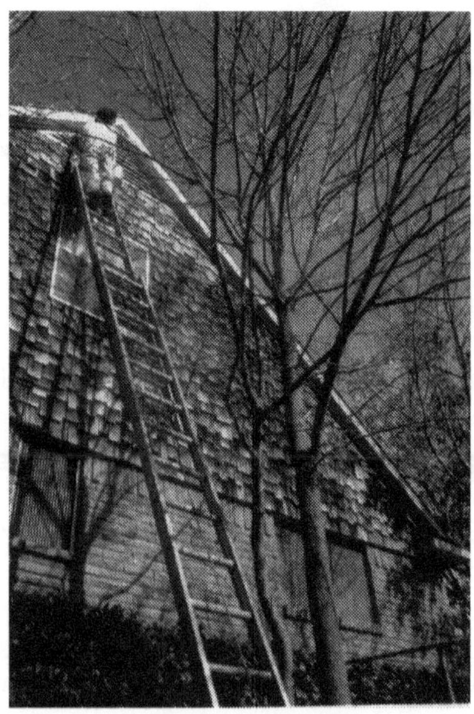

Austin – November 1977

Continuing Education

The 1977 Texas State Board of Examiners of Psychologists Renewal Application requested information about hours of continuing education. Continuing education was not yet mandatory, but came shortly thereafter.

Response for the year, 1977: "Jan. 5-7, 1977 (32 hours) - attended VA Conference in Training in Chronic Care Concept of Long-Term Chronic Psychiatric Patients, Dallas, TX. I attended SWPA, APA, and TPA in 1977 for estimated total of 30 hours of seminars, papers, etc. Dec. 5-7, 1977 (32 hrs.) attended VA Conference of VA Chief Psychologists reviewing Peer Review, Privileges, Documentation and Evaluation of Programs."

Psychology Annual Christmas Party

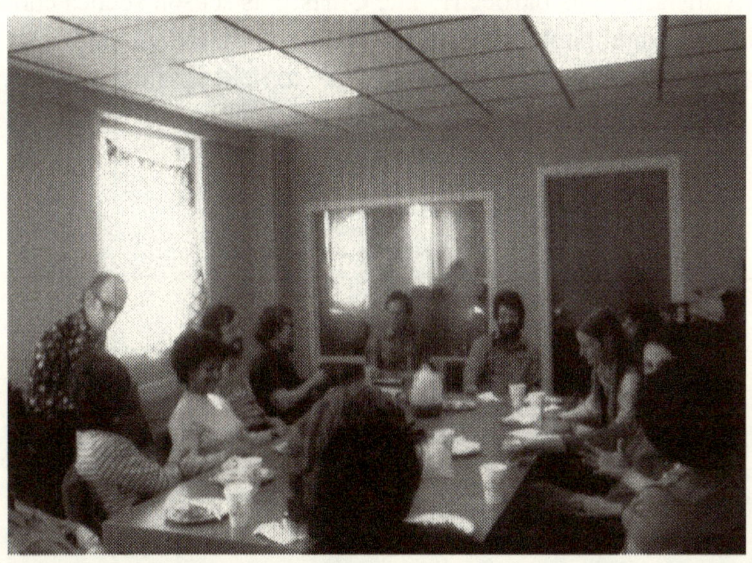

Buzz Tucker (talking) to Mrs. Gallo, Rozen Patmon, Earl Patterson, Reagan Andrews, Royce Scrivner, Trainee (Jack Gold?), Ardith Zander and Kathy Meyers.

VA Psychology held the annual Staff Christmas party in the 9th floor conference room. Those present in photographs: Buzz

Tucker (retired), Kathy Meyers, Rozen Patmon, Rutha Waters, Ivoune Widows, Regan Andrews, Mrs. Gallo, Artie Zander, Ron Kidd and an unidentified trainee.

Christmas 1977

We visited Jamie and his family at Christmas. The festive occasion ended with Jamie at the electric ice cream freezer dipping out a big bowl of homemade ice cream.

Our family Christmas tree was surrounded with gifts including a new bicycle tire for one of the boys. "Opening of presents" photos: Austin with a picture puzzle, and Lisa with an inflated kite that encompassed the den. The kite was later photographed in the sky over the grounds of Browne Junior High School. Outside, Cornish hens turned on the rotisserie of the newly installed gas barbecue. The Christmas season scenes ended with the annual photograph of Lisa and grandfather at side of the growing Christmas tree. I was still able to hold Lisa in my arms.

Chapter 21 - 1978

Letter

Stewart wrote in early January 1978, ". . . thank you for all the work you have done for us." His "work" reference was to the transfer of deed of the 129+ acre farm and property to the Jernigan Brothers.

Mary and Stewart spent the Christmas Holidays in Washington with their son David and his wife, Pat. Stewart told of some of their experiences. He concluded with:

". . . We also enjoyed two fine performances - National Ballet (doing Nutcracker) at Kennedy Center and James Earl Jones in the monodrama about Paul Robeson. Jones sings well enough to be credible, and he is a fine actor. Also we had some good meals eating out."

Professional - Psychology Trainees

Psychology Trainee John Ubersax announced he would not resume his projected training assignment. This created a question whether the trainee should reimburse the Federal Government for overpayment, and a telephone call was placed to Central Office on a crisp, clear January 13, 1978. Following are excerpts from Memorandum I dictated that day to Chief, Employee Accounts Fiscal Service (04).

"1. Dr. Dana Moore, Coordinator of Psychology Training in VA Central Office was contacted on January 13, 1978 regarding the obligation of former Psychology Trainee John S. Ubersax who has been paid for approximately one-half of his third year level stipend but has accomplished only 296 hours of training. Dr. Moore conferred with Dr. Charles Stenger, Acting Associate Director of Psychology in VA Central Office . . . it was the decision that if Mr. Ubersax has changed his graduate degree program from Clinical Psychology and the University will give the Veterans Administration a letter to that effect, then Mr. Ubersax does not owe either hours or money.

"2. Dr. Stenger suggested the Dallas Psychology Training Committee request a letter from the University of Texas in Austin giving the exact status of Mr. Ubersax's current training plan. Dr. Joseph M. Horn, Director of Clinical Training, Department of Psychology, the University of Texas at Austin was contacted and said he would confer with the Clinical faculty and inform the Veterans Administration about the exact training status of Mr. Ubersax."

Final decision: Mr. Ubersax did not owe hours or money.

Intern William Alexander came to the VA Hospital in early 1978 following completion of a six month's rotation at the Health Science Center, and assigned to Drs. Patterson, Day Hospital and Toland, MHC. In May he rotated to Psychiatry under the supervision of Dr. Andrews and continued to carry patients at the MHC.

All supervisors gave consistent praise to Mr. Alexander's attention to training assignments, e.g. Dr. Toland: "A unique strength observed was his ability to use his clinical skills in a versatile manner in different therapeutic situations." Dr. Fougerousse (Medical School) observed: ". . . an extraordinarily good teacher in addition to being a good clinician." In August, Bill was offered an attractive teaching position at Wichita State University in Kansas. My final summary statement, "This man has many skills to offer the profession of Psychology."

Likewise, Michael McGrath completed a six months rotation at the Health Science Center and came to the VA Drug Dependence Treatment Center on March 1, 1978 under the supervision of Dr. Ardith Zander, and later under Dr. Earl Patterson at the Day Hospital in June. His special research interests brought him into contact with Dr. Walter Penk, Research Psychologist, with whom he collaborated on a research project with drug dependent patients.

Mr. McGrath's multiple interests resulted in an active schedule and supervisors counseled him on spreading his energies over many training activities. With his strong research interests it was recommended his professional future might best be served in the research-academic field rather than a pure clinical setting.

Level IV trainee Thomas Harrell completed the second half of his six months rotation at the VA Hospital under the supervision of Dr. Earl Patterson. His second six months was at the Health Science Center with assignments at the Dallas Children's Medical Center and Dallas Mental Health Clinic. Mr. Harrell had achieved 963 hours of experience with the VA Medical Center at the expiration of his internship appointment on August 30, 1978.

Mr. Harrell was able to effectively utilize and respond appropriately to supervisors. He was rated in the upper quartile of interns in the joint internship training program.

Three new trainee appointments were made during 1978, but there are no extant summary documents since they were still in training status when I retired in 1979. The following interns were joint appointments to the VA-Health Science Center program and came on duty in the fall of 1978 at the beginning of the new academic year:

Theodore Kent Olson, University of Kansas, Level III, 1978-1979. Alvin Smith, University of Georgia, Level III, 1978-1979. Arthur R. Tarbox, Emory University, Level IV, 1978-1979.

Rozene Patmon, Oklahoma State, Level III-IV, began her appointment in 1977, and was on duty when I retired in 1979. I remember with fondness each of these trainees. Ted Olson was married and there are nice photos of him and his lovely wife.

Rozen Patmon and Alvin Smith were African-American, pleasant, inquisitive individuals - good students.

Arthur R. Tarbox is one of the few trainees from whom there is post-graduation correspondence. He appeared on or was referred to on a Dr. Red Duke PBS program in 1990. Art's reply to a letter of congratulation:

"November 7, 1990

"Dear Jack:

"Thank you so much for your letter last week. It was delightful for me to have one of my old mentors 'reinforcing my behavior.'

"My training at the hand of my mentors has certainly stood me in good stead. My life, both professionally and otherwise, has gone extremely well and in a very fortunate direction since I left you and Dallas. My academic career went extremely well at the University of Texas Medical School [Houston], to the point that I was promoted to Associate Professor with tenure. Because of numerous changes within the medical school itself and especially in my department, I resigned my tenure a couple of years ago and went into private practice, although I still retain my academic connection in terms of being a Clinical Associate Professor.

"Private practice has been an extremely good move for me, and I have had the good fortune to continue to do much of the same work that I was doing when a full-time faculty. That is one of the reasons that I know Dr. Red Duke, as he continues to refer patients to me. I do specialize, more or less, in the treatment of trauma and stress-related disorders, as you probably have guessed.

"Sheila and I have recently moved into a new house and we have some beautiful godchildren. Our lives have been blessed in many ways.

"I am so happy for you and Jean as you are both enjoying your 'semi-retirement.' I am particularly excited about your book, so let me know when it comes out [Albert's Hidden Treasure]. My very best regards to you both."

VA Sponsored Training

Hospital Director, C. Wayne Hawkins invited many hospital staff to attend: "TIGER Workshop, January 24, 25, 26, 1978. . . The workshop is designed to promote a meaningful group experience among those who attend . . . sessions will be at the Holiday Inn-Duncanville, 711 E. Camp Wisdom Road."

We were divided into participation groups covering topics titled: "Ursula and the Alligators", "Jo-Hari Window", "Group Painting", "D-Groups", etc. We began at 8:30 AM, took an hour lunch-break, and concluded at 4:30 PM. I was not an eager participant, but as a Service Chief was required to attend and endorse. However, I identified with the workshop objective, to promote a meaningful group experience among employees.

Labor Relations

As Management's representative to Employees Labor Union hearings (Union contract negotiations and like matters), I was required to attend a Labor Relations Workshop conducted by the Department of Labor in February 1978 at Holiday Inn in Garland. The Garland workshop began February 8, 1978 with an all day training session.

I recall one lengthy Employee Union Contract negotiation with Nursing Service. A key issue was Nursing Service's 24 hour problem in establishing three patient-care shifts.

Psychology Staff

The Chairman of the TIGER Steering Committee, J. B. Sprenkle submitted a Memorandum February 16, 1978 announcing a workshop to be conducted by "Dr. Ron Kidd who has been the key figure in the development of the V. A. Dallas TIGER Program. Dr. Kidd is transferring to V. A. San Antonio at the end of this month and this workshop is intended to reap the benefits of his many years of experience." Ninth floor conference room photographs also documented a staff party prior to Ron's departure.

Ron Kidd made multiple contributions to the Dallas VA Psychology Programs. He and Kathy Meyer worked together on evaluation of research data gathered from hundreds of patients through the Group Assessment Program as well as other research projects. Ron divorced his wife. Kathy Meyer divorced her husband. Ron and Kathy eventually married.

Dr. Pamela Walker joined the staff upon completion of her Ph.D. at the University of Texas in January 1978.

In late spring 1978, I met Dr. Kenneth E. Rylee at D/FW Airport and brought him to the hospital for a series of interviews. Dr. Rylee, a military psychologist at Wilford Hall U.S.A.F. Medical Center, Lackland (formerly San Antonio Aviation Cadet Center) was in search of a civilian position. 1

Dr. Rylee identified with the evolving discipline of neuropsychology. He independently requested a white laboratory coat, his attire at Wilford Hall. It was pointed out psychology staff wore street clothes, usually a dress suit, but Ken insisted he wear a white laboratory coat.

Dr. Rylee worked closely with Dr. Walker, the most recent staff addition. The two psychologists covered Medical and Surgical Services and had frequent need to confer about patient care.

Dr. Mike Dolan, a University of Kentucky Ph.D. was selected in 1978 as a Staff Psychologist for the Drug Dependence Treatment Center. Details are vague, but as recalled, Mike's appointment and marriage dates overlapped. A Catholic from Pennsylvania married a strong willed young Baptist lady from Kentucky. We met his attractive bride for the first time in November 1978 when we entertained the staff.

Hogg Foundation - Captain Kangaroo

I drove to Austin Friday, March 10, 1978 to attend a "University of Texas Hogg Foundation Meeting." The jovial, insightful Captain Kangaroo (Bob Keeshan) was the featured speaker. It was a pleasant experience to hear him speak and to watch his interaction with the children surrounding him.

Austin, Richard and I had lunch together as was the custom during a quick trip to Austin.

VA Regional Psychology Training Committee Meeting

The Dallas VA Hospital was host to a VA Regional Psychology Training Committee Meeting held in the 9th floor conference room March 31, 1978. Those present: Regional Training Secretary, Joe Rickard, Temple VAH, Pat Kuekes, Oklahoma City VAH, Rodney Baker, San Antonio VAH, and the Psychologist stationed at Bonham VAH whose name is not recalled. Stations included in the Training Region identified by Chairman Joe Rickard were: Temple, Oklahoma City, San Antonio, Bonham, Houston, Waco, and Dallas.

It was a pleasant day with friends, all of whom were interested in the advancement of psychology through training and continuing education. Rodney Baker became a TPA advocate for continuing education and submitted the subject and peer review as agenda topics for our VA meeting.

Letter from Richard

Richard wrote April 23, 1978 that the house in which he and Austin were living had a new tenant and they were to move.

"Dear Mother and Dad,

"I've been working for nearly two weeks now at the mailroom and it's coming along pretty well. It's all busy work, - picking up mail, sorting out, delivering. But I'm enjoying the routine and the physical workout and, of course, the $235 a month.

"I haven't done anything about looking for a house to live in with Austin. Spring is here in all its grandeur. All the windows in the house are open. Every now and then a hot day arrives and the fans come on. All the folks here at the house are waking up after winter hibernation. It gets harder and harder each day to think about moving. I feel that I've got the best view in the city. The sunsets are always beautiful. It's awfully hard to give up.

"We had a party Friday night. It was mostly given by Charles, the new tenant, and Keith. Charles supplied barbequed chicken and sausage which was prepared in big oil drum pits outside and I fixed about thirty pounds of potato salad. Charles is already about to move out so I guess this was a welcoming and going away party for him.

"My film production class has split-up into film crews and our group has been shooting the past week. I'm going to do a film sometime this week. The purpose of the assignment is to learn how to shoot synchronous sound. I'm going to shoot a dialogue from Plato's Republic with Ed Lowry as Socrates and Austin as Adeimantus, disciple of Socrates whose lines consist of comments like "Indeed" and "How correct you are" in response to his leader's long-winded expositions.

"As you might expect, I'm broke. I've drawn money from my savings account to cover the costs of the film, but I believe I'll need extra money at the end of the month to pay off rent and phone bills.

"I've been thinking about summer school. I may take some more photography for the darkrooms, and I would also like to get into some kind of RTF course where I could have access to the studios and equipment. I've also thought of government courses which courses to take, which I think is a pretty good record as I don't have to worry about foreign language and sciences or any of that other stuff that tends to suddenly appear unstudied with the approach of graduation.

"The camera is working great. I really am enjoying it. I'll send you some photos when I get the chance. Austin bought a non-reflex 35mm the other day. He's shooting color slides. He's being forgetful on remembering to remove the lens cap and that brings big laughs every time he goes to shoot a group portrait.

"Thanks for the postcard!

Love, Richard"

Some Hospital Activities

Mrs. Rutha Waters, Psychology Technician at the Drug Dependence Treatment Center became ill one day in April, and I drove her to her home in Waxahachie. It was a temporary illness. Rutha was an active member of the VA Hospital Labor Union and Hospital Credit Union and a leader among her fellow African-Americans. She was also a lady with a beautiful singing voice.

The Veterans Administration Volunteer Service Committee sponsored a cook-out late in the afternoon of May 15, 1978. I attended as member of the Committee, and photographed the Chaplain and other members of the committee cooking hamburgers at the Day Treatment Center Building. The building was the former Nurses Quarters of the 1940's.

Two First Ladies

The Hogg Foundation sponsored a National Mental Health Meeting in Austin, Texas May 25-26, 1978, titled, "The Robert Lee Sutherland Seminar in Mental Health." The keynote speaker was the First Lady of the United States, Rosalynn Carter. Former First Lady, Lady Bird Johnson was also one of the featured speakers. I felt privileged to have an invitation from host Wayne Holtzman of the Hogg Foundation.

Multiple photographs documented the conference speakers that included Dr. Holtzman, Mrs. Carter and Mrs. Johnson. Other photographed guests were: Phil Roos, Al Burstein and wife, Bob Anderson, and Eddie Bernice Johnson, former Dallas VAH Psychiatric Nurse and future Congresswoman.

The two-day seminar was named in honor of the first Director of the Hogg Foundation, Robert Lee Sutherland. In 1946 WWII Veteran, Captain James C. Jernigan visited Dr. Sutherland about employment possibilities. Bob Sutherland informed Jamie of a staff opening at Texas A & I.

The following letter was mailed Wayne Holtzman June 16, 1978:

"Dear Wayne,

"It was a privilege to be a participant in the First Robert Lee Sutherland Seminar in Mental Health. The information and material gathered at the seminar have been shared with staff at the Dallas VA Hospital and discussed informally with staff at the Medical School.

“Having been assigned to the work session on Adulthood and Aging rekindled my thoughts about some of the dormant data of the 1966 State Survey. Specifically, I have been considering a review of the data using Daniel Levinson’s outline from his new book, The Seasons of a Man’s Life, as an organizational guideline. Clinical assessment and the aging process is a subject of personal interest and perhaps the State Survey has potential pilot norms which could be further explored.

“Thought you might like some samples of candid photographs I took at the seminar.

“Thank you for inviting me.”

There were some well focused, close-up photographs of Wayne escorting Mrs. Carter among a horde of invitees as she answered questions from individual participants. Also included in the group of photos mailed to Dr. Holtzman were copies from close-up slides of Mrs. Johnson.

Family Happenings

Jamie and Frances held a reception for Laura and her fiancée, Ken Espensen., May 21, 1978, at the Canyon Creek Country Club in Richardson. Among those friends and relatives present were: Kermit and Mozelle Rosser, Alton and Beulah Hoyle, Swain and Anita Tidwell, Gene and Elford Lane, Agnes Coffey, Jones Pierce and wife, Jay, Beth and Lisa Fain. It was a joyous Sunday afternoon visit with old friends and relatives.

A Letter from Lisa – Houston Alert

Beth addressed the envelope postmarked, Dallas, Texas 5 June 1978, but eight year old Lisa wrote the letter:

“Dear Grandma and Grandpa,

"I liked my presents very much. They'll give me something to do on those rainy days in Houston. Its so fun to draw on that little board. I liked spending the night with you last night. It was a lot of fun.

"Bye.

Love,
Lisa"

Proctor and Gamble transferred Jay to Houston, Texas. Soon after Lisa's letter, she and her parents moved to their new home at 14910 Beechmoor in Houston.

Farm-log

For a brief time, Jamie and I were able to fulfill Mother's wish that her children enjoy the "old home place after I am gone." Unfortunately Stewart had little opportunity to visit the farm, especially after Alzheimer's began its insidious course. Jamie placed a notepad at the farm to record our "coming and going", henceforth identified as Farm-log. The first entry:

"Farm-log: 6-10-78 Jack and Jamie picked up potatoes, 3 1/2 Bu., and onions, strung 26 bunches of onions in barn; mowed graves @ Highland, some squash, bean and beets. Jamie"

"Farm-log: 6/19 & 6/20 Spent Monday and Monday night at farm; slept under blanket, a full golden moon. Trimmed hedge, repaired picnic table, front porch rocker, mowed garden (broke mower). Jack"

Conservation Summit

Jean and I made plans in March to attend the National Wildlife Conservation Summit, Black Mountain, North Carolina June 24-30, 1978. We flew to Atlanta, and transferred to Piedmont

Air Lines for the flight into North Carolina. We drove a Budget-Rent-A-Car from the airport to the Summit's stately YMCA Blue Ridge Assembly grounds. And once again enjoyed its mansion-like headquarters building nestled among majestic trees.

It was a relaxing and educational week. We listened to educators from the South lecture on a variety of subjects, and walked about the beautiful grounds identifying trees, birds, and flowers.

Dr. Jolly from one of the Carolina Universities presented a lecture on the "mountain man" that helped better understand our collective heritage. He asked if we sometime surprised ourselves by being able to do a task with our hands for which we had received no training. Dr. Jolly proposed that it came from our ancestors, "the mountain people," who subsequently migrated west into Tennessee, Kentucky, etc. Dr. Jolly also had a room filled with tools and instruments of all types and shapes collected from the mountain people era and asked us to identify the, "What Is It?"

We rediscovered old friends and lecturers from previous Summits and made new friends. One afternoon we drove down to Asheville, North Carolina to visit Carl Sandburg's home, a signal event. One could almost feel Sandburg's presence in his study and home filled with photographs, walls of books, and his guitar beside Sandburg's favorite chair, waiting to be played.

While in North Carolina we visited the home of Thomas Wolfe and the cemetery where he was buried, "1900-1938." And in the same cemetery we visited the grave-site of William Sydney Porter, "1862-1910."

We concluded the Summit with a drive along the breath-taking Blue Ridge Mountains Sky Line Parkway, pausing frequently to take photographs, occasionally crossing paths with some Summit friends. Jean and I had a great time together.

Texas

"Farm-log: 7/2/78 After an excellent lunch w/ JCJs came to farm. Corn, okra b. peas and squash. Man is it warm. Thundering in northwest. Jack"

"Farm-log: 7/15/78 Jamie and I gathered okra and tomatoes. He edged. 98 on porch. Jack"

Laura and Ken

We drove toward Kingsville in late July 1978, picked up Richard and Austin, then on to Kingsville to attend Laura and Ken's wedding July 29, 1978. We stayed at Holiday Inn with a host of other relatives. A member of the A & I faculty hosted a luncheon for the families. Stewart was active with his camera.

It was a lovely wedding. Afterwards Jamie became ill as told in the Farm-log.

"Farm-log: 8/5/78 Jean and I were up to pick tomatoes. Jamie in hospital in Kingsville - pains in stomach - so far Doctors have not found cause. [For Edgar]: Call when you cut the maize if it's near the weekend. Jack"

Edgar Edwards continued to monitor the house and buildings much as he did when Mother was alive. Our log book was left in the kitchen and Edgar kept up with our coming and going.

Jamie remained a few more days in Kingsville. His problem was food and stress.

VA Hospital

I met each week at the Mental Hygiene Clinic with a group of WWII Veterans. It pleased the men when I asked permission to take their photograph. In fact, it was therapeutic.

A Day at Work

Beth wrote requesting, "Write down some of your life experiences." On August 10, 1978, I wrote a summary of the day, excerpts follow:

"Perhaps this need occurs in each generation. As I mowed the lawn I began to formulate a variety of memories which could possibly be of interest to others, and suddenly thoughts began to flood through my head, rapidly picking up anecdotes which in the space of 50 minutes, if recorded through the written word would have filled a small monograph.

"Later, I had the idea an hour by hour recall of this day might be an outline for a start on a biographical sketch.

"Going to bed about 10:45 last evening I quickly dropped off to sleep soon as is my pattern. I woke about 2:00 AM and went to the bathroom. Return to sleep was not too difficult - but some restlessness. Then up at 5:00 AM, again to bathroom, but quickly back to sleep, awakened by the alarm at 5:52 AM. Shaved, and turned on the radio, lay on floor to take 'back exercises.' Caught the ABC news with a direct broadcast from Rome describing the long line of mourners filing past Pope Paul's body as it lay in state. The weather report from Dallas registered temperature of around 70 with a high of 95 expected.

"Waked Jean, completed dressing and went out to pick up the August 10, 1978 Dallas Morning News. The head lines repeated an earlier heard summary of Congressional Committee's conclusion that Oswald had an accomplice when he shot President Kennedy in 1963.

"We had fruit juice (orange), dry cereal and banana (Heartland Natural Cereal) and 1/2 of a piece of blueberry Pop-Tart. After going to bathroom, placed breakfast dishes in dishwasher and made a lunch of bologna, cheese, lettuce, Fritos and an apple.

"Finished dressing and backed out Jean's car for her while she gathered objects to carry to work including a banana cake baked the night before to take to the office for a girl retiring.

"Fed the birds and cut 3 blossoms from the [unnamed] bush to take to office. Drove by the cleaners [Lancaster Rd.] to pick up a suit and listened to Paul Harvey on car radio. Left home at 7:25 and arrived at the VA parking lot about 7:45.

"As I walked in saw ahead of me a group of 5 strange employees exiting from a Govt. Vehicle - all dressed as if visitors, and as one carried a calculator I gathered they were an audit team. Arriving at separate elevator exits so that I came face to face, one called me by given name, 'Jack" and I immediately recognized Ches Howell, Fiscal Officer at Waco. He was here today for a regional fiscal officers meeting. . . We exchanged information about families and I invited him to have lunch which he declined because the group was leaving before noon.

"Arriving at the office about 5 minutes later than usual, I completed my outline of tasks for the day and placed on Mrs. Gallo's desk. Began work on an evaluation of a former patient for a company in Fort Worth asking for information, as person was an applicant for employment.

"Interrupted at 8:05, Dr. Andrews calling from New Orleans saying would not be on duty. . . About 8:30 had a call from Dr. Robinowitz about Alcohol Conference of 9th and other related matters.

"Had a visitor from Library, a young female employee inquiring about a Psych Tech vacancy. . . I encouraged her to apply and referred her to Personnel, Jim Turner, calling Jim for an appointment.

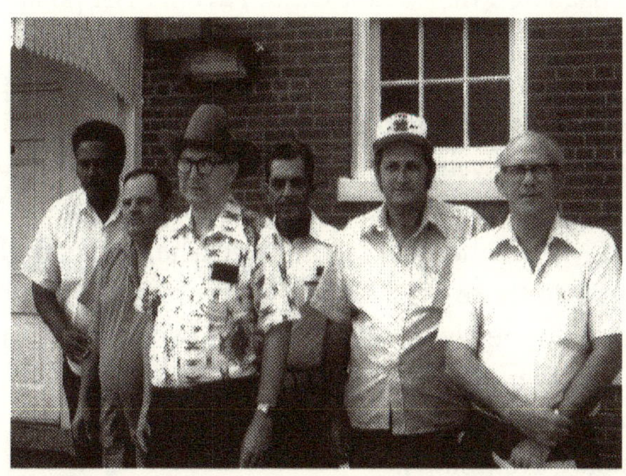

"Now being 9:05 went to Canteen for coffee. Sat with Tom Ford [Laboratory Supervisor - we were employees together in McKinney] who told of his daughter's new teaching position in Houston. We also discussed arthritis.

"Bought 4 pair of socks, and a package of panty hose and chocolate Orio cookies to surprise Jean.

"Back to office 9:45 - spoke to Walter Penk about patient evaluation, had he known him in 1971?

"Mrs. Gallo asked about Form 52 on Bill Alexander. Bill and I talked about closing date of his Internship. Mrs. Gallo went to zerox. I completed work on patient report.

"Mail arrived - letter from Don Carver asking for internship verification for California State license. A call from Dr. Edward's office [Chief of Staff] on request for appointment at 10:45.

"Spent approximately one hour with Dr. Edwards. Discussed I. T., one year limitation for 3 patients; space for Family Service; 3 position vacancies; low census at DDTC. Gave details of a patient's death and the service. He sought counsel on medical retirement. Discussed the vacant Chief Psychiatrist position.

"Now noon. Mrs. Gallo tells of problem with Supply on MMPI forms and asked me to call company. Ate lunch. Jim Turner came up to discuss Psych Tech series. Mrs. Gallo goes to lunch. I work on Dr. Carver's form. Called Psych Corporation on MMPI forms. Asked Mrs. Gallo how feeling as earlier she complained of pains similar to those prior to heart surgery in '77. Said had about subsided. Reviewed form on clinical privileges. Completed form on Don Carver. Received call from TRC employee asking about position. Received call from St. Louis Psychologist on APA Symposium on Gerontology.

"Called Dallas Post Office about register to locate when Sedalia had a Post Office. Worked on administrative audit. . . Left work at 4:40.

"Read Beth's letter, mowed yard."

New Car

We purchased a 1978 four-door, red Plymouth Volarie from Fred Oakley of Dallas August 29, 1978 with a check for $6,000 and began monthly repayments to savings of $98.20 a month. One of our first trips in the Volarie was to Houston to visit the Fains in their lovely new home on Beechmoor. There is a photograph of the red Plymouth and Jay's cream "company" Ford parked in the driveway.

"Farm-log: 9/28/78 Jamie and I were up. The place looks mighty pretty. All three sons will be up to Westminster Church,

Sunday Oct. 1, 1978 for the ground breaking for the Blanche Coffey Jernigan Education Building. Jack"

"Farm-log: 9/30/78 "Dear Edgar,

"The farm is in beautiful condition. I don't when we've had it this ready for next year so early. Sorry Jamie and I didn't get to see you today. We did talk to Norman. Stewart"

Blanche C. Jernigan Memorial Building

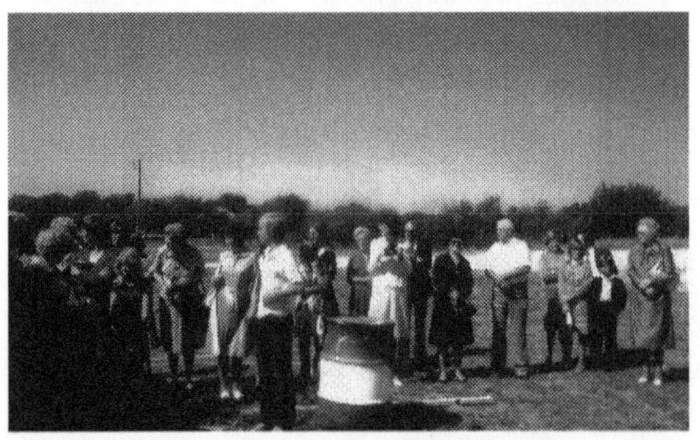

Ground-Breaking at Westminster

Rubye Hill submitted an announcement to the McKinney Courier-Gazette for publication Wednesday, September 27, 1978, "Building set as Memorial."

"The groundbreaking for the Blanche C. Jernigan Memorial Building will be held on Oct. 1, [1978] at 11 a.m.

"This is an education building which will be constructed on the north side of the Baptist Church.

"Mrs. Jernigan was a member of this church since childhood. She had ties with the Westminster Academy.

"Her Christian life, her interest in music, her service to public education and her faithful stewardship were exemplary.

"The Jernigan family will be present, along with several other families who had great admiration for Mrs. Jernigan."

Four church deacons, the pastor, and Anthony Geer, former member of the church, and President of Anna National Bank participated in the groundbreaking. Anthony gave the principal remarks. Approximately twenty five church members and guests were identified in twenty photographs as well as the following Jernigan family members: Stewart, Jamie and Frances, granddaughter Susan, and her two children, Lisa and Rip.

All the family returned to the farm for a visit. Stewart and Mary said they wanted to take the sewing machine Mother promised to Susan. All agreed, but later Jamie commented Mother also promised the sewing machine to Laura.

There were many instances of Mother's dual or triple "willing" an object to a grandchild or child. A personal example: Jamie took Daddy's mandolin for his son, Jim, and had it restrung. Mother wrote a letter to Richard and enclosed a photograph of Daddy playing the mandolin. On the back she wrote: "Richard this will be yours when I die." Jamie graciously passed the instrument back to Richard.

State Fair

The State Fair of Texas check to Creative Arts/Special Events Department mailed on August 30, 1978 for $3.00, indicated three photographs were entered. Jean and I went immediately to look for the display of photograph winners in the Women's Building on opening day of the 1978 State Fair of Texas. Prominent among the group was the portrait submitted of Mrs. Standridge with an honorable mention award.

The wall of "winners display" did not include an entry of a photograph taken during the 1977 State Fair of a group of square dancers in their colorful dance routine. It won first place! We neglected to look in every cubicle of creative art. We later learned that some photographs were selected each year to supplement or enhance another art subject. The first place winner became known when the entries were retrieved.

The 1978 annual meeting of the Texas Psychological Association was held in Dallas November 2-4, 1978.

Recent VA Psychology staff members Pam Walker and Ken Rylee attended the convention. Others friends seen at the Convention were: Naomi and David Meadows, Ralph Robinowitz, Joe Kobos, and Joy Anderson.

Staff Party

A few days later, November 13, 1978, we hosted our VA staff at 4012 Fountainhead. Fourteen staff and trainees plus their spouses or escorts were present.

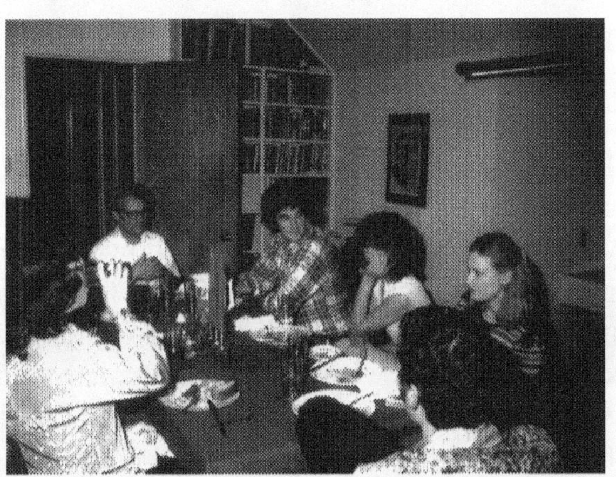

Ralph R. – Mike Dolan and wife- Pamela W.
Pamela's husband and Yvonne Widows

Photographs were taken of people eating in the dining room, den and the boys' upstairs theater (above photo). Some of the identified individuals: Rutha Waters and husband, Mike Dolan and wife, Ken Rylee, wife and son, Pamela Walker and husband, Arthur Tarbox, Ardie Zander and husband, Ralph and Hanna Robinowitz, Reagan Andrews and wife, Royce Scrivner, Rozene Patmon and male guest, Jean, etc. Each individual offered to bring a dish. Royce contributed a special punch.

The Gibson Family Gathered

Jean's Mother, Mary Gibson was bed ridden with a stroke (1976) at Wysong Nursing Center. Several members of the Gibson family met at the Gibson home place November 24, 1978. Those present reminisced about times past. Marian recommended that Mrs. Gibson's old refrigerator be removed. Austin and Richard transported it in their VW Bus to the farm at Sedalia.

Beth wrote December 10, 1978. She began with descriptions of the decoration of their new home, and concluded with thoughts about their Christmas schedule in Dallas. The middle paragraph is quoted:

"Dear Mother and Daddy,

"I want to tell you that Jay and I went and saw a counselor last week. I'd really been unhappy most of the time since I'd been in Houston and couldn't seem to get out of it. Most of it, I believe, was my job and the way it gets me down, and part of it was resentment and anger (that transferred to Jay) that I felt about leaving my happy life in Dallas and moving to Houston. She was recommended to me by the mother of a friend in Dallas who is active in mental health somehow; the friend's husband is having problems and going through therapy. I didn't want to go to anyone who knew you, Daddy. I hope you understand that that's the reason I didn't talk to you about it first. I was embarrassed and put out that I couldn't get over being depressed by myself; it was the scariest move I ever made. I have never been so anxious about going somewhere in my life. The counselor is in H. SW in an office with a psychiatrist and psychologist - a kind of family counseling clinic, I suppose. Her name is ----- --------. I liked her quite a bit. I feel better this week than I have since we came to Houston. I feel through some kind of pretending, acting out, whatever we did that I have finally resolved the move to Houston and am finally feeling at home here. I was concerned that she would be using counseling 101 techniques with me; I know enough that there are things she could have done that I would have resented. I'm going back alone tomorrow night and I don't feel I need to go back much more often There's one other problem that I need help working through. I hope it doesn't bother you to talk about it before hand, but it was just too painful. However, it is the best move I've made since coming here and I am <u>finally</u> feeling like my old self.

Love, Beth"

Christmas 1978

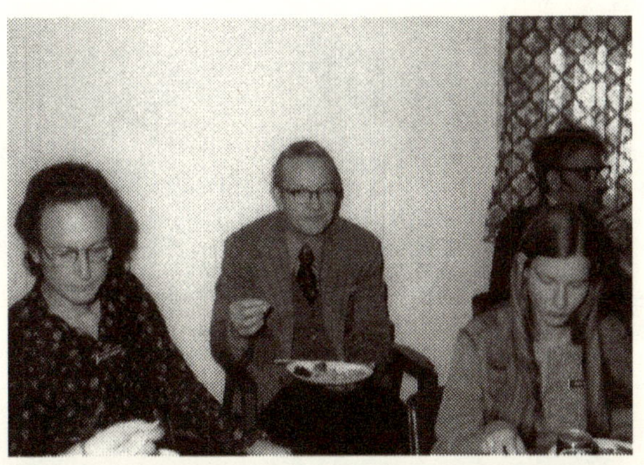

Royce Scrivner –AJJ – Ardie Zander – Ralph Robinowitz

We held the 1978 VA Staff Christmas party in the 9th floor conference room the afternoon of December 21.

Christmas 1978 at 4012 Fountainhead found the family opening presents in early morning: Lisa - Jean and Lisa - Jack and Lisa - Jay sitting on hearth of fireplace with fire in background, Austin, Richard, Lisa, and an inquisitive cat. Jamie, Frances,

Laura, and Ken joined us for lunch. Lisa and I posed for our annual "living Christmas tree photographs."

The year ended with 4012 Fountainhead's ice laden-trees bent to the ground as if in prayer.

Chapter 22 - 1979

Retirement Thoughts

North Texas was covered with ice January 1, 1979. In spite of the cold-gray, icy weather, Alpine Aluminum Co. began the installation of storm-doors and windows at 4012 Fountainhead as contracted in November 1978 ($1800). The Alpine salesperson predicted the gas and electric bills would decrease with the added insulation.

The New Year brought new thoughts of retirement. The Federal Civil Service Retirement Act allowed an employee to retire on reaching age 55 with 30 years of Federal Service. That goal was reached in 1976 with 34 years of Federal Service, but retirement was not seriously considered until 1979. 1

Letter from Austin

Austin settled down to a job at Half Price Books. He helped organize a commune like residence atmosphere at 1900 San Gabriel, Austin, TX. Austin wrote from his new residence January 12, 1979,

"Dear Dad and Mother:

"I'm having a fine time this year. Last night I was going to start showing movies at Half Price Books (Angel, Three Stooges, etc.) at 8:00 and made three pots of popcorn and made it out of the house at 8, only to find the bus would not start. (It began starting again New Years but the starter quit again today and now there's no connection at all.) So Jennifer was going to give us a ride but couldn't find her key, so I ended up calling it off 'til tonight. Walked over anyway and distributed the popcorn. Saturday and possibly Sunday we're having musicians and other guests over for a jamboree and New Year Celebration.

"The most used Christmas gift so far is the thermos, keeping plenty of hot coffee. Next is the TV set - we've seen lots of great movies (Sergeant York, Spellbound, You Only Live Twice, Rio Lobo) and night before last took it to the Laundromat to watch a show. I've shot four rolls of film so far but haven't seen any results yet. Really like the overalls, too.

"We have 3 cats now, Walter, Lucy and Buzz. Buzz is big now and a sterling example of cathood, but Lucy is a mess - we finally took her to a vet over at the pound and she may turn out OK - and Walter is a little kitten and hasn't learned everything yet, tho she's smart and cute and smells rather like oatmeal cookies.

"There's plenty more happening, but that would involve too many pages if started, so good cheers and see you later.

Love, Austin"

Funerals

"Farm-log: 1-16-79 Jamie and I came to Urb Downey's funeral at Whitewright - burial @ Elm Grove. A few limbs are broken but no other apparent damage from the ice storm. Jack"

Mr. Downey's funeral came on a bleak Friday afternoon. We stopped at a McKinney florist for a pot plant of red flowers, and attended only the graveside service. We visited with a number of Sedalia folks at Elm Grove Cemetery: the many relatives of Urb Downey, his wife, Eula Downey, son, Joe Urb Downey, Burl Shields and son, Vinson, etc.

"Farm-log: February 12, 1979 Jamie and Frances came by after Weldon's funeral to check on everything. Frances"

Although I had a large backlog of annual leave at the Veterans Administration, it was not always possible to take leave to attend a funeral. Frances' farm-log entry was the only extant note of the passing of long term family friend, Weldon Lane.

Professional Activities

Federal Income Tax record for 1979 documented many pre and post-retirement professional activities. The first declared expense occurred February 16-18, 1979 to "attended Executive Committee meeting Texas Psychological Association" in Austin. A weather change brought icy streets to Austin on the night of February 16. I spent the evening of the 16th at Howard Johnson and invited Austin and Richard to meet there the next morning for breakfast.

A call came to Howard Johnson Coffee Shop where I awaited their arrival to say they skidded on an icy overpass and flipped the VW Bus. Thankfully, neither was injured.

By the time I reached the overpass, the officers, Austin, Richard, and other motorists had up-righted the VW Bus, and waited for the arrival of a tow-truck. A photograph captured the I-35 scene of the VW Bus on the bank of the overpass with Austin and Richard waiting for the tow-truck. The tow-truck arrived, but the driver required $50 cash to move the vehicle. Fortunately, Richard had $50 in cash. The bus was not seriously damaged.

My heart really went out to our two sons that day. Austin and Richard were shivering from the cold weather and the harrowing experience. To warm their bodies, raise their spirits and fill their stomachs, we drove to the reopened Coffee Shop at the Driskell Hotel for breakfast.

Afterwards, I went to my meeting, and later found time to do "Albert's Hidden Treasure" research before starting back toward Dallas in the afternoon. The roads became so dangerous that it was necessary to spend the night at Stagecoach Inn at Salado, February

18, 1979. While snowed in at Salado, I transcribed tape recording of "Albert notes" taken that day in Austin.

None of the other 1979 professional meetings had such dramatic associations. I attended a "Rehabilitation Conference" at Airport Hotel, Dallas February 28, 1979. The conference was for state and federal agencies involved in rehabilitation. 2

Sedalia

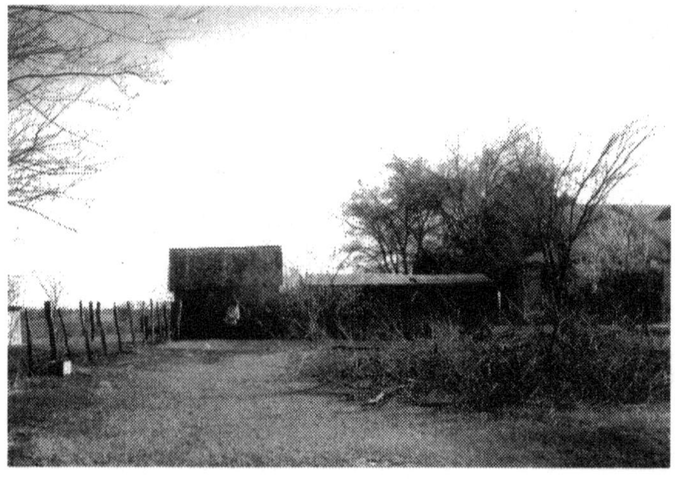

Jean stacking brush

Jean and I began making frequent Saturday trips to Sedalia to trim trees and prepare for a vegetable garden.

"Farm-log: 4-7-79 Jean, Edgar and I planted 4 rows of Topcrop Beans + 3 kinds squash. Took dining table.

The dining table was a "loan" to Mother of the walnut dining table we bought at a Waco estate sale in 1951.

"Farm- log: 4-14-79 Planted 2 rows sweet corn next to potatoes. Enjoyed relish. Jack, Jean, Beth & Lisa (Jean)"

Letter from Beth

Excerpts from letter dated April 19, 1979.

Dear Mother and Daddy,

"We all arrived home safely with no difficulty about 1:00, this morning. Katie had her kittens Easter night in a basket of broom-weed - 3 white kittens & one gray. I was hoping for a calico cat like Petulia, oh well! She's being a good mother & we have had a steady pilgrimage of children to see our new arrivals.

". . . The tennis racket Lisa wanted at 'the club' was $14 - unstrung. We will be making a visit to Houston Jewelry (owned by Sterlings) one night this week, I'm sure. Lisa doesn't need that expensive a racket.

"The humidity is bothering Chen Tai's [dog] back - he is creeping around & not himself. I feel for him - I may try giving him some asprin.

"Wednesday

"I'm waiting for the plumber to day. There's a leak under my sink in the bathroom. Our plumbing was really thrown in - glad that we've got warranty until July 1. The carpet in Lisa's bathroom is coming apart and the linoleum is coming up in the kitchen. I'm having much trouble getting that company to come fix things. It's great having a new house & having the builder repair things, but it's a hassle when the builder's agents don't follow through!

"Thanks again for your warm hospitality.

Love, Beth"

After Swain Tidwell's death, Anita recommended Swain's early model garden tractor with cultivator, planter, mower, and other attachments would be useful at the farm. I agreed, paid her $100, and took the tractor and equipment to the farm and stored it in the old garage.

Dedication of VA Research Building

Representative Ray Roberts was principal speaker at the dedication of the VA Research Building on April 21, 1979. Several community leaders spoke including Dean Sprague of the Medical School and Hospital Director Wayne Hawkins. After the ribbon cutting ceremony I visited briefly with Mr. Roberts, who quickly mentioned Stewart whom he remembered from their days together in McKinney.

The Research Building was a significant addition to the hospital system. Walter Penk and his staff of research technicians were given a suite of offices in the new building.

Professional Meetings

Four days later I flew to San Antonio to attend the 25th anniversary meeting of the Southwestern Psychological Association. April 26 was a clear day, as captured in a photographic scene of Mountain Creek Lake as the Southwest Airline plane lifted into the air out of Love Field. Scenes along the San Antonio River included photographs of a number of psychologists strolling along the River Walk. Betty Cleland invited me to photograph all the living SWPA past-presidents. I was well acquainted with most all the psychologists in the group photograph, and had intimately worked with many of them over the years.

There was a delay in route on returning to Dallas at Pease Park in Austin the afternoon the University celebrated "Eeyore Day." Many of the students were in costumes of cloth and bare skin painted to demonstrate a few hours of freedom from academia. Richard, a student, and ex-student Austin were in the midst of the fun and frolic.

On June 6, 1979 I attended a "Mental Health Association Meeting at Loew's Anatole, Dallas, Texas." Dr. Kenneth Altschuler, the new Chairman of Psychiatry, Southwestern Medical School was one of the participants.

A Family Gathered

"Farm Log: 6-15 & 16 Came Friday night, ate at Van Alstyne Dairy Queen. Jack and Norman mowed and trimmed. Jean cleaned, washed curtains and picked beans and squash. Beets and squash should be ready the 22nd, onions are ready. [Jean]

The Westminster Baptist Church's projected educational building named in Mother's memory was completed in the spring of 1979. Sunday, June 24, 1979 was the designated day of dedication, the 100th anniversary of the founding of the church. Mother's life spanned 90 of those years. 3

VA Hospital - Trainees - Staff

The following trainees were on duty during 1979: Kay D. Bullock, University of Texas, Level III, Counseling; Theodore Kent Olson, University of Kansas, Level III, Clinical; Rozene Patmon, Oklahoma State University, Level III-IV, Clinical; Alvin Smith, University of Georgia, Clinical; and Arthur R. Tarbox, Emory University, Level IV, Clinical.

The following clinical trainee applicants were selected to begin training in the fall 1979-1980: Milton L. Gearing, II, University South Carolina, Level III; D. Carol Smith Murthy, Baylor University, Level III; Stephen T. Skiffington, University of Georgia, Level III; and Michael E. Wolf, Oklahoma University, Level III.

Retirement began before these individuals came on duty. I had no contact with three of the four trainees other than having been a participant in the selection process and signed their appointments. However, I interacted later with Dr. Milton Gearing when he became Director of Psychological Services at the Plano Child Guidance Clinic.

I participated with Ralph Robinowitz in the hiring of Dr. Gray Atkins for the Drug Dependence Treatment Center. Gray did not remain long with the VA, and soon went to work for one of the commercial drug treatment centers.

An August 8, 1979 membership application for the Society for Personality Assessment, Incorporated noted that my "Duties" included the supervision of ". . . of 13 Ph. D Staff, 4 Technicians, and 5 Psychology Interns."

Family

Richard wrote July 2, 1979, and a young lady named "Leslie" appeared in Richard's letter. However, he referred to Leslie and their weekend trip as though we were probably acquainted with Leslie. Richard also enclosed five photocopied pages from a religious book he discovered at Half-Price Books.

"Dear Mother and Dad,

"Thought I'd write an annual letter! We're all sweating it out down here but everyone's doing well. Leslie and I drove to her grandparents' house on Sunday out near Kingsland (near Burnet). They live on a small lake and have a garden. We brought back lots of vegetables, peaches, and tomatoes. They're real fine people and we got along well.

"I haven't been up to a whole lot other than my bookstore job. I found another old TV set which I plan on building another aquarium with. What you want for Christmas?

"Valentine had some pups under the house - part Valentine but mostly a Doberman name Radar that was bothering her back in April.

"I've about 90% decided to go back to school this fall. I'm not exactly sure what to take or how to take it. I don't know if I want to go full time and work part time, or work full time and attend part time. I do want to keep my job, I like the incentive it gives me and I like the balance. I want to take a whack at calculus again it's something I feel I need training in. I'm considering taking silk screen printing in the art department, I know the professor through Mike. I'm also thinking about some psychology courses see what sort of agreements and disagreements I'll get into.

"Leslie and I are going to Washington in late August. I've made train reservations which I have to answer to before July 21st.

"Here's some pages I xeroxed from the Urantia Book. I thought you might find it as interesting as I have.

"Hope you all are doing well!

Love, Richard." 4

We met the attractive, personable Leslie Harden two weeks later. She and Richard came in a truck filled with books for delivery to the home store of Half-Price Books. These two University of Texas Seniors seemed more than fast-friends. And we were glad.

Vacation on the Farm

We enjoyed our freedom to come and go at the old Sedalia homestead. Following are summer '79 "Farm-logs" including a description of a rest-work vacation.

"Farm-log: July 4, 1979 Jack and Jean spent night and canned beets. Picked few Blackeyed peas, lots of sweet corn (will freeze), squash and finished pulling onions.

"Jamie, Frances, Laura and Ken just back from Kansas City to see Lindseys. Took them some produce.

"Beth, Jay and Lisa in Washington, DC with David J. & Pat this week. 4th at the Pentagon. Jean took samples of all [vegetables] to Mrs. Standridge. Jack"

"Farm-log: July 21 [Saturday] - Jack and Jean began vacation. Arrived @ 1:00 PM - called Mr. Stewart to repair GE Refrigerator. Promised to call at 8:00 PM. We will see. Jean canned 5 pints of peaches; 4 from the delicious JCJ's tree and one from the original stock tree at farm. Jack mowed fence rows, around barn, etc. Just before dusk, Jean and I walked down to south row of trees [original Aunt Belle land]. Weather cool. July 22 Had a good nights rest. Up at 7:00 AM to hear Dr. Elliot's sermon [retired pastor, Dallas' First Presbyterian]. Jean picked okra. Jack sprayed poison-ivy with Weed-Be-Gone. His experiment of two weeks ago proves this product will at least "stun" the plant. We are on way to church [Westminster] and then to Bill's for lunch.

"July 23. Picked Blackeyed peas, hoed garden, took 2 sacks of trash from smokehouse, measured kitchen, bedroom, bath and windows for size. Left for McKinney, Richardson, Dallas @ 12:15 PM.

"Returned afternoon 24th. Brought bicycles, rode over to east side of farm. Looking for hole to bury old refrigerator. Pulled the corn sheller from barn, front legs rotted away; rat odor is significant. Cleaned as best we could and put in garage. Wind in northeast, but cooled down well for sleeping by 11:00 PM. Put out rat poison in Barn. [July] 25 - Just before sunrise some bee-like creatures came in for about 15 minutes (this is second morning this phenomena has occurred). Trimmed hedge; Jean cleaned the bath room closet. Phone out - must go call - because Mrs. Standridge wants to go to beauty shop. Went to Edwards' to call on phone; promise to be in by 5 PM (and was). Called Tom Bean for appointment for Mrs. Standridge. Checked with PM Furniture floor layer - will come Thursday PM. Visited Mrs. Standridge - feels unable to ride to Tom Bean. Jean and I went to McKinney, selected pattern (6.50 a yard). Then to courthouse to determine who owns Chambers home-place (Owen Estate). Then to see Aunt Sally - a most rewarding experience. She served "Three in One"- 3 oranges, 3 lemons, 3 bananas plus water and sugar - all frozen. Came back, began preparing for laying rugs. Had two dead rats in barn.

"7-26-79 Woke up - raining- prepared for "layers." Jean and I went down to Mrs. Standridge to cut and wash her hair. The Baileys (Cecil) a father (57) and two large sons came at 2:00 to lay carpet. Had completed job by 3:15. Jean and I went to Van to get pipe compound for installing cook stove. Ate supper at Bill Barretts.

"July 27. Edgar arrived at 8:00 AM to take us on tour of Burlington Mills at Sherman. An educational tour which makes one appreciate [bed] sheets. (We were permitted to buy a set.) Jack"

The "week" at the farm-homestead reintroduced us to the serenity, hard work and pleasure of rural life. However, we would not have predicted pioneering five years later, twenty miles to the southwest on a Chambers homestead site. But that is another story and another book.

Veterans Administration - Conclusion

Extant data concerning the last few weeks at Dallas VAH are limited primarily to a photographic slide diary. Retirement count-down began with a visit to Charlton Methodist Hospital in southwest Oak Cliff to discuss the possibility of part time consulting when their projected Drug Treatment Program opened.

The opportunity for a late 1979 Charleton appointment seemed promising.

I asked Personnel Office the possible cost to add to the Retirement Fund for those VA years when retirement was not deducted. Personnel's detailed worksheet suggested a repayment cost of $3, 000+, and on that basis purchased a bond ($3163) in August 1979 from Paine Webber as a reserve or alternative for payment into the retirement fund. (Kept the bond and paid into Retirement Fund, which proved to be a much better investment.)

Beth and Jay came from Houston August 9, 1979 for Beth's 10th year graduation anniversary from Kimball High School. Austin arrived August 19, 1979 and spent time at the farm, picking peas and plowing the garden with the Tidwell tractor. A thief came shortly thereafter, stole the tractor and all equipment, and a 5 gallon GI, Army surplus gas can.

Dr. Dana Moore, made an official Central Office visit to VAH Dallas on August 21-22, 1979. I met her plane at Dallas-Fort Worth Airport and returned her next day to D/FW. Dana came to survey our program to help determine what changes were necessary for Dallas VAH Psychology Training Program to be approved by the American Psychological Association. For over thirty years the Veterans Administration Psychology Training Program served as a role model for the nation. APA no longer gave blanket approval to the Psychology Internship Program, and required each hospital be individually approved.

Under the leadership of Acting Chief, Dr. Ralph Robinowitz and Royce Scrivner, the Psychology Service began the tedious documentation process. The Dallas VAH Psychology Training Program became an approved internship program, and so listed by the American Psychological Association.

Following are the staff left behind that helped meet APA criteria for our well established Psychology Training Program: Dr.

Walter Penk, Dr. Mary Louise Toland, Dr. Ralph Robinowitz, Dr. Jack Fudge, Dr. Royce Scrivner, Dr. Reagan Andrews, Dr. Earl Patterson, Dr. Mike Dolan, Dr. Gray Atkins, Dr. Pamela Walker, Dr. Ken Rylee, John Carpenter, Sally Condor, Yvonne Widows, Rutha Waters, and Sue Gallo. A great team!

INSTRUCTIONS FOR DR. JERNIGAN'S PARTY
(7:30 P. M., August 28)

Royce Scrivner planned and coordinated the Psychology Staff's special dinner at the McKinney Avenue Restaurant, "Crackers." Royce sent instructions to each person with a map for directions to Crackers, 2621 McKinney Avenue, and for dessert afterward at the home of Kay and William Allenworth.

I carried the camera and recorded a number of scenes as the staff, trainees, technicians and spouses gathered on the restaurant's upper deck veranda. One informal photograph included some twenty-two or more individuals. Among those present were Drs. Buzz Tucker and Joy Herod McCreary. Joy was in Dallas to conduct an Echner-system, Rorschach workshop. Royce or one of the staff took several photographs of approximately two dozen friends seated around a U-shaped dinner-table arrangement with the overflow at an adjacent table. It was a delightful gathering of staff, trainees, spouses, and former staff.

As scheduled, after dinner we drove ". . . north on McKinney, turn right on Hall, follow Hall to Swiss, turn left; the Allenworth's home is between Collett and Munger." The exquisite old Swiss Avenue home of former trainee Kay Bullock (now Allenworth) and lawyer husband William Allenworth added immensely to the memorable evening.

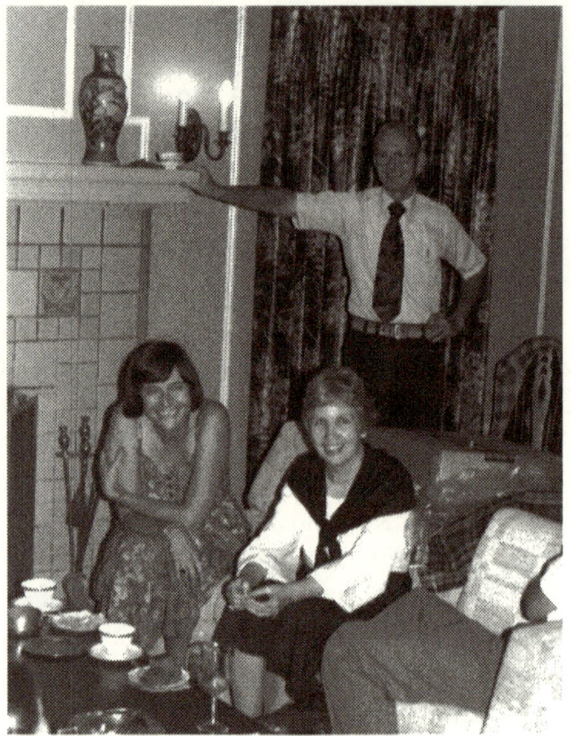

Joy Herod McCreary – Jean – Jack

Royce took many photographs and later presented a treasured photo album of the evening festivities at the dinner party and the Allenworths. The staff and trainees presented an embossed leather brief case. It proved to be an excellent gift as the brief case became most useful in post-retirement, consulting and counseling activities.

Former Waco VA Hospital trainee Pat Kuekes came to Dallas later that week, not in his capacity as Chief, Psychology Service, Oklahoma City VA Hospital, but as a participant in a Barber Shop Quartet convention. We visited briefly at the hospital and I took Pat out to the house to see Jean. Somewhere during his stay I took a photograph dated August 30, 1979. We spoke of Pat's being present at the beginning and conclusion of my career as a Ph.D. Clinical Psychologist with the Veterans Administration Hospital System.

The following day the hospital recognized the retirement with an afternoon "drop-in and goodbye" party. Jean and I greeted and visited briefly with many old friends. Over sixty five people from all walks of the hospital signed the "Guests Book." The psychology interns presented a gift certificate to Texas Highways. Many greeting cards were received from fellow employees. Dr. George Edwards sent an elegant card with "Best wishes on Behalf of the Entire Staff - George Edwards." And a card of special meaning came from the Mental Hygiene Therapy Group I led for several years. Each member of the group signed the card. (See photo in Chapter 21.)

Two framed certificates were presented by Hospital Management, "Retirement Service Award" and "Commendation" for "36 years of faithful service to the United States Government." It was 37 years of service: August 5, 1942 to August 31, 1979.

Commendation

"This certificate is awarded to Austin J. Jernigan, Ph.D. GIVEN IN RECOGNITION OF OUTSTANDING CONTRIBUTIONS TO PATIENT CARE AND THE VETERANS ADMINISTRATION IN HIS CAPACITY AS CHIEF, PSYCHOLOGY SERVICE. HIS 36 YEARS OF SERVICE HAVE BEEN CHARACTERIZED BY PROFESSIONAL SKILL, CONCERN AND COMPASSION. AS A DEDICATED LEADER, WISE COUNSELOR AND ESTEEMED ADVISOR HE HAS EARNED THE RESPECT AND FRIENDSHIP OF MEMBERS OF HIS OWN SERVICE, HIS FELLOW SERVICE CHIEFS AND OTHER EMPLOYEES WHO HAVE BEEN FORTUNATE ENOUGH TO WORK WITH HIM.

THESE DEDICATED EFFORTS ARE HEREBY GRATFULLY ACKNOWLEDGED BY THE UNDERSIGNED ON BEHALF OF THE ENTIRE STAFF OF THIS VA MEDICAL CENTER.

C. Wayne Hawkins, Medical Center Director, August 29, 1979." It was time to go.

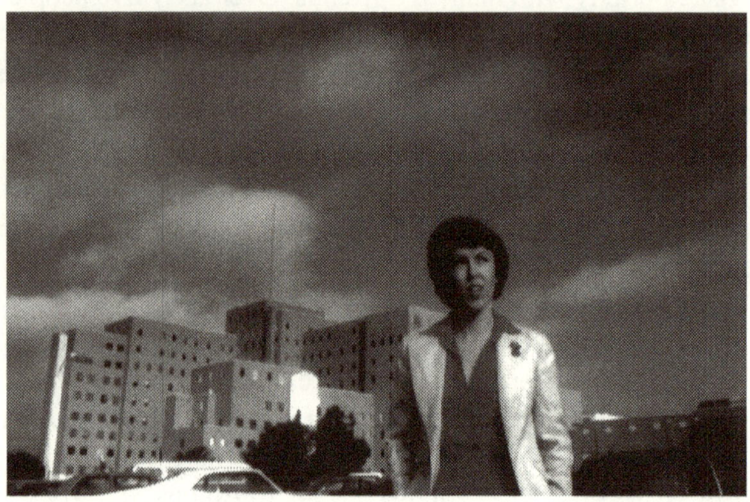

Dr. Dana Moore's official Central Office visit was my last official administrative training action. The above is an early morning photo of Dr. Moore and a view of the "backside" of the Dallas VA Hospital. I drove away from this parking lot for the last time as Chief, Psychology Service on August 29, 1979.

A Few Post Retirement Thoughts

There was less than a two month break between service in WWII and the beginning of service to some of the millions of WWII veterans through the Veterans Administration Hospital system.

It is difficult to summarize thirty-three years of learning, responding and assisting in the rehabilitation of Veterans of five wars, and teaching and supervising others in the same efforts. (Stretched it a bit - saw only one Spanish American War Veteran.) The identification with the Veterans Administration Clinical Psychology Training Program was a gift that enabled me to help in the rehabilitation of Veterans, and also enjoy the work of learning and serving.

Many years later the discovery of two verses in Paul's letter to the Colossians gave me special thought about those years: "Whatever you do, work at it with all your heart, as working for the Lord, not for man, since you know you will receive an inheritance from the Lord as a reward. It is the Lord Christ you are serving." 5

If I had consciously identified with those words earlier, my service to veterans might have been more effective. As Dad would say during World War II, "Jack is a lucky fellow."

Although my Curriculum Vitae listed a number of publications, and presentations, none resulted in a new Psychological theory or discovery. I became an innovative leader in group assessment of psychologically disturbed individuals. The development of the procedure reached its peak as the computer age began and retirement neared. It was not unlike building a better rubber-tired buggy at the time Henry Ford came out with the Model T Ford.

But it was fun building the group assessment buggy. The system proved its contribution to Clinical Psychology in the 1966 Texas State Survey of Hospital Patients, and to veteran patients at Dallas VA Hospital.

There was sadness on leaving the Veterans Administration. Yet, there was an eagerness to move on to the (semi) retirement "season." The Veterans Administration routine was soon replaced by the desire to increase time with the Holy scriptures, be more available to family, find new avenues for sharing my psychological skills, and develop the Albert story.

Jean left early each morning by city bus for her Social Security office in downtown Dallas, leaving me home to adapt as an unemployed husband. A few days after retirement I drove out to the VA Hospital and upon return to the parking lot discovered all wheel covers missing from the '78 Plymouth. For 33 years I parked as an employee without loss, and on the first visit as a veteran to a VA Hospital, someone stole wheel covers worth $157.88 (reimbursed by insurance.)

Continuing Education

I attended two seminar-workshops during September 1979. The first, a three day - "University Affiliated Center, Adolescent Conference" led by Dr. Sol Gordon in downtown Adolphus Hotel. During a break in the conference I visited Jean in her downtown office.

The second September educational meeting, held at the Scottish Rite Hospital, was led by members of the Southwest Family Institute. And later in the fall I attended a "Professional Meeting at the Medical School." I drove to San Antonio in November to attend the annual meeting of the Texas Psychological Association. Sid Cleveland was also registering at the Gunter Hotel for the convention as I registered, and we chatted about my present and his future retirement.

A week later I drove to Waco and rode with Mac Sterling to a part of Texas never before visited, the Howard E. Butts' sanctuary of magnificent views. Mac, Director of Clinical Training at Baylor University, invited me to a two day doctoral graduate student retreat. The experience was reminiscent of a National Wildlife Summit as the HEB setting offered nature walks, bird walks, photography, good food and fellowship. It was a rich opportunity to be with doctoral students, and Dr. Mac Sterling a classmate, fellow psychologist, and good friend.

The post-retirement continuing educational interests focused on marketable alternatives to traditional clinical psychology experiences. As the search continued for part time professional employment, it was soon discovered that although only 58, being past middle age was a detriment. I ordered a "Bill Moyers Journal" transcript on the subject, "How to Get a Job."

Thankfully the Charlton Methodist Hospital lead proved successful and fulfilled the desire for part time professional work.

The camera was always with me wherever I traveled, be it the farm, professional meetings, on walks and bike rides to view abundant wildflowers and nature scenes, or at the 1979 State Fair of Texas.

Jean was not with me on an October Friday when I toured the grounds of the State Fair. Some of the scenes I saw and photographed: Groups of people riding the ancient, wood constructed Lightening that Uncle George and I rode when I was a lad; a man shoeing a horse; youth grooming their sheep to show; a young girl receiving a first prize for her beautiful calf.

There was much to be done at Sedalia and many days and some nights were spent there in the fading 1979 months. Uncle Albert research continued in libraries at Austin and Dallas as I explored possible manuscripts to tell his story. Dr. Dan Griffin and Gayle Bone helped bring new growth to my spiritual life through a multitude of training seminars at Cliff Temple Baptist Church.

Richard and Leslie announced their engagement to be married. I met Leslie Harden's father, Retired Naval Captain Thad Harden in December. We had lunch just off Central Expressway at Northwest Highway. It was a pleasant discussion about the pending union of our children. We talked of them and of our retirements. When I expressed reservation about the imminent part time work in a Drug Addiction Program, Thad strongly encouraged me to take the challenge. As a former Commander of a Naval Base in Greece he witnessed the need for such treatment programs.

We entertained our "42" Group on December 22. Austin or Richard took the annual Christmas photo of Lisa and her Grandpa beside the outdoor Cedar tree. The living Christmas tree was planted the year Lisa was born. I could still hold Lisa.

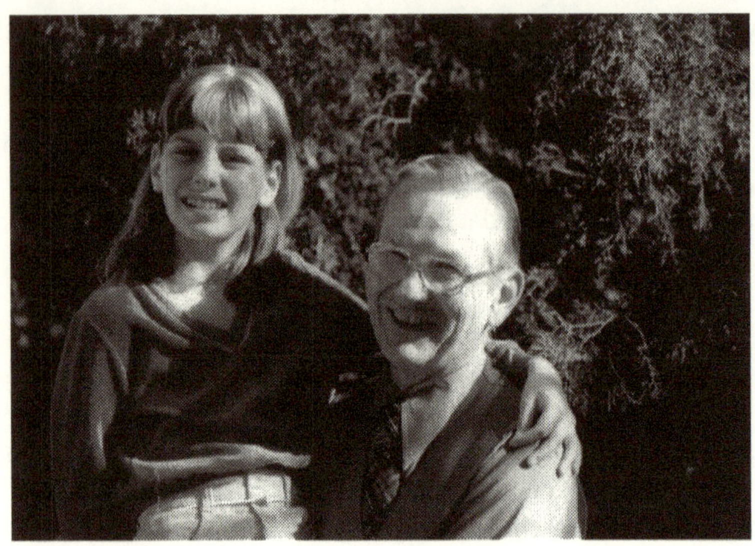

Lisa and her Grandpa – 11th photo of the annual series

Great days lay ahead. Suddenly the retirement daily schedule became full time. It was good to be alive, and that leads to another story to be later told.

Notes

Chapter 1 – 1947 – McKinney VA

1. Elizabeth Jean Gibson was introduced in the Epilogue, Selecting The Best - World War II United States Army Air Forces Aviation Psychology, the story of my World War II years 1942 - 1946.

Three Jernigan brothers left Texas in the fall of 1947 to attend graduate schools under the GI Bill of Rights: Stewart resigned his faculty position at Oklahoma A&M to work toward a Ph.D in English at the University of California; Jamie was granted a leave of absence from Texas A&I as Dean of Student Life to study for his doctorate in Education at the University of Chicago; and Jean and I drove toward Lexington, Kentucky to enter graduate school at the University of Kentucky.

2. I came out of the Air Force with $1600 in U. S. Savings Bonds, money in the bank, and anxious to buy a car. Demands for new automobiles greatly exceeded supply. Thus, I continued the WW II pattern of riding the Interurban and walking, making specific plans with Daddy to meet me at the Van Alstyne station. My parents did not have telephone service so the meeting was arranged by mail or a message left for Dad at the Sedalia store.

3. Letter of recommendation from Dr. Glen Finch:

3 June 1947

TO WHOM IT MAY CONCERN:

A. J. Jernigan worked under my supervision or in close association with me for approximately four years at various AAF Aviation Psychology Research and Testing Units. His work was always of the highest caliber and he was regarded as one of the most capable men assigned to these Units.

At Medical and Psychological Examining Unit No. 5, Miami Beach, Florida, Mr. Jernigan was non-commissioned officer in charge of individual testing (psychomotor). In this capacity, he was responsible for the administering of six tests to as many as 10,000 Aviation Cadet Candidates per month. He supervised the work of about 50 Psychological Assistants.

Mr. Jernigan was signally honored by being chosen as a member of a small cadre of Psychological Assistants and Aviation Psychologists sent to the Philippine Islands to set up an Aircrew Selection Program.

I believe that Mr. Jernigan's best qualifications are centered in his leadership abilities. He is an indefatigable worker, extremely conscientious, cheerful, and intelligent. I recommend him with enthusiasm and without reservation.

Glen Finch
Chief, Aircrew Equipment Unit
Psychology Branch, Aero Medical Laboratory
Wright Field, Dayton, Ohio

Letter of recommendation from Dr. Arthur W. Melton:

THE OHIO STATE UNIVERSITY
Howard L. Bevis, President
COLUMBUS 10

COLLEGE OF EDUCATION
Department of Psychology

June 8, 1947

TO WHOM IT MAY CONCERN:

Mr. Austin J. Jernigan served with distinction on the staff of the Department of Psychology, AAF School of Aviation Medicine, Randolph Field, Texas, for a period of more than one year in 1944 and 1945. It is my opinion that he has superior intellectual ability, an excellent personality and character, and an extraordinary talent for organization and leadership.

While attached to the Department of Psychology, Mr. Jernigan acted as 1st Sgt. in the organization, immediately responsible to the undersigned, as Chief of the Department of Psychology. In this capacity he kept records of the assignment of personnel to the various research projects of the Department, recommended the assignment of personnel in line with their talents, supervised the conduct of experimentation with human subjects, and on numerous occasions took part in experimental studies involving the psychological evaluation of aircraft instruments and controls, selection tests for pilots, etc. Prior to his assignment to the Department of Psychology, he had become thoroughly familiar with the routine processing of aviation students in the Psychological Section of the Aircrew Selection and Classification Program of the Army Air Forces, and had been given duties carrying major responsibilities in that Program. In 1945 he was relieved from duty in the Department of Psychology at the request of the senior officer, Colonel Frank A. Geldard, of a Psychological Detachment to the Philippine Islands, and was given major responsibilities in that detachment.

No real opportunity to observe Mr. Jernigan's knowledge of general and experimental psychology was presented by his duties in the Department of Psychology. However, I do not hesitate to recommend that he be admitted to graduate study in that field. His sincerity of purpose, stable and attractive personality, and excellent work-habits and work-attitudes lead me to expect his success in any chosen field of endeavor.

Arthur W. Melton
Professor of Psychology
The Ohio State University

I am grateful for such glowing letters of recommendation, somewhat embarrassed to record them here, but do so because they added much strength to my weak academic qualifications for graduate study at the University of Kentucky.

Chapter 2 – 1947-51 Lexington VA

1. The Introduction to <u>Albert's Hidden Treasure - The Study of a Texas Civil War Veteran</u> referred to the 1950 dissertation idea. Many assessment projects, this, and other manuscripts stem from the 1950 observation that letters are a storehouse of personality data.

2. We viewed scenes in Ohio, West Virginia, the Pennsylvania Turnpike where for seventy cents one traveled without interruption for seventy miles. We returned toward Lexington through parts of the Allegheny Mountains to Gettysburg, Washington, D.C., to Shenandoah National Park, to Lexington, Virginia - Washington & Lee University and VMI, and White Sulphur Springs, West Virginia. We drove 1600 miles and spent $85.

3. I recall a Washington APA convention - a midnight coffee shop sharing of pie and Baptist heritage. Fillmore Sanford's father was a prominent North Carolina Baptist minister. In Fillmore's teenage eagerness to witness his faith, he felt his father's discouragement, believed he had treaded on father's territory. Dr. Sanford later moved to UT, Austin and paid a consultant visit to Dallas VAH.

4. The Proposed Ph.D. Thesis handout given to students and faculty:

Nature of Problem:

A study of the Rorschach Test in a situation of stress. Stress is defined in this problem as the forcing of a subject to repeat the Rorschach without repeating any of the original percepts.

Significance of Problem:

1. Current theories of adjustment to stress and the need for further exploration.

2. Clinical importance of a method for determining how an N. P. patient will react to a stressful situation.

Previous Investigations:

1. Review of literature on variations in Rorschach procedure.

2. Review of literature on experiments conducted to measure reaction to stress.

Procedure:

1. Subjects - A group of N. P. patients who on the basis of admission notes and screening tests are tentatively diagnosed as psychotic; a comparable group of normal veterans.

2. Szondi Test to be administered as a buffer test.

3. Alternate subjects will receive one of two levels of stress:

Level A: Subject asked to look at the Rorschach cards a second time, everything he sees, etc., but told not to repeat any of the original percepts.

Level B: Procedure same as Level A except the subject is told his original performance was inadequate.

4. A verbal report of subject's reaction to the experiment.

5. A group of questions designed to probe further into subject's reaction to the experiment.

Treatment of Results:

1. Hypotheses - Two general hypotheses are proposed from which additional hypotheses evolve.

2. A number of comparisons are projected: Level A (Psychotic) versus Level A (Normal); Level B (Psychotic) versus Level B (Normal); Level A (Psychotic) versus Level B (Psychotic), et. cetera. These comparisons are to be made on various Rorschach factors, such as form quality, color percepts, experience balance.

5. From the Kentucky Alumnus, Spring 2001, Vol. 72, Number 1, p. 47: "Violin virtuoso Jascha Heifetz presents a concert in Memorial Coliseum . . .The UK Radio Arts department conducts a survey of 102 of the 300 television set owners in Lexington. Owners report that the number of visitors to their homes has almost doubled since they acquired a television . . . Red Skelton and Arlene Dahl appear in the movie "Watch the Birdie" at the Ashland Theatre on Euclid Avenue . . . The first book by Dean of Men A. D. Irwin, 'The Revolt of the Rednecks,' is published by the University of Kentucky Press. . .The annual UK Religious Week is held by its sponsors, the YM-YWCA and the Interfaith Council. Dr. James M. Schreyer, professor of chemistry, is voted 'most popular professor' in a Newman Club sponsored election . . . The Tootsie Roll is advertised as a 'campus favorite' . . . Priscilla Hancher

is selected the 'colonel of the Week' by the Stirrup Club. . . Bill Spivey is named the top ranking collegiate basketball player by a United Press poll of the nation's sports writers and broadcasters."

6. Significant findings summarized in the one hundred and forty-nine page dissertation, "A Rorschach Study of Normal and Psychotic Subjects in a Situation of Stress" delivered to the graduate school committee August 9, 1951:

Six Rorschach factors discriminated between the reactions to stress of 32 normal and 32 psychotic male veterans. The most significant factor was the Beck System of measuring F+%, form quality thought to be an index of ego strength. Normals tended to increase in form quality under stress but psychotics decreased significantly.

The final paragraph stated: From these conclusions on the behavior of normal and psychotic persons under stress, it is not to be inferred that an absolute dichotomy exists between the two groups in reactions to stress. Even in those areas in which the two groups differed significantly, similarity of functioning was found between some members of the groups. However, in general, the study indicated that under stress psychotics become more psychotic and normals retain their normality.

Chapter 3 – 1951-56 – Waco VA

1. Dr. Keyes, Jean's Kentucky obstetrician did not suggest a Waco physician. A member of the Waco VA Hospital staff referred her to Dr. Traylor who was somewhat reluctant to add another expectant mother to his list. We will be ever grateful for his professional attention.

Limited insurance paid the flat fee of $35 doctor and hospital care. Dr. Traylor's fee was $135, Hillcrest Hospital, $51.85. Dr. Jack W. Flowers became Beth's pediatrician.

2. Our check stub "diary" indicates we paid monthly utility bills of $1.90 for water, $4.00 for electricity, and $1.50 for gas. Milk and eggs were delivered to the house, averaging $9.00 a month.

3. Dr. Ruth Hubbard's letter to Dr. Buckholts, July 10, 1956: "We should be exceedingly sorry to lose Dr. Jernigan from this staff, but it is appropriate that he have advancement and further responsibilities."

"In every way he is a valuable and effective psychologist. He is a thoughtful and skilled psycho diagnostician, a patient and imaginative psychotherapist, and can teach these skills to others. As our Supervisor of Training he has been particularly successful in maintaining a friendly learning attitude in trainees even while he taught them new and broader ways of viewing their cases.

"His relationship with everyone in the hospital setting, with patients, with colleagues of this and other professions, with supervisors and administrators, have been uniformly productive. Not only are his relationships friendly; they are growth-producing. He is active and progressive in ways that are accepted by others.

"As the Chief of a department he will be a leader, a participator in group projects, an easer of tensions, a real catalyst for constructive interdepartmental developments. His organizational thinking takes account of the task but even more of the personalities who are carrying on the task."

"Sincerely - Ruth M. Hubbard, Ph.D. - Chief Clinical Psychologist."

4. Sold to Charles and Mary Miles on September 6, 1956 for $8900 with agreement to pay agent 2% ". . . . discount or brokerage fee."

5. Total fees for down payment, abstract, etc. were $1258 for the $15,150 "Model House." The Veterans Administration stored our household effects at Texas Fireproof Storage, Dallas.

Chapter 4 – 1956-59 – Dallas VA

1. The number "179" was the nation-wide Veterans Administration routing code for Clinical Psychology. Counseling Psychology became a designated service some years later, and received the routing code "175."

2. "On August 19, 1940, the first patient, O'Byrne Cox was admitted to the Dallas VA Hospital, a 300 bed facility managed by Charles Magruder, MD." Brochure written by Shirley Campbell, Library Service, Dallas, August 2000.

3. Paragraph 1, Minutes: "At seven-thirty p. m. the following people met at the Lisbon Veteran's Administration Hospital to form a new investment club: Drs. T. W. Wade, Earl B. Ross, J. B. Geers, A. J. Jernigan, Ben Cohen, W. H. Barris, A. W. Osborn. W. B. Hesselbrock, Mr. M. W. Williams, Mr. C. E. Young, J. Owen Dodd, Pauline Cromer, Elizabeth Brown, Doris Freberg, and Mrs. Gwen Selby."

Dr. Osborn, Chief, Dental Service was elected President, Marshall Williams of Registrar, Vice-President, Doris Freberg, Secretary, and Carl Young, Assistant Finance Officer was elected Treasurer. We voted to purchase ten shares of Pure Oil and ten of Bethlehem Steel.

Three new members joined at the May 5 meeting: Drs. Henry Lanz and D. W. Maas, and Margaret Younger. We bought six shares of General Motors.

4. The five page appraisal outline covered the following areas: General Qualifications; Performance Characteristics that included Assessment and Evaluation, Behavior Modification,

Research, Training, Consultation, Administration and Community Relations; Interests, Capacity and Potential; Personal-Interpersonal and Professional-Interprofessional Relationships; and Recommendations. The document was signed by Earl B. Ross, M. D., Director of Professional Service.

Some excerpts: ". . . began his duties . . . with most acceptable background of technical training. His performance over a period of three years has justified hopes held for him . . . has found it necessary to function in an atmosphere not entirely ideal. . . Friction was notable by its absence. . . active in areas in the hospital having to do with other employees. . . served as a discussion leader in the orientation of nurses. . . has discharged his duties of alternate deputy fair employment officer for the station. . . very active in establishing the Federal Credit Union. . . served as its first president. . . consistently been called upon to interpret to residents and interns and member of the Nursing Service the psychological factors involved in problems which they have with patients. . . has shown unusual ability in planning, organizing and developing a psychological program. . . has taken an active part in the fund drives of the Community Chest, Red Cross, and other groups approved by his supervisor [Ross]. . . a wide breadth of interests. . . civic affairs, religious affairs. . . non-technical activities in his hospital. . .this young man possesses and has demonstrated unique abilities in leadership. . . an outstanding ability to get along with his fellows and to influence them. Any program with which he is associated would be most benefited by having him."

Chapter 5 – 1960-62 Patients from Waco

1. Virginia Chancey, a member of the Program Committee wrote an excellent "Summary of the Programs for 1958-159." Some excerpts:

"October: The membership <u>demonstrates</u> shared decision making and group action. The membership <u>observes</u> its own process of working together as a group. Dr. Al North serves as observer. Some wishes: more closely knit group, wish for more social activity, interchange of idea, need for knowledge about psychological work in areas other than one's special interest, and occasional outside expert.

"November: Desired Outcomes in Academic Training by Dr. Jack Strange and Dr. I. J. Knopf. Areas covered: requirements for the master's degree; the problem of generalization vs. specialization; internship; post-doctoral; APA accreditation; that master's level should be called technician rather than psychologist.

"December: Problems of Communication with Related Disciplines with Kathleen Varner representing education, Dr. Jerry Lewis, medicine, and John Burst from industry. Dr. John Bowen served as process leader and John Geers as observer. Concluded: . . .guests stated that they believed the psychologists function more adequately than the psychologists themselves believe they do, that the necessary qualifications are due to dealing with man and his complexity and that for the most part the psychologist's predictions are accurate.

"January 1959: Principles of Consultation led by Virginia Chancey and Bob Stoltz with guests: Ruth Shorter, Social Work Consultant of the U. S. Public health Service and Dr. Bob Leon, Assistant Professor of Psychiatry at Southwestern University Medical School. Some points mentioned: obligations to clients and the community; how far does the consultant's responsibility go; how organizations can be encouraged to recognize their needs; one time vs. continuous sessions.

"February: Problems of Evaluation. Panel discussion by Drs. Maurice Korman, Earl Wilkinson, Joe Siegel and Mrs. Genette Burrus. Dr. Korman posed five questions for consideration; Mrs. Burrus oriented the group to clinical work in the 30's as to tests available and prevalent concepts; Dr. Siegel reviewed Holzberg's article, 'Clinical and Scientific Methods,

Synthesis or Antithesis;' Dr. Wilkinson discussed the flexibility of the clinician in the areas of prediction. Summary: Modifiability (qualifying predictions), continuing critical attitude, and feasibility of refusing to answer questions that one is unqualified to answer.

"March: Questionnaire prepared by program committee, 'Standards in Operational Procedure' filled out by group in beginning. Dr. Gladfelter gave a summary of Questionnaire. Discussion, how one arrives at the fee. One member, 'what New York charges' [probably Joe Siegel]; another, expectation of medical profession; another, same as psychiatrists; consultation in industry is universal throughout country [probably Bob Topper]. Rates different for evaluation and therapy, etc.

"April: Psychologists in Community Service led by Dr. Carmen Michael. Introduced articles of the last two years in the American Psychologist and the Psychological Abstracts to clarify what is meant by community service for psychologists. The group thought an individual's community service depended on his psychological field, if he felt he served the community more by taking time away from his work or not, and the most general service could be rendered by giving of advice through speeches and general contacts and by making adequate referrals."

2. Psychological Report, dated 10-29-59: "This patient was seen in group psychological screening on 10-27-59. Patient is neat in appearance, well groomed, his face is flushed. During the testing proper he expressed many feelings of inadequacy toward the task at hand, and this was especially true on the human figure drawings. He made one aborted attempt to draw a person, then destroyed the production and carried the scrap of paper with him from the testing room. His performance was unusually slow, and when he reached the Sentence Completion Test which is designed to elicit feelings, attitudes, etc., there was extreme blocking, and finally the patient gave up after he had completed approximately one-third of the items.

"The patient rates within the high average range of intelligence on the Kent Verbal Intelligence Test. There is evidence to suggest a potential for functioning at a higher level than this. His present performance is probably best described as constricted. The rumination on an internal basis along with the performance given would suggest an obsessive compulsive adjustment. His visual motor coordination tests, for example, were extremely slow and meticulous and accurate, the latter, of course, being a favorable sign. There is no indication on his performance of any breaks in reality testing.

"The patient gives clues that he is obsessed with thoughts of a disturbing nature. He gives no clues as to the content of the thinking disturbance, or perhaps more accurately described as fantasy. This man may be beginning to use the mechanism of projection as a defense. His extreme guardedness in performance would indicate that the condition may be moving beyond the neurotic level; however, on the surface there is no evidence to support this, the evidence being that the patient is so reluctant to allow anyone to go below the surface, at least through the medium of the [group] psychological tests.

"Test Administered: Kent E-G-Y Scale D; Grayson Perceptualization Test; Bender Gestalt; Human Figure Drawings (attempted); Sentence Completion Test.

A. J. Jernigan, Ph.D.
Chief, Clinical Psychological Section"

Over forty years later: The report indicates there was need for more detailed psychological assessment, e. g., Wechlser (WAIS), Rorschach, T.A.T., etc. If a psychologist had been assigned to the ward to follow up on the group assessment report, a tragedy might have been prevented.

3. Charles E. Bounds, Ph.D., Walter E Penk, M.A (Psychology Trainee), and I presented in July 1965 to the Hospital

Research Committee a "Report of Research Project" titled, "Psychological Assessment of Behavior: A Longitudinal Study". The "Significance of Project" section of Report is presented here:

"In March 1961, 83 psychiatric patients were transferred to the Dallas VAH from the Waco VAH. Immediately after the transfer, a battery of psychological screening measures was administered to the patients in small groups. In July 1964, this screening procedure was replicated and comparable data were obtained from 43 of the original 83 patients. There is a need to know the extent present behavioral indication of level of adjustment could have been predicted on the basis of psychological data obtained in 1961; and further, the extent to which behavioral adjustment is correlated with, or reflected in subsequent psychological measures."

4. Jack Wheeler's letter is no longer extant, but his enclosed copy of the Board minutes for 29 October 1961 was retained. There is a historically interesting paragraph concerning a registered letter to Dr. Austin Foster to "request an accounting of the Board's funds, both income and expenditures, by the 16th of November 1961."

Texas Psychologists adopted the BYLAWS of the Texas Board of Psychological Examiners, Incorporated at their annual meeting on December 7, 1962 at the Statler-Hilton Hotel in Dallas. Bylaw X stated: "The Board shall create an Advisory Committee composed of leading psychologists of this state to advise the Board on its various functions. The Advisory Committee shall be terminated one year after the date of the adoption of the bylaws of the Board. The original members of the Advisory Committee shall be issued certificates of certification."

My earliest extant Certificate, Diploma Number 18 was issued 6th day of April 1963, signed by Harold A. Goolishin, Chairman; Gordon T. Anderson, Vice-Chairman, and Glen V. Ramsey, Treasurer, valid until December 31, 1964.

5. An undated map gave the name and location of each tree: Bartlett Pear; Alberta Peach; Belle of Georgia; Gerber Pear; Hale Haven; Belle of Georgia; Yellow Delicious Apple; Early Alberta; Elberta; Red Delicious Apple; Early Alberta; Hale Haven; Burbank Plum; J. H. Hale: Indian Cling; Allred Plum; J. H. Hale; Early Wheeler.

Chapter 6 – 1962-63 November 22, 1963

1. See Chapter 6 pages 123 and 144 - Albert's Hidden Treasure for additional details.

2. Telephone conversation with Dr. Ralph Robinowitz, November 8, 2000 confirmed that Jack Sandt was appointed Chief of Psychiatry probably in late 1961; Dr. Sandt was not on duty when Ralph arrived in June 1961. Dr. Sandt resigned sometime after February 18, 1963 because in telephone conversation with Walter Penk, November 19, 2000, Walter recalled Dr. Sandt was there at time of Walter's February 1963 appointment as a Trainee.

Jack Sandt's letter from his home in South Hadley, Mass. on September 16, 1963 suggests he resigned from Dallas VAH in late summer 1963.

"Just a line to thank you for your help and support over the past 2 years as well as for your kind farewell gift. . .Please remember me to the other members of the psychology group, too. . .I hope you have continued success and satisfaction in your work at the hospital. . . If ever there is anything in which you feel I might be of help, do not hesitate to write me - and should you ever be in this area, please look me up. --- Best of luck -- Sincerely, Jack"

3. Fox, Emmet, The Sermon on the Mount, A General Introduction to Scientific Christianity in the Form of a Spiritual Key to Matthew V, VI and VII, New York: Grosset & Dunlap, p. 190.

"The method of forgiving is this: Get by yourself and become quiet. Repeat any prayer or treatment that appeals to you, or read a chapter of the Bible. Then quietly say, 'I fully and freely forgive the whole business in question. As far as I am concerned, it is finished forever. I cast the burden of resentment upon the Christ within me. He is free now, and I am free too. I wish him well in every phase of his life. That incident is finished. The Christ Truth has set us both free. I thank God.' Then get up and go about your business. On no account repeat this act of forgiveness, because you have done it once and for all, and to do it a second time would be tacitly to repudiate your own work. Afterward, whenever the memory of the offender of the offense happens to come into your mind, bless the delinquent briefly and dismiss the thought. Do this however, shorter or longer, the old trouble may come back to memory once more, but you will find that now all bitterness and resentment have disappeared, and you are both free with the perfect freedom of the children of God."

4. "Dr. James C. Jernigan was inaugurated Monday [March 25, 1963] as president of Texas A&I College and called for additional highly-trained scholars on its staff so that the college may assume a rightful role in research, academic excellence and intellectual leadership.

"Gov. Connally was guest speaker at the inauguration. Dr. James C. Matthews, president of North Texas State University, spoke at a luncheon honoring Jernigan.

"Jernigan who has been president of A&I since September stressed higher quality in education and academic freedom for faculty members.

". . . He said the college is on the threshold of taking its rightful place among the leading institutions in the country.

". . . In an address during the ceremonies, Connally said that Texas stands at the educational crossroads.

"'We have had a good system of higher education always, and we have a good one now. But being good is not enough if we are to fill the major role destiny has assigned to us in this new and wonderful age,' Connally said.

". . . Matthews, who once taught Jernigan at North Texas State, gave his views on a college presidency and future problems of higher education.

"He told Jernigan, 'your specific job is to build a fence here at A&I of such dimensions that the students and the faculty can participate in the fullest in the zest for learning so that none inside shall fail to be led to the very threshold of his own mind.'

"Matthews said since Sputnik I, science has taken over the place of prominence in education. He said laymen are now more aware of the need for brainpower but science does not have a corner on it."

5. Wayne R. Carroll: "The differentiation of organic and non-organic hospital patients by the use of the Wechsler Memory Scale." Don A. Nelson: "Group vs. individual administration of the Kent E-G-Y." Gerald L. Clore, Jr.: "Differential scoring on the Kent E-G-Y and its relationship to the WAIS." David Andre: "Some important variables in Grayson Perceptualization ability."

Dr. Donne Byrne, Associate Professor of Psychology, University of Texas, served as discussant.

6. Return of the 8 mm roll sent to Kodak came after an anxious and unusually long delay. A note in the box stated the FBI was to be contacted if anything of significance to the assassination was on the film. The FBI had no interest when told of the film's content. There were many calls from a group in Dallas wanting to sell Kennedy film.

Chapter 7 – 1964-65 – National Archives

1. It is assumed Dr. Baugh did not get the position. A 10 July 1964 letter received from the Chief Clinical Psychologist for the National Security Agency, Ft. George S. Meade, Maryland requested ". . . full and frank appraisal of Dr. Baugh's qualifications." Do not know if he was accepted at Ft. Meade.

2. Jean, Beth, Austin, and I visited the American History Center (formerly Barker Texas History Center) August 21, 2003 to donate, preserve and make available to historians the Civil War Diary of Elijah W. Chambers.

3. I wrote the National Archives and Records Service on May 3, 1964 and outlined the confusing data re the two Andrew Jackson Jernigans and asked for a photocopy of an original document with the signature of the 30th Regiment Jernigan, believed to be our grandfather. I quoted an anecdote given by one of the surviving daughters: "At the time of Dad's capture, all officers of his company had been killed, and Dad stepped forward to surrender the company to the federal troops. Thereafter his friends nicknamed him 'General.'" I began reading books about the fascinating saga, the tragic Civil War.

4. Powell, Larry, Dallas Morning News, Monday, April 15, 2002.

5. Requested the Muster Rolls for Elijah Chambers and received from archivist: War Department Collection of Confederate Records - Record Group 109 - Confederate Pay Rolls and Muster Rolls - Company K, 16th Regiment Texas Cavalry - March 11, 1862; August 31, 1862; February 29, 1864.

6. An effort was made to identify the service record of James M. Griffin born November 22, 1813 - died January 6, 1880 (approximately 48 when the Civil War began.). Uncertain whether he served with Alabama or Georgia troops, I searched, and located

six James and James M. Griffins in Alabama military rosters and thirteen James and James M. Griffins in Georgia rosters. I did locate his death record: "J. M. Griffin, 65 [66], male, white, born in South Carolina, both parents born in Virginia, a farmer, died in January of 'Bilious Fever,' lived in Texas 10 years, name of certifying physician. Dr. Holmes."

Chapter 8 – 1966 – Collecting Mass Data

1. Pokorny, A. D. and Frazier, S. H. Report of the Administrative Survey of Texas State Mental Hospitals, 1966, prepared by Texas Foundation for Mental Health Research, Austin, Texas, 1967.

Chapter 9 – 1966 – Rating Mass Data

1. Charles Joseph Whitman, 25, shot and killed 15 people at the University of Texas on August 1, 1966 before he was gunned down by police. Dallas Morning News "Sound Notes" August 1, 2004.

2. Jernigan, A. J. Large Scale Assessment of State Mental Patients. Journal of Clinical Psychology, 1967, 23.

Chapter 10 – 1967 – Reporting Mass Data

1. Attached to Hook's letter and other participants was a final draft of a paper submitted to the American Psychologist, reviewed and supported by Maurice Korman and Wayne Holtzman. The paper was rejected but accepted for publication by the Journal of Clinical Psychology. (See previous chapter)

Also published in 1967, a paper titled: Rotation Style On The Bender Gestalt Test. Journal of Clinical Psychology: Vol. XXIII: No. 2, 176-179, April 1967.

Bill Hales expanded the 1963 report of demographic and diagnostic facts about the Psychiatric Consultation Program. Dr. Hales replicated the research and added additional data in a paper titled: "Hales, W. H., Jernigan, A. J., & Fuller, D. S. "Demographic Study of Referrals for Psychiatric Consultation over a 5-year Period." Paper presented at Southwestern Medical School Grand Rounds, 1967.

2. Crossan, The Birth of Christianity, p. 113. For a fascinating discussion on the subject "filtered distant memories" read Crossan's review of "Memories" and especially his review of the studies by Bartlett.

3. Obituary: "Funeral services for George A. Coffey of 8023 Woodhue Road, retired owner of George A. Coffey Construction Co., were at Shamrock Shores Church of Christ, 8822 Angora at 2:30 p.m., Wednesday. Interment - Hillcrest [Dallas].

"Mr. Coffey, 78, died in Dallas Tuesday. Born in Westminster, Collin County, he had lived in Dallas 62 years. He attended Westminster Baptist Academy. He was a member of Shamrock Shores Church of Christ in Dallas. He is survived by his wife, Mrs. Gladys A. Coffey; a [step] son Vernon J. Dunn of Houston, two [step] daughters, Mrs. Gordon Fagg of Irving and Mrs. Charles Groves of Dallas; two sisters, Mrs. R. L. Johnsey of Dallas and Mrs. A. W. Jernigan of Van Alstyne; 10 [step] grandchildren and four [step] great-grandchildren." [George and first wife, Bernice had only the one daughter, Evelyn Mae, deceased.]

4. Dr. Kimball was on duty April 10, 1968 as documented in letter to Bill Hales. See Chapter 11.

5. Excerpts from Larry Powell's, December 25, 2000 Dallas Morning News.

Chapter 11 – 1968 – New Beginnings

1. The 1968 had a "V-8, 318 cu. in. engine, Torqueflite Trns., Air Cond., Radio, Power Steering, Tinted glass, Mirror Left outside, Under coat, Wheel Covers, List $3924.25. Trade diff $2143.00 Tax 52.00 - Balance $2195.00." The balance was drawn from our "loan-to-self account" at Dallas Federal Savings. Wrote a check for the car, and began monthly payments of $59.58 to Dallas Federal Savings.

2. A tax record entry for Saturday, April 6, 1968 stated: "Trip to Ft. Worth - School business - 33440 - 33520 [Corvair] 80 miles - 8.00; Lunch - 3.10 - Tollway .90, transported Kimball H. S. Annual Staff to workshop.

3. A family folk-saying: Ernest Hale a hermit-like person, of low intelligence lived east of Westminster. When his mother died it is reported some of the neighbors invited him to view his mother's body and he responded: "Naw, I've seen her a thousand times."

Chapter 12 – 1969 – Penk Research Grant

1. We drew up the following contract: "Selling 1964 Corvair for $475 to be repaid in payments of $20 or $25 a month [Beth penciled in, starting Feb. 1] at the wish of the buyer, Jay Fain. Seller (A. J. Jernigan) agrees to pay 1/2 of charge to get air conditioner going and will during the 1st year pay any major repair (not accident) in excess of $50. Buyer agrees to purchase adequate insurance. Signed - Seller - A. J. Jernigan 1-4-69"

Buyer- Jay Fain.

Our plan was to put payments in a savings account to be turned over later to Beth and Jay. Don't recall the amount accumulated.

2. Stewart was "Director of Texas A & M University EPDA (Education Professions Development Act) Institute for Advanced Study in English." Stewart's February trip to Washington was probably orientation for the six weeks Institute scheduled for June 2 to July 11, 1969. This was an "Educational Personnel Development Program under a grant from the U. S. Office of Education, as authorized under Part D of the EPDA." The Institute was "for experienced teachers, grades 7-12."

3. The Dallas Morning News, page 6A, Friday, November 21, 1969.

4. I became acquainted with Mayor Jonsson through Natalie. Mayor Jonsson's interest in Natalie Murray and Sandy Swain's Lamplighter School on Churchill Way began when the Mayor's grandchildren enrolled. Mayor Jonsson became one of their great patrons, and encouraged Natalie and Sandy to build the beautiful institution just off Inwood Road. The Mayor frequently visited Natalie and Sandy and told them they had the "best bar and grill in Dallas." I last spoke to the Mayor at either Natalie or Sandy's funeral.

Chapter 13 – 1970 – Conservation Summit

1. Don shared this story soon after he was hired: Don attended Dr. Criswell's First Baptist Church Dallas and did not agree with a sermon comment made by Dr. Criswell. He asked for an audience with the noted pastor, and was graciously received by Dr. Criswell. I complimented Don on his effort to gain theological clarification with Dr. Criswell. Dr. Smith attended a Unitarian church when he wore the Peace Pin.

3. Jernigan, A. J. "Judging Whether a Patient Is White or Black By His Draw-A-Person Test." Journal of Projective Techniques & Personality Assessment: Vol. 34: 1970, No. 6: 503-506. The summary read in part: The modest success . . . adds minimal evidence to the body image hypothesis." The

paper generated some interest in the professional community as measured by the number of requests from psychologists across the nation for a copy of the paper.

4. The narrative summarized analyses prior to October 1970:

"Hubert Reese and Bob Humble, a statistical review of the Psychological Ratings carried as Table 40 of the Report of Administrative Survey. They also gave partial distributions of scores and frequency counts of seven tests.

"Dr. Wayne Holtzman selected 699 of the 1464 patients and completed a correlation matrix of 50 variables of 9 of the 12 sets of psychological data. Findings were presented at SWPA Symposium in April 1967.

"In February 1967, Dr. Donald Gorham of the VA Psychology Research Laboratory, Perry Point prepared computer scored Holtzman Inkblot Test summaries for 725 records.

"In September 1968, Wayne Holtzman and Don Witzke presented a Summary Report: Multivariate Analysis of 123 variables for 685 patients. The report excluded three of the eleven tests.

"In July 1969, the Federal Data Processing Center, Ft. Worth prepared format lists from ten card decks that included all 12 sets of psychological data, the NOISE 30 deck and the Biometrics deck. These data were placed on magnetic tape and forwarded to Mr. Robinette in Arkansas."

Chapter 14 – 1971 – State Board

1. Our 1971 Income Tax records state, "As member of the VA Hospital-Medical School Research Committee, made eleven trips to attend meetings at the Medical School; twelve trips to

Planned Parenthood Board meetings; and seven trips to D/FW to pick up consultants and prospective employees."

2. I declared my portion of the tuition, food and lodging ($155) a deductible expense with the explanation: "This was a 5-day lecture series on topics of pollution, conservation, family planning, etc.; member Dallas Board of Planned Parenthood and a professional psychologist."

3. Some of the data collected and mailed included, biographies of James, W. M. and T. W. Jernigan and John F. Gibson found in: History of Tennessee, Goodspeed, biographies of: p. 1162 James A. Jernigan; p. 1163 W. M. Jernigan; p. 1163 T. W. Jernigan. And from Biographical Souvenir of the State of Texas, R920 Chicago, 1869: Captain John F. Gibson; Andrew J. Jernigan.

Chapter 15 – 1972 –Drug Treatment Program

1. Celia F. Fields, wife of G. H. Fields Nov. 25, 1809 - July 17, 1888; and Green H. Fields: Nov. 4, 1804 - June 30, 1866. The Fields family puzzle was solved at the Collin County Clerks Office. Michael Fields, with whom Grandpa Jernigan lived briefly when he moved from Tennessee to Texas in 1874, died intestate, and the state carefully reviewed and documented all eligible relatives subject to proceeds from Mike's minimal estate. Copies of the findings re "Fields & Jernigan" were mailed to Mother, Anna Lou Brown, Mrs. Linvle Anderson, Burl Shields for Dovie Hunter, his sister-in-law, and to Nina Sparks.

2. Later Paul McReynolds invited me to present a chapter on group assessment in his projected Psychological Assessment, Vol. 3. The chapter was titled: Jernigan, A. J., "Use of Group Tests In Clinical Settings," Chapter 8 in Advances in Psychological Assessment:, Vol. 3:, Paul McReynolds, Editor, Jossey-Bass Publishers, 1975, 313-351.

Chapter 16 – 1973 - 25th TPA President

1. The 1973 Income Tax professional expense justification statement: "As President of Texas Psychological Assn. attended 16 Executive Committee and Task Force meetings incurring the following expenses."

2. Samples of other Notebook entries: " February 17, 1973 in Dallas Library, located Biographical Directory of Congress and the identity of (Col.) Giddings, DeWitt Clinton." p. 32.

"March 16, 1973, Travis County Library, notes on election of 1888." p. 33.

"April 13, 1973, located article of 8-22-80 of interview of Albert re Arkansas Post and his head wound received." p. 34.

"June 2, 1973, visited old Thaxton house, Mrs. W. O. Karcher. A Mrs. Cage then lived in Old Sneed house. That evening visited Mary Belle and Col. and Mrs. Williams." p. 18.

"July 20, 1973, visited Cousin Laura and her husband Richard Congdon." p. 36.

3. Check book entries: Ft. Hays Motel, $7.42 Saturday night; the next day, July 1, 1973 paid YMCA - Rockies the balance due, $259.56; total fee for the four of us was $465. We returned July 7, 1973.

4. Excerpts from "Looking Back: 1973, Report from the President," in the December TPA Newsletter summarized remarks to convention:

"The Executive Committee of TPA has taken action on a wide array of TPA matters. . . The Ad Hoc Committee established . . . to study psychology in Texas public schools has, with the support of the Hogg Foundation, conducted a number of working meetings and is gaining new insights in three areas: 1. current models of delivery of psychological services in schools; 2. models to be proposed for delivery of such services; and 3. implication for improvement in school psychology services through training, certification and legislation.

"Without exception, each Committee has accepted its constitutional charge and many have gone far beyond the minimum requirements. Effective communication with the membership has been maintained through four informative issues of the Psychology newsletter, supplemented by the work of the Council in the meetings and contacts with local psychological groups. A number of people have participated in the deliberations and actions taken by the Legislative and Insurance committees for maintaining the interests of the public and the profession. The Ethics Committee has been especially active in its study and preparation of more specific guidelines of professional conduct by the membership.

"The association has taken a position on a variety of social and political issues and has attempted to voice its concern where indicated. TPA in the case of Morales v. Turman, Federal District Court in Tyler, Texas, supported members who testified as expert witnesses and advocated the right to adequate treatment at issue in this case. Again, when the Governor and the Lieutenant Governor took firm action against the deplorable situation at Artesia Hall in Liberty County, TPA sent a strong letter of support and commendation to these state officials.

"Of concern is the small voice of the association in communication with the public. Maintenance of an active, viable membership is the first step and committees work to this end is evident. There have been some creative inroads in dissemination of information by the Division of Psychological Associates, School and Applied, as well as by the Committee on State Agencies. The proposal that TPA consider a paid public relations consultant should be studied further. The annual Meeting in December is the time to exchange information and hopefully each of us will serve as a public relations expert as we present psychology's image to the public."

Chapter 17 – 1974 – Management Seminar

1. Tax return for 1974 documented seven professional trips to Austin and/or San Antonio; five trips to Southwestern Medical School; two trips to Texas Employment Commission; and also within city of Dallas, to Goodwill Industries, Dallas Psychological Association meetings, a "TSVC Conference," and VA Office at Santa Fe Building.

2. Leo Luka, Chief, Personnel Service, VAH, Houston asked me to send him a copy of the slide of the group, and Houston's Medical Illustration made copies for each participant. Identified in the photograph by rows: (1) Archie Walker, Alvin Malloy, Dr. Michele Meyers, Dr. Paul Golliher; (2) Edward Ballard, Earl Guyer, James Sullivan, Dr. Leonard Duce, Wesley Murphy; (3) Jack Jernigan, Gene Clobfelter, Patricia Irby, Madge McGregor, Marie Saunders, Marguerite Butt; (4) Amy Shimopsu, Jack Adams, Charles Sevac, James Hinton, Jerry Dozier; (5) Leo Luka, Charles Nesbit, Joe Schenkel, George Cook, Frank Quintan, William Graham.

3. The Freemantle Diary Being the Journal of Lieutenant Colonel Arthur James Lynon Tremantle, Coldstream Guards, on His Three Months in the Southern States. Editing and Commentary by Walter Lord- Published by Little, Brown and Company, Boston, 1954. . . reprinted September 1954.

See Albert's Hidden Treasure. Chapter 4, pp. 105-108 for excerpts from Tremantle's description of Texas.

4. Dr. Profant went on duty 9-30-74 at Dallas VAH and resigned 11-29-77. Personal correspondence with Dr. Patricia M. Profant, Baldwin, MO 63011, dated July 2, 2002. In 2002 Dr.

Profant worked for Magellan Behavioral Health, a managed care company, reviewing all requests for psychological testing.

Chapter 18 – 1975 TIGER

1. Obituary - McKinney Courier-Gazette, April 1975:

"William Marvin (Jake) Gibson, 91, of Melissa, died 10 p.m. Thursday at his residence. He was born March 29, 1884 in Melissa, the son of J. F. and Miranda Frances Graves Gibson, and lived on the same farm all his life. He was a retired farmer and cattleman; member of Melissa Masonic Lodge 569; past president of Texas Jersey Cattle Club; past chairman of A.S.C. [Agriculture & Soil Conservation Service]; past director of Production Credit Association; and director of Highland Cemetery Association.

"He was married July 5, 1911 in Melissa to the former Mary Windsor Chambers, who survives.

"Other survivors include two sons, John Windsor Gibson of Oklahoma City, Okla., William Marvin Gibson, Jr. of Salt Lake City, Utah; four daughters, Mrs. Frances Waller and Mrs. Marian Wysong of Melissa, Mrs. Margaret Tilton of Plano, Mrs. Jean Jernigan of Dallas; a number of grandchildren, great-grandchildren, and one great-great-grandchild; one sister, Mrs. Aurel Belden. He was preceded in death by his parents, two brothers, three sisters, one daughter, Doris Virginia Gibson.

"Funeral services will be held 3 p.m. Saturday in Melissa Baptist Church with Rev. Richard Ivy officiating. Interment will be in Highland Cemetery, Horn-Harris-Crouch in charge.

2. I included a reprint of, "Large Scale Assessment of State Mental Patients" with the paper requested by Dr. Tolar, and this explanation:

"This paper describes a project never adequately analyzed because of depleted funds and time that included the Bender Gestalt as one of many assessment techniques used in the testing of 1475 psychiatric patients. . . I have returned to the original worksheets and pulled together some facts which may be of interest to you: (1) 1081 of 1475 patients gave scoreable Benders; (2) approximately 300 patients were not testable; (3) 71 patients gave unrateable Benders (no recognizable design reproduced); (4) of the 1081 patients with scoreable Bender records, 249 (23%) rotated one or more designs; (5) the rotation style for the 249 patients using the '67 paper classification system' was: Counter Clockwise (CC) 31%; Clockwise (C), 41%; Indeterminate (I), 22.5%; Mixed (M) 5.5%.

It is of interest to make a cursory comparison with the data reported in 1967 on the subject of rotation style and note there does seem to be a distinct pattern difference between general medical and psychiatric populations. . . Thank you for including my work in your survey. I look forward to your published comprehensive review."

3. Telephone conversation with Reagan Andrews March 13, 2001.

4. These details of an intern's assignments are given so that the interested reader can obtain a glimpse into the variety of training opportunities available through the joint Dallas VAH and at UTHSC program.

5. The documentation was recorded in Family Land Heritage -Registry Volume 2, 1975.

> "JERNIGAN FARM* - 1875 - Eight miles east of Van Alstyne at Sedalia
> Founder: Andrew Jackson Jernigan of Robertson County, Tennessee
> 1975 Owner: Mrs. A. W. Jernigan, Van Alstyne

"Andrew Jackson Jernigan came to Texas in 1874, following an uncle, Green Fields, who already owned land in Grayson County, and together with his cousin Michael Fields, bought 203 acres next to the uncle's land. Cotton, oats, wheat, hogs, horses, and cattle were raised on the founder's land to which were added some 229 acres over the years. Jernigan, who built his home on the site of an old stage coach route to Bonham, was active in local church and school development. The Jernigans were a peace-abiding family and the large parlor of their home, which is still standing, was the site of many gay social functions. All of the children were trained on one or more musical instruments and the family emphasis on education was shown by the fact that all the Jernigan children entered Grayson College in Whitewright.

"Jernigan and his wife, Laura Stewart, had seven children, and a son, Austin Wallace Jernigan, assumed possession of 76 acres of the family land upon the death of his mother in 1922. Austin, who served as administrator of the land after his father's death in 1912, was a quiet community leader who raised cotton, corn, wheat, millet, oats and hogs, and, over the years, added 53 acres to his inheritance. Along with his work in encouraging sound farming practices, Austin, with his wife, Blanche Coffey, continued the furtherance of educational opportunities for his family and members of the community. Three sons born to the second generation of Jernigans included Stewart, James, and Jack. Today, Mrs. A. W. Jernigan, 89-year-old widow of the founder's son, lives on the family acreage which she inherited upon her husband's death in 1956. She consults on a daily basis with Edgar Edwards who now farms the land on which maize and corn are grown."

"JERNIGAN FARM* Registry*" indicates a structure at least 100 years old remains on property. This *designation was in error as Mr. and Mrs. Standridge owned the land and the original structure.

Chapter 19 – 1976 – Psychology Trainees

1. Wyatt Griffin inherited the property. Wyatt delivered butane to the Standridge family and recalled Mr. Standridge would come outside the house with the checkbook in hand to pay. He would tell Wyatt to fill out the amount. After complying with the request, Wyatt asked Mr. Standridge to sign, and he would inquire, "Where?" and when told asked, "What is my name?" Mrs. Standridge indicated her awareness of this confusion, but stated that Lester had desired so much to continue taking care of "his business I just couldn't remove the privilege." (Interview with Wyatt, January 25, 1998.)

2. I wrote her insurance carrier and attached the diagnostic statement by Physician Karen Pennington, "Primary Diagnosis - Basal Cell Ca. of Left Ear; Secondary Diagnosis - Cerebral Arterio Sileroscis [sic]."

3. Those from Sedalia: "Mrs. Dennis Garner and Tommy and Mandy, Mrs. W. R. Wallen, Mrs. Eula Bush, Mrs. Coffey Hunter, Linda Terry, Mrs. C. R. Presley and Riley, Mrs. Glynn Presley and Jena, Mrs. Alfred Loftice, Kim and Amy, Linda Loftice and Cheryl Loftice."

Chapter 20 – 1977 – Continuing Education

1. Letters preserved by Blanche Jernigan ended in October 1976. Other extant correspondence, residual financial records including income tax returns, and hundreds of photographic slides were available.

2. "Mrs. Blanche Coffey Jernigan, 90 wife of the late A. W. Jernigan, died Thursday, March 24 [1977], at the Wysong Hospital in McKinney. She was a longtime resident of the Sedalia community, east of Van Alstyne. Funeral services were held Friday at the Westminster Baptist Church with burial at Highland Cemetery.

"Rev. Joe N. Smith, pastor of Westminster Baptist Church; Rev. Mac Pope, First Baptist Church, Melissa; and Rev. Larry Rolison, First Baptist Church, Milford, conducted the service. Music was provided by Glynn Presley, soloist; Mrs. Joe N. Smith, pianist; and the Westminster Baptist Choir.

"Pallbearers were Bill Barrett of Van Alstyne, Elford Lane of Plano, Edgar Edwards and Russell Presley of Sedalia, Henry Griffin and Everett Sparks of Westminster.

"Mrs. Jernigan is survived by three sons: J. Stewart Jernigan of Bryan, professor of English at Texas A&M University; James C. Jernigan, retired president of Texas A&I university and currently visiting professor and consultant with the University of Oklahoma, and A. Jack Jernigan, Chief of Psychological Services at the Veterans Administration Hospital. There are also seven grandchildren and three great grandchildren.

"Mrs. Jernigan began her teaching career at Pike, Texas; then after a year or two teaching at Westminster, she began a long career at Sedalia, interrupted only by the birth of her three sons. After the Sedalia school closed, she taught again at Westminster ending her professional career in 1948 to spend full time with her husband. Education was very important to Mrs. Jernigan and her husband, and this influence carried over into the lives of her three sons and their families. At the time of her death twenty-two college degrees had been earned in her family with three grandchildren still pursuing college work.

"Although Mrs. Jernigan was recognized as a great teacher, the dominant characteristic and love of her life was an unshakeable and living faith in God. She was active in her church until a few months before her death. Her husband died 21 years ago.

"Mrs. Jernigan placed her full faith in God and never once expressed fear of continuing on alone following her husband's death. She even learned how to drive a car at age 69 in order to maintain her independence.

"Through the years, she was an important segment in the lives of many families. Not only did she teach public school and Sunday School, but she also played the piano for many weddings, funerals, revivals, and other functions. She wrote many letters on behalf of others, as well as articles for the news media.

"She had hoped to live all her years in her own home. She almost made it. She left her home on October 20, 1976, to enter Wysong Hospital and later the Wysong Center in McKinney. On March 25, 1977, five months later, her body was laid to rest by the side of her late husband in Highland Cemetery." [No date on copy.]

3. I transcribed the symposium in August 1994 and gave a copy to the Archives of the History of American Psychology, University of Akron, Akron, Ohio 44323, under the subject, "The Geldard Papers." A detailed review of the symposium is in Chapter 19: Selecting The Best - World War II Army Air Forces Aviation Psychology, titled "Thirty Years Later."

4. A copy of Dr. Melton's letter is in the Notes - Chapter 19, Selecting The Best - World War II Army Air Forces Aviation Psychology.

5. Mother's goal was to set aside $1,000 in a trust with interest each year to go to the annual Lottie Moon Christmas offering. She reached the goal. Each year Jean sends an additional check to Westminster Church in her memory.

6. Following are the professional trips reported in the 1977 Federal Income Tax return: 9 trips to Southwestern Medical School; 4 trips to attend Dallas Psychological Assn. meetings; 1-5-77 through 1-7-77 attended VACO meeting at Sheraton Hotel, Dallas; 4-13 and 4-14-77, Austin, Texas to confer on VA Psychology training; 4-21 through 4-22-77, attended Southwestern

Psychological Assn. annual meeting, Ft. Worth, Texas; 5-4-77 and 10-20-77, to Duncanville High School to present VA Psychology Program; 7-27 and 8-16-77, to pick up prospective staff to VA Hospital and return to Dallas/Ft. Worth Airport; 9-4-77, Austin Texas, attend Psychological Assn. Business meeting as committee member;10-31 to 11-3-77, Austin, Texas confer with Hogg Foundation and Dept. of Psychology on programs; 12-1 through 12-3-77, attended annual meeting Texas Psychological Association.

Chapter 21 – 1978 – A Day at Work

1. Federal Income Tax return for 1978 documented four trips, February 22, May 1, December 4, and December 11, 1978, to "airport to pick up a candidate applying for staff position."

Chapter 22 – 1979 – Count Down

1. Inquiry was made in 1974 about "paying in" to the retirement fund for those years when a percentage of my salary was not deducted for retirement, e.g., McKinney VA Hospital and the four years of VA Training time at Lexington VA Hospital, 1946-1951. Personnel advised the pay-back be made at time of retirement.

2. Two other tax documented meetings attended in the spring of 1979 were, "To represent Veterans Administration" Mountain View Community College, Dallas, Texas, February 28; Presbyterian Hospital, April 18.

Tax records identified four other "Professional Meetings" without clue as to purpose: Texas Woman's University, Dallas, Texas (School of Nursing), April 12, and again May 7, 1979; Methodist Hospital, Dallas, Texas, June 6, and again July 3, 1979. The meetings probably included "net-working" with the staff as I explored post-retirement employment opportunities at both of those institutions during 1979.

3. Excerpt from the celebration program for the day:

Westminster Baptist Church
Westminster, Texas
Sunday June 24, 1979

1979 - Our 100th Year

IN MEMORY
BLANCHE C. JERNIGAN

* A member of this church approximately 80 years
* A good witness for Jesus Christ
* A devoted life of service in the Christian faith.
* An excellent example of devotion to her husband, Austin, and to her family.
* An excellent example of Personal Stewardship
* A link between the church and Westminster Baptist Academy.
* A career as a public school teacher.

4. The "Urantia Book" is a story to be told later. It became an impetus to the post-retirement study of the Holy Scriptures so that I could come to say and write emphatically, "This I believe." Soon after Richard wrote of his discovery at Half-Price Books, Austin wrote, "I hope you'll look at the Urantia Book so we can discuss it."

5. Colossians 3: 23-24. (NIV)

Bibliography

Books

Allport, Gordon W. The Use of Personal Documents in Psychological Science. New York: Social Science Research Council, 1942.

Biographical Souvenir of the State of Texas, R920 Chicago, 1869

Crossan, John Dominic. The Birth of Christianity. Discovering What Happened In The Years Immediately After The Execution of Jesus. Harper: San Francisco, 1999.

Fox, Emmet, The Sermon on the Mount, A General Introduction to Scientific Christianity in the Form of a Spiritual Key to Matthew V, VI and VII, New York: Grosset & Dunlap, 1938

The Freemantle Diary Being the Journal of Lieutenant Colonel Arthur James Lynon Tremantle, Coldstream Guards, on His Three Months in the Southern States. Editing and Commentary by Walter Lord- Published by Little, Brown and Company, Boston, 1954. . . reprinted September 1954.

Jernigan, A. Jack. Selecting the Best – World War II Army Air Forces Aviation Psychology. Bloomington, Indiana: 1st Books, 2003. www.SelectingWWIIAircrew.com

Jernigan, A. J., "Use of Groups Tests In Clinical Settings", Chapter 8 in Advances in Psychological Assessment:, Vol 3:, Paul McReynolds, Editor, Jossey-Bass Publishers, 1975, 313-351.

Levinson, Daniel J. with C. N. Darrow, E. B. Klein, M. H. Levinson, B. McKee. The Seasons of a Man's Life. New York: Alfred A. Knopf, 1978.

“50 Years of Pride in Serving America’s Best, Our Veterans” 1940-1990 – Department of Veterans Affairs Medical Center Dallas, Texas, undated publication by VAMC, Dallas, Texas.

Unpublished Manuscripts

Jernigan, A. Jack. Dissertation: A Rorschach Study of Normal and Psychotic Subjects in a Situation of Stress, University of Kentucky 1951.

Jernigan, A. Jack. “World War II Letterbox – Letters to Austin and Blanche Jernigan – 1942 – 1946,” 1977.

Jernigan, A. Jack. “Autobiographical Diary” (1470 + pages), September 2002.

Pokorny, A. D. and Frazier, S. H. Report of the Administrative Survey of Texas State Mental Hospitals, 1966, prepared by Texas Foundation for Mental Health Research, Austin, Texas, 1967.

Circulars -Journals

Veterans Administration Washington 25, D. C., Circular No. 105, May 2, 1946, “Training Program for Clinical Psychologists Associated with Part Time-Work in V. A. Stations where Neuropsychiatric Cases are Treated.”

Jernigan, A. Jack. Rotation Style On The Bender Gestalt Test. Journal of Clinical Psychology: Vol XXIII: No. 2, 176-179, April 1967.

Jernigan, A. Jack. Large Scale Assessment of State Mental Patients. Journal of Clinical Psychology: Vol XXIII:, No. 4:, 504-506, October 1967.

Jernigan, A. Jack. Judging Whether a Patient Is White or Black By His Draw-A-Person Test. Journal of Projective Techniques & Personality Assessment: Vol 34: 1970, No. 6:, 503-506.

Newspaper Articles

"Tribute to a Father." Van Alstyne Leader, February 17, 1956.

"Foreman Fatally Shot by Ex-Mental Patient." Dallas Morning News, Section 4, March 25, 1960.

"Scholars Need Seen by Jernigan – Gov. Connally Speaks at Inauguration of A&I President, Kingsville." Corpus Christi Caller March 26, 1963.

"Many Add to Pleasure of Open House for Mrs. A. W. Jernigan Sunday." Van Alstyne Leader September 6, 1963.

Jernigan, Dr. J. C. "Jernigans at Trade Mart While President is Shot." Kingsville Record, November 1963

"Jernigan-Coffey Reunion Held Sunday." Van Alstyne Leader, December 6, 1963.

Hill, Rubye. "Building Set as Memorial. McKinney Courier-Gazette, September 27, 1978

The Dallas Morning News, page 6A, Friday, November 21, 1969.

Dallas Morning News "Sound Notes" August 1, 2004.

Powell, Larry, Feature Writer, Dallas Morning News Highlights of News article, May 21, 2001, "May 21, 1958."

Powell: April 15, 2002: "April 15, 1964."

Powell: December 25, 2000: "December 25, 1967.

Appendix

Following is information I reviewed and discussed at University of Texas Seminar in Clinical Psychology March 13th, 1970:

"Certification of Psychologists: The Case Example of Texas"

1. One of the distinguishing features of a profession is that it "polices" itself; it develops standards of conduct for its members and claims to enforce them.

Two historical issues are pertinent for discussion: (1) development of Code of Ethics by American Psychological Association and (2) evaluation of American Association of State Psychology Boards.

2. In 1938 - with 2,318 members (2,333 psychologists were elected to membership on Jan. 1, 1969) - the American Psychological Association formed a committee to draft a Code of Ethics. Little support was generated until after WW II, when demands for application of psychological knowledge was so greatly accelerated. In 1948, its 7500 members were asked to describe a situation in which a psychologist made a decision having ethical implication and to indicate the ethical issue involved. One thousand reports were received, edited, and classified. The Code of Ethics, developed over a period of four years, was adopted in 1953. (Feb. 1970, American Psychologist - page 206.)

3. The next large scale effort to "police" self began in late 40's regarding certification of psychologists. By 1950, four boards had been established: Connecticut, Virginia, Kentucky, and Ohio. By 1960, there were 32 boards (including Canada). In 1970, there are 58 boards - 47 laws plus 11 non-statutory laws. Forty-one states have laws, 9 states have non-statutory. Six Canadian provinces have laws - British Columbia has non-statutory provisions as does District of Columbia.

Need for association of Boards became apparent. Constitutional convention held in Chicago 1960 and approved Constitution and By-laws of American Association of State Psychology Boards (AASPB).

AASPB has following major functions:

(1) Provides forum for discussion and information exchange.

(2) Publishes newsletter.

(3) Has set guidelines for telephone listings.

(4) Assisted in developing greater uniformity in application forms to Boards.

(5) Studied difficulties encountered by psychologists moving from one jurisdiction to another.

(6) Published Manual on Legal Issues.

(7) Handbook for all State Boards.

(8) Under contract with Professional Examination Service of the American. Public Health Association - constructed standard objective test: Examination of Professional Practice in Psychology.

4. Recommendations - APA regarding Legislation - 14 areas concerned:

A. Type of Legislation. Custom is to speak of licensing and certification laws.

<u>Licensing Law</u> defines the practice of psychology and restricts the function to qualified persons, who may be

psychologists, or who may be members of other professions using psychological techniques.

Certification Law on the other hand, limits the use of the title "psychologist" to qualified persons: it may or may not have a definition of practice. Licensing covers practice of psychology no matter what the person wishes to call himself; certification covers the practice of psychology only when the person wishes to call himself a psychologist.

Three critical issues: (1) Preemption - make certain our regulatory efforts do not have a preemptive effect upon other professional groups; (2) Innovation - more restrictive the regulatory law, the more potential there is for inhibition of innovative developments; (3) Legal definition of vocation. It may be impossible to cite vocations that are not legally defined in state law. That is, psychology laws cannot exclude a vocation that has not also been legally identified.

APA takes position: State seeking legislation regulating the practice of psychology should attempt to develop laws falling in the category of licensing legislation (28 laws contain definition of practice of psychology). Of the 47 laws in the U. S. and Canada, 17 are licensing laws. (See page 30 for series of definitions of psychology AASPB Handbook.)

B. Level of Certification or license.

Recommend - restricting to one level, Ph.D. - accredited school - primarily psychological - not less than two years of experience, one of which is post-doctoral. Below this level - title should include adjective "psychological" followed by noun such as technician, assistant, etc.

Above this level - designate "consulting psychologist" and require competence equivalent to ABEPP diploma.

C. Specialty. Does not recommend specialty listing.

D. Exemption for psychologists. Institutional psychologists exempted. Institutional psychologist in part-time practice not exempted. Organizations that sell psychological services to public not exempted (i.e., psychologists who work for them). Students are exempted. 1959 agreement between APA and American Sociological Association not to restrict sociologists. Lecture services for fee not excluded for psychologists exempted by virtue of institutional employment.

E. Offer for fee - money or otherwise.

F. APA Code of Ethics.

G. Accreditation. Degree person has from accredited institution - each state defines its accrediting body - but, not to require the registration of departments of psychology as a part of the law.

H. Examining Boards. Consent of representatives from various fields of psychology.

I. Examination. Should, after grandfather clause, have waiver for examination. Also recommend that waiving the examination for diplomates of ABEPP be included in law.

J. Reciprocity. Where requirements are "no lower than" those in present state.

K. Out-of-State Consultant. Allow for psychological consultation on short term basis.

L. Privileged Communication Provision. "When appropriate, psychologists assist in obtaining general 'across the board' legislation for privileged communication."

M. Injunction authority (to restrain an unlicensed person from unlawful practice of psychology).

N. Review of Proposed Legislation by national committee concerned with legislative principles.

5. Now let us return to Texas. A Legislative Committee was first established as a part of TPA at the 1949 annual meeting in Austin. A sample bill - a tentative draft of a licensing bill was presented. The Legislative Committee was authorized to draw up legislation to be submitted at the next annual meeting.

For the next several years, the topic of legislation was discussed at every annual meting. A bill was presented to TPA in 1956 based in large part on the New York bill, written by Dr. Millard Rudd, Professor of Constitutional Law at the University of Texas. The bill was approved for submission to the 1957 Legislature, sponsored by a representative from Galveston. It cleared the House, but died in Senate Sub-Committee.

Members voted at the 1957 annual meeting in San Antonio to continue attempts at legislation, but the Legislative Committee was also directed to prepare a self-certification proposal at the 1958 Houston meeting. There was considerable discussion regarding the merits of self-certification versus legislation at the 1958 meeting. Decided to approach in a dual way: If legislation should prove possible, the self-certification scheme could be abandoned; if legislation was not possible, then move for self-certification.

Legislation was again attempted with the 1959 Legislature. Members received letters requesting support. "News Bulletins" of progress were mailed to all members. Liaison was attempted with TMA and TWPA. Several members of TPA appeared before the House Committee. This time, the bill did not even reach the floor.

There was no immediate need for action at the 1959 annual meeting in Ft. Worth. President Carl Hereford stated: "The old problem of what to do about regulation of psychologists rests squarely before the membership with our same three choices: Do nothing; attempt to get statutory certification once more; the third is non-statutory certification." (The 1958 Houston proposal for self-certification was still available.) Members voted to continue to strive for legislation. Those opposing the 1959 bill strongly implied that if psychologists would regulate themselves, this would demonstrate professional maturity and warrant legal regulations.

With this thought in mind, the Committee on Certification and Standards in cooperation with the Legislative Committee proposed and presented a plan to the 1960 TPA that met in Abilene. Members of TPA supported the plan and the Texas Board of Psychological Examiners was established. The Board was incorporated as a separate organization from TPA. However, only a small sample of total membership was present at the 1960 meeting, and discontent was voiced by many members. In January 1961, the Board met in Austin and established an Advisory Committee of 30 Texas psychologists to assist the Board.

The Advisory Committee met in Austin in April 1961 and recommended the By-Laws be submitted to all psychologists in the state (TPA and APA members). Thus, much activity took place prior to the Dallas 1961 annual meeting. At that meeting, recommendations were made regarding revision of By-Laws. A series of regional meetings were held across the state during 1962 with all psychologists were given a voice in the development of Self-Certification-By Laws.

By-Laws were refined in 1962 and a procedure outlined for ballot election of the Board. By-Laws and new Board were approved at the 1962 San Antonio annual meeting.

Self Certification was approved for 413 of 491 individual applicants during the period 1963-1969. As of April 1, 1969, 325 certified psychologists were on the rolls.

The Legislative Committee of TPA continued its search for Statutory Legislation. Some additional background:

President Carson McGuire wrote in the March 1963 Newsletter to membership about a meeting between Drs. Oliver Bown, Gordon Anderson and Ira Iscoe and Mr. Philip Overton, General Council for Texas Medical Association. Mr. Overton spoke about the 1959 bill being declared unconstitutional by the Attorney General because of the definition of psychologist. Mr. Overton was skeptical about the possibility of writing a definition of a psychologist that would not conflict with the Medical Practices Act.

The Legislative Committee sought legal counsel to clarify psychology's position.

President Ira Iscoe took a new attack in 1964 with the appointment of a Professional Development of Psychology Committee with sub committees ranging from academic to industrial psychology. This was a long range program designed to upgrade the professional and academic development of psychologists in Texas, and to eventually obtain legal certification.

An informal poll of TPA membership in 1968 indicated unanimous approval to move toward legal certification in 1969. New rumblings had taken place in Texas the previous year. The Governor vetoed a bill which would have expanded use of sub-doctoral level psychologists in 20 Regional Centers involving psychological services and indirectly affecting the school psychology program. Thus, it was only a matter of time (1969) until a law would be passed identifying the minimum qualifications of such sub-doctoral psychologists.

A second event, peripheral to this development, took place in 1968, adding fuel to the fire for need to press for legal recognition. The Texas Education Agency as coordinator of disability determination claims for Social Security Administration informed psychology that examiners would be required to submit psychological test data to TEA. The Texas Board of Psychological Examiners took issue and informed all certified psychologist to refrain from complying with the sending of psychological test protocols to any agency.

This issue was resolved in November 1968 and surely had its impact, in that a large body of psychologists were reminded of need for legal backing.

Dr. Larry Smith, Chairman, Legislative Committee began the 1969 drive which led to successful passage of certification bill. A new version of the bill vetoed by the Governor in 1967 regarding School Psychologist was again introduced. The history of the 5 hectic months of 1969 have not been written and there seems to be very little recorded. I can only talk from my own limited experience.

When the Texas Board of Psychological Examiners met in mid-March 1969, work had begun toward legislation which the Board supported. Larry Smith wrote March 22, 1969, "Monday, March 17, 1969, a bill was entered in the Texas Senate for licensing psychologists. It is Senate Bill No. 667, entered by Senator Kennard of Ft. Worth. It has been referred to the Senate Committee on State Affairs."

Senate Bill No. 230, sponsored by Texas Education Agency, re school psychologist had already passed the Senate. Each psychologist was assigned a senator to contact. My contact was Sen. Akins of Paris.

Senator Akins first response was: "What do the medics think of the bill?" (At that time we knew they were opposed.)

A follow-up letter from Legislative Committee urged two points: (1) The licensing bill is essential to the program being established in the Texas Education Agency under Senate Bill 230, called the Special Education Bill; and (2) the fact that Texas is now surrounded by states which have licensing laws.

All psychologists received a letter from TPA President McCrary reporting a meeting between Legislative Committee and Mental Health Committee of the Texas Medical Association on Saturday, April 19, 1969. TMA reported they would oppose licensing bill, but would support certification. Each psychologist was asked to vote whether to go for licensing or certification. Result: push for certification law.

The bill was subsequently passed by Senate and House. The Governor delayed signing up to last moment and there was considerable anxiety generated by this delay, but in time the bill was signed and became law.

Another waiting period began for those of us on the Texas Board of Psychological Examiners. In late May all Board members received requests from the Governor's Office for biographical data and willingness to serve on the new Board. The bill became law in September 1969. The State Board was to be appointed in 90 days. The Board was fully appointed in December 1969. [A dramatic story.]

The following Psychologists served as members of the Texas Board of Psychological Examiners 1963-1969:

Gordon Anderson
Theodore Andreychuk
Richard B. Austin
Gladys Guy Brown
Wayne S. Gill
Harold Goolishian
Carl Hereford
Ruth Hubbard
Ira Iscoe
A. Jack Jernigan
Irwin Jay Knopf
Earl Koile
Maurice Korman
George Kramer
John MacNaughton
Harry Martin
Glenn Ramsey
Laurence Smith
Joseph Thorpe
John Wheeler
Harold Weiner

Photograph of Dallas VA Hospital supervisory staff in front of Building No. 2 was taken in 1957 or 1958. Those identified by author and Ms. Shirley Campbell, current (2005) Librarian, Dallas VA Medical Center:

Front Row: [?] Chief Nurse; Dr. Earl B. Ross, Chief of Staff; A. L. Gaubert, Assistant Director; Dr. W. H. Buckholts, Director (1955-1965); Mr. Moran, Hospital Administration; Dr. T. W. Wade, Chief Medical Rehabilitation; Mr. Modisett, Veteran Claims Representative.

Second Row: Merle Walker, Finance Officer; Mr. Williams, Chief of Volunteers; Chaplain George Nelson; Burton King, Audiologist; Douglas Torrie, Chief of Social Service.

Third Row: Dr. Seymour Eisenberg, Asst. Chief of Medicine; W. R. McCullough, Chief of Personnel; Dr. John Geers, Chief, Vocational Counseling; Dr. Ben Cohen, Chief of Neurology.

Fourth Row: Walter Sullivan, Chief of Medical Illustration; [?]; Chief of Housekeeping [?]; [?]; Dr. Robert (Red) Hayes, Asst. Chief of Surgery; [?]; [?]; Author.

The photograph is presented in Chapter 4, page 76.

The cover was suggested and designed by Richard Jernigan.

Name Index by Chapters

www.ingramcontent.com/pod-product-compliance
Lightning Source LLC
Chambersburg PA
CBHW031810170526
45157CB00001B/19

* 9 7 8 1 4 2 0 8 6 4 5 0 2 *